PROGRESS IN PATHOLOGY

PROGRESS IN PATHOLOGY

Provisional Contents of Volume 2
Edited by N. Kirkham, N. Lemoine

Prion-related diseases

Cell adhesion molecules and cancer

Transgenic models of disease

Molecular pathology of renal neoplasia

Confocal laser microscopy: applications in pathology

In situ polymerase chain reaction: research and clinical application

Pathological prognostic factors in colorectal carcinoma

The lung biopsy

The Spitz naevus and spitzoid melanoma

Ductal carcinoma in situ

Structure and function of intermediate filaments

Apo E and human disease

Oestrogen receptors, the history, the relevance and the methods

Animal models in experimental pathology

Death and apoptosis

Pathology literature review

Look out for *Volume 2* (ISBN 0443 0   ) in September 1995

You can place your order by contacting your local medical bookseller or the Sales Promotion Department, Churchill Livingstone, Robert Stevenson House, 1–3 Baxter's Place, Leith Walk, Edinburgh EH1 3AF, UK

Tel: (031) 556 2424; Telex: 727511 LONGMN G; Fax: (031) 558 1278

PROGRESS IN PATHOLOGY
Volume One

EDITED BY

NIGEL KIRKHAM MB ChB FRCPath

Consultant Histopathologist and Cytopathologist,
Royal Sussex County Hospital, Brighton, UK

PETER A. HALL BSc PHD MD MRCPath

Professor of Pathology, Ninewells Hospital and Medical School,
University of Dundee, UK

CHURCHILL LIVINGSTONE
EDINBURGH LONDON MADRID MELBOURNE NEW YORK AND TOKYO 1995

CHURCHILL LIVINGSTONE
Medical Division of Longman Group Limited

Distributed in the United States of America by
Churchill Livingstone Inc., 650 Avenue of the Americas, New York,
N.Y. 10011, and by associated companies, branches and
representatives throughout the world.

First published 1995

ISBN 0 443 05013 9
ISSN 0968–896X

British Library Cataloguing in Publication Data
A catalogue record for this book is available from the British Library

Library of Congress Cataloging in Publication Data
is available

The
publisher's
policy is to use
**paper manufactured
from sustainable forests**

Produced by Longman Singapore Publishers Pte Ltd
Printed in Singapore

Contents

Preface

This is the first volume in what will be an annual series that is intended to provide current reviews of topics at the growing edge of histopathology. *Progress in Pathology* is aimed at a readership that will include histopathology trainees working for the MRCPath, or equivalent professional qualifications, as well as consultants aiming to keep abreast of developments. The volume is also intended to interest and inform other laboratory staff and the scientists working in the subject.

The volume covers a variety of topics that will be relevant to a wide range of readers. As well as contributions describing issues of everyday diagnostic relevance there are chapters reviewing some of the molecular mechanisms underlying development and metastasis. Elsewhere there are discussions of the difficulties encountered in achieving good immunohistochemical staining, and of controversial problems such as the dysplastic naevus and the place of aspiration cytology in the diagnosis of thyroid disease. A further chapter reviews the growing area of clinical audit in histopathology. Finally, there is a selection of recently published papers as an aid to further reading.

We trust that our readers will find this first volume to be both interesting and informative. We look forward to offering many similar feasts in the years to come.

Brighton   N. K.
Dundee   P. A. H.
1995

Contributors

Sir Colin Berry DSc MD PhD FRCPath FRCP FFPM
Professor of Morbid Anatomy, The Royal London Hospital, Whitechapel, London, UK

Dennis W. K. Cotton BSc PhD BM MD MRCPath
Reader in Pathology, University of Sheffield Medical School; Honorary Consultant, Department of Pathology, Royal Hallamshire Hospital, Sheffield, UK

Michael F. Dixon MD FRCPath
Reader in Gastrointestinal Pathology, University of Leeds, Leeds, UK

N. M. Gibbs MB MRCP FRCPath
Consultant in Histopathology, Royal Sussex County Hospital, Brighton, East Sussex, UK

Ian R. Hart BVSc PhD MRCPath MRCVS
Richard Dimbleby Professor of Cancer Research, St Thomas' Hospital, London, UK

Ruth F. Jarrett MB ChB
Deputy Director, LRF Virus Centre, University of Glasgow Veterinary School, Glasgow, UK

Nigel Kirkham MB ChB FRCPath
Consultant Histopathologist and Cytopathologist, Royal Sussex County Hospital, Brighton, UK

A. S. Krajewski PhD MRCPath
Senior Lecturer, Department of Pathology, University of Edinburgh Medical School, Edinburgh, UK

James Lowe BMedSci BM BS DM MRCPath
Reader and Consultant in Neuropathology, University of Nottingham Medical School, Nottingham, UK

Keith Miller FIMLS
Senior Chief Medical Laboratory Scientist, Department of Histopathology, University College London Medical School, London, UK

Euphemia McGoogan MB ChB FRCPath
Senior Lecturer, and Honorary Consultant Cytopathologist, Department of Pathology, University of Edinburgh Medical School, Edinburgh, UK

Kathryn M. McLaren BSc MB ChB FRCPath
Senior Lecturer, and Honorary Consultant, Department of Pathology, University of Edinburgh Medical School, Edinburgh, UK

Julia A. Newton Bishop MD FRCP
ICRF Senior Lecturer in Dermatology, London Hospital Medical College, London, UK

Neil A. Shepherd MB BS MRCPath
Consultant Histopathologist, Gloucestershire Royal Hospital, Gloucester, UK

Nalini Singh FIMLS DMS
Chief MLSO, Department of Histopathology, University College London Medical School, London, UK

Richard G. Vile MA PhD
Research Fellow, Biology of Metastases Laboratory, Imperial Cancer Research Fund, London, UK

Bryan F. Warren MB ChB MRCPath
Lecturer in Pathology, University of Bristol, Bristol, UK

Bridget S. Wilkins BSc DM MRCPath
CRC Clinical Research Fellow, University Department of Pathology, Southampton General Hospital, Southampton, UK

Andrew C. Wotherspoon MB BCh
Lecturer in Histopathology, University College London Medical School, London, UK

1. Death: the individual

D. W. K. Cotton

You can always tell that a subject is poorly understood or intellectually uncomfortable when it is defined by negatives. Death is a particularly good example of such a subject in that the United Nations Health Statistic defines death as the permanent disappearance of all signs of life. Death is very prone to these types of evasion since even people with an academic interest in the subject may be humanly concerned about the concept of their own non-existence.

For those of us who are interested in the living world and in the phenomenon of life, death is the great 'natural experiment'; it shows us what biological material is like when life is absent. The difference between a living organism and a dead one is life itself and it does not matter if our model of life is mechanistic or theological, the interesting part of an organism that is lost in death is life. It is therefore a very valid study for a biologist and it is surprising that there is so little direct literature on the subject of death at the level of the whole animal. There is rather more material on cell death and we will approach this via the concepts of organismal death and organ death.

At the gross somatic level it may seem that death is a fairly obvious state, at least at the extremes. However, is someone who has just been decapitated dead? By what criteria? Is their heart still beating? Yes. Is there recordable brain activity? Yes. Could you culture their cells just as well as those from a healthy control? Yes. So they are not dead. What they are is in a condition incompatible with the continuation of life; they are dying. But not all death is preceded by dying and not all dying is inevitably followed by death. Someone who is crushed in an automobile accident was not necessarily dying up to that point and someone with ventricular fibrillation is certainly dying but can, sometimes, be resuscitated.

Even allowing for these uncertainties, there are still several kinds of death. Obviously people may die of disease and accident but just as obviously, particularly to the practising pathologist, many people just seem to die of old age. What is actually meant by this becomes a little less clear when we examine it closely. To die of old age must signify that the individual is free of any disease of sufficient severity to result in death, otherwise they have died of that disease and not old age. However, many elderly people have a burden of disease, such as atheroma or cerebral atrophy, which, if present in a

1

younger individual, we might be willing to accept as sufficiently abnormal to be classed as a cause of death. But even in elderly patients we sometimes see individuals who have no discernible reason to be dead; they are just old. Also we frequently see people who are killed in accidents but who have sufficient disease to have accounted for death at any time even in the absence of accidents. If we try and dissect out that group which are free from disease and accident the modal age of death seems to be around 75 years; a little more in women, a little less in men. We also see that this is the age of death in most societies and in most historical populations. Of course this does not refer to the average life span in any one population but just to the age that individuals would reach if all disease and accident were eliminated. This figure is always likely to be an underestimate since there will always be a small residuum of undetected disease lowering the apparent life expectancy. Therefore the apparent increase in age in advanced societies will appear to further increase as the occult causes of death in the elderly have less effect, but this does not mean that the true age at which people die is being increased, only revealed.

All of this suggests that there is an 'inbuilt' or 'programmed' life expectancy, something that is determined genetically, the so-called 'clonal senescence theory'. There is certainly some good evidence for this. Simple observation shows us that most animals have a characteristic life span and that many human families seem to inherit longevity or a tendency to early death. There are also some remarkable natural experiments that seem to support the concept of a mechanism for ageing and death built into the human genome; these are Werner's syndrome and other progerias. These conditions manifest as individuals who show all the appearances of old age at young chronological age and who die very early of diseases that we commonly associate with senescence.

An alternative theory of ageing and death is the so-called 'replicative senescence theory'. This suggests that ageing is due to accumulations of damage that cannot be adequately repaired and thus ageing is essentially a process of wear and tear. However, the reason why wear and tear is not effectively repaired by the body depends upon the concept of stem cells with replicative limitations, which is essentially the same concept as the 'clonal senescence' theory. At root, both theories appear to imply the inbuilt nature of the timing of death.

Many observations that are either clinically familiar or familiar to comparative physiologists lend support to this. There was a recent vogue for the idea that the indicator for life span was the number of heart beats in a lifetime. In fact there is quite a good correlation between the total number of heart beats and the age to which various mammals live. Small creatures with short lifetimes such as voles have a very rapid heart beat and a generally very rapid metabolism; large long-lived animals such as elephants have a slow heart beat and a generally gentler pace of life. But this correlation does not necessarily imply a causal connection: both heart beat rates and dying may be two independent aspects of the same process.

A more difficult problem arises from the fact that the literature on death is inseparable from the literature on ageing; authors writing on the latter topic tend to make the tacit assumption that death is the end-result of ageing processes and it is therefore necessary to trawl the literature on ageing to locate studies that are directly relevant to the study of death.

CAUSES OF DEATH: EPIDEMIOLOGY AND MORTALITY STATISTICS

The various causes of death in a particular society at a particular time are collected, if at all, in various ways that may render direct comparison almost impossible. In times of national disasters such as wars and famines, accurate data collection may cease entirely or be manipulated for political or tactical reasons. Even in societies at peace and living in relative affluence it may prove very difficult to obtain comparable death rates; in Belgium and The Netherlands infants dying the first 3 days of life are registered as 'presented dead' and do not appear elsewhere in the statistics, whereas in Italy they are counted as 'live births' and 'infantile deaths' for statistical purposes. In England and Wales the data are collected by the Registrar General via the Office of Population Censuses and Surveys (OPCS) and are published regularly as a series of books. These use the International Classification of Disease (ICD) codes and rely upon death certification for their raw data. Death certification has been shown to be a very poor descriptor of actual causes of death in the absence of an autopsy even in highly investigated hospital populations (Underwood 1993); its reliability in the general community is presumably even lower although there are far fewer studies of this. One survey compared death certification by hospital house officers and general practitioners and revealed that 18.5% of the sample of general practitioners and 3.4% of house officers would alter the cause of death statement on the death certificate so as not to distress relatives (Maudsley & Williams 1993). Numerous other factors were also shown to reduce the reliability of death certification both in hospital and in the community in spite of reported high regard for the importance of accurate death certification. A remarkable population study was carried out in East Germany in 1987 in which 96.5% of people dying in Goerlitz during that period received a full autopsy (1023 individuals). Overall the authors reported a 47% discrepancy rate between death certificates and subsequent autopsy findings; in 30% of the total the discrepancy crossed a major disease category (Modelmog et al 1992). The problems associated with such findings and with the reporting habits in England and Wales have been discussed at length by authors from the OPCS (Ashley & Devis 1992) and in the joint report from the Royal College of Physicians and the Royal College of Pathologists (1982). The overall major discrepancy rate in hospitals has been extensively investigated and runs at about 15–30% (Underwood 1993).

With this degree of difficulty in obtaining accurate epidemiological figures, the use of epidemiology to try and dissect out the nature of programmed death is very unlikely to be profitable. What we can say is that even when the great mass of data is examined, and even if we were to believe that it was totally accurate, there still remains a large portion of any community that does not die of disease (Lancaster 1990).

DEFINING DEATH AND THE DETERMINATION OF DEATH

This area has been brought to prominence by the transplant programme in which the need for fresh tissues may be in conflict with the desire to be sure that death has occurred by leaving a reasonable delay time, and with the problem of turning off life-support systems in patients who would be dead were it not for the artificial maintenance of life. In order to deal with these problems it has been necessary for doctors, lawyers and administrators to examine very closely the concepts of life and death as applied to such cases. It is just as difficult to determine when life begins as it is to say with confidence which criteria must be used to say that life has ended. Those involved in the abortion debate have found it impossible to do so and have settled to the position of ignoring the problem ('no abortion is legitimate' versus 'all abortions are a woman's right to choose') whereas the legislators have settled to a middle position that also avoids the definition-of-life problem by basing their rules around the possibility of independent existence for the abortus.

The legal arguments regarding the decision to terminate life support are very complex and highly technical and have been substantially reviewed by Ikuta (1989). From the pathologist's point of view the definition of death, in a legal or even a medical sense, is less of a problem than the legal requirement or an opinion on the mechanism of death, and Gordon (1968) goes so far as to say 'It may be stated categorically that the forensic pathologist is not entitled to speculate about the mechanism of death on the basis of findings at necropsy . . . or on the basis of conventional microscopic or other laboratory investigations.' This may seem to be an extreme view but several points of interest arise from it. At the moment we do not have any clear idea of the terminal mechanism of dying even if the cause of death is fairly dramatic and obvious, such as massive trauma. It is clear that many different organs have very different thresholds for hypoxic damage; the more tolerant can be 'kept going' when other, more sensitive, organs have passed the point of irreversible damage and are effectively dead. Presumably other causes of organ death have a similar range of organ-critical levels, and it follows that in different modes of death one organ may be a more sensitive indicator than another.

From the practical point of view the law tends to defer to medical opinion in determining whether or not death has occurred and the end-point remains the definition that death has occurred when medical opinion states it. There have been various codifications but the law in this country accepts the opinions of the relevant Royal Colleges who, between them, have drawn up a Code of Practice issued by the Health Department which accepts that the diagnostic feature of significance is that all functions of the brain have permanently and irreversibly ceased. This is based on the view that even if other organ systems are still functional, as they must be for transplantation purposes, such a function is irrelevant to the definition of death since no meaningful quality of life can exist without brain function. Mant (1984) quotes a series of diagnostic tests for death set out in the Code of Practice:

1. The pupils are fixed in diameter and do not respond to sharp changes in the intensity of incident light
2. There is no corneal reflex
3. The vestibulo-ocular reflexes are absent
4. No motor responses within the cranial nerve distribution can be elicited by adequate stimulation of any somatic area
5. There is no gag reflex or reflex response to bronchial stimulation by a suction catheter passed down the trachea
6. No respiratory movements occur when the patient is disconnected from the mechanical ventilator for long enough to ensure that the arterial CO_2 level rises above the threshold for stimulation of respiration.

However, various conditions such as the presence of drugs and the body temperature can modify this. The tests are also required to be repeated before they can be accepted as satisfactory. Further, if brain death is to be the criterion then the code of practice imposes further restrictions. The tests must be carried out by a consultant, preferably the one in whose care the patient is, together with another consultant or senior registrar clinically independent of the first. They must have a suitable level of expertise and neither should be a member of the proposed transplant team.

Another conceptual problem arising from the new technology is the case of cardiopulmonary resuscitation. If the diagnosis of death is made on cardiopulmonary grounds then those patients responding to such interventions may be considered to have been brought back to life after clinical death. Their subsequent clinical problems form a very discrete clinical entity described as postresuscitation disease or syndrome (Safar 1988), but in either case the findings are likely to be a mixture of the extreme ends of the spectrum of their original condition and the results of the methods used to resuscitate them and cannot be expected to shed specific light on the process of death in any general sense. The situation has been subject to several experimental studies and these are reviewed by Safar, who claims that the longest normothermic non-flow times yet observed in which good functional survival of heart, brain and entire organism is 15–20 min rather than the 5 min or so usually quoted. However, this is in animal studies and needs careful evaluation before it can have any relevance to the human situations in which death usually occurs.

Prior to death one might expect to see metabolic derangements of increasing severity terminating in an inability to reverse this process, thus leading to clinical death, although none of these observations could be said to be specific for death itself. Such situations are difficult to monitor in spontaneous or programmed death since this is so unpredictable and most human studies have therefore been carried out on patients dying with various diseases or on animals being unnaturally killed.

A final common pathway in much human death is 'shock', although the unifying name covers a number of clinical syndromes. Shoemaker (1976) makes an interesting point regarding this when he distinguishes between the structural and functional aspects of shock in terms that might well be applied to death. He points out that, although we believe that structure and function must be two different aspects of the same problem, there is often a practical disparity between them: 'Until such time as structure and function are more fully reconciled, the two must be regarded from an operational point of view as separate but interrelated aspects of a biologic state; that is, the clinician must clearly distinguish in his own mind diagnostic procedures from monitoring procedures that are designed to assess the physiologic defect. These two distinct activities should proceed along relatively independent pathways.'

A related area is that of multiple organ failure and this too has arisen out of various technological developments. As life-support systems have become more elaborate and successful critically ill patients can be maintained for a longer time before entering a recovery phase or dying. As a consequence this type of patient tends to develop sequential organ failure rather than the solitary organ dysfunctions that were identified before such support systems were available. Fry (1988) points to the sequential development of support technologies as the support time lengthens and the progressive revelation of new organ failures. This lends support to the concept that various organs have, in a general sense, a gradation in their tolerance of critical conditions and the length of time that they can tolerate these before changes become irreversible.

Reviewing the whole field of premortal biochemical changes, Kirk (1968) came to the conclusion that the limiting factor in survival is the integrity of the central nervous system. Even though this does not mean that death is determined by the state of the nervous system there are data and a hypothesis that go some way to supporting this. The terminal drop hypothesis originates with Kleemeier (Siegler 1975) who stated that, '. . . the factors related to the death of the individual cause a decline in intellectual performance, and that the onset of this decline may be detected in some instances several years prior to the death of the person.' This has generated a large volume of literature, most of it well outside the general pathology literature, which has been extensively reviewed by Siegler. On the whole there is support for the terminal drop hypothesis, but even better correlations are produced when other factors such as general health status and age at death were also taken into account.

In conclusion it is interesting to see that the clinical, ethical, legal, biochemical, experimental and psychological viewpoints all seem to converge on the central nervous system being the significant determinant of spontaneous death, but this is still a long way from proof.

DETERMINING THE TIME OF DEATH

It is a staple of crime fiction that a pathologist can determine the length of time that has elapsed between death and examination of the body, as with most fond beliefs, reality is a lot less satisfactory. As in the case of multiorgan failure, there is also a sequence in which organs and tissues retain some vitality and can be used for the determination of time elapsed since death. The classic triad of forensic pathology consists of rigor mortis, liver mortis and algor mortis and these have been used and criticized for many years in determining time of death. Obviously they depend on ambient conditions of temperature, the physical condition of the subject, the manner of death, the age, sex and nutritional status. To further complicate matters, some drugs may influence these gross physical signs and postmortem handling of the corpse may further modify such appearances. Dissatisfaction with these methods has led to a long search for other techniques that might be more reproducible and reliable; included in these are measurements of intraocular pressure, fundoscopy, the responses of various muscles to electrical stimulation and of sweat glands to chemical stimulation and the motility of spermatozoa. Biochemical studies are beset by similar problems to those encountered in premortem studies of dying and in fact seem to be an extension of these. Suffice it to say, as yet there are no reliable methods for timing death and none that throw any light on the basic mechanism of natural death. The various methods used in determining time of death have been reviewed by Van den Oever (1976) and more recently by Knight (1991).

MECHANISMS OF AGEING

There is some inevitable overlap between studies on somatic ageing and cellular ageing which is to be expected since, ultimately, somatic ageing is most probably a function of some cellular process. However, in as far as possible we will restrict ourselves here to somatic aspects of the process.

Three distinct syndromes are usually described under the heading of progerias: Hutchinson–Gilford, Cockayne and Werner's syndromes (Goldstein et al 1990). These are all autosomal recessive conditions in which young individuals show marked signs of senescence and die of age-related diseases at chronologically young ages. Human diploid fibroblast-like cells derived from the patients with either of the first two syndromes only undergo ten doublings in culture compared to the 30 or so seen when using similar cells from normal individuals. The potential for doublings of cells is often taken as a model for the ageing process since normal human cells only show a maximum of 50 doublings in culture and then they start to die. This phenomenon first described by Hayflick (1965) suggests an inbuilt limit to the lifetime of cells and is often used as a model for the inbuilt ageing process. Cells from patients with the progerias also show restricted mitotic activity, DNA synthesis and DNA repair efficiency (Davies 1993). Interestingly, patients with Down's syndrome also show early signs of senescence and often die very young of age-related diseases.

Manipulations of the ageing process have not been very successful and the only reproducible way of significantly lengthening lifespan experimentally has been by juvenile caloric restriction. Laboratory rodents fed a fully balanced diet but with caloric restriction have shown increases in longevity of up to 50%; the animals were also 'fitter', the onset of age-related diseases is delayed, as is the development of the immune system and reproductive ability. It seems that the animals are switched to a new metabolic track, one of whose features is longevity, rather than the diet having a specific effect on lifespan. But of course this still implies that lifespan is inbuilt but with the added possibility that different programmes are available each with its own predetermined lifespan (see Davies 1993 for review).

A gene for longevity in mice has been demonstrated by taking six inbred strains with known, different lifespans, and mating them. The gene appeared to be a single locus inherited as an autosomal dominant. It is postulated that the gene modifies a number of other genes that themselves were responsible for the animal's death (Goodrick 1975). In cell fusion studies genetic analysis reveals genes concerned with cellular senescence and normal growth regulation on chromosome 4 and these genes were able to reverse the immortality of various human cell lines in culture (Ning et al 1991). Another genetic element is the strong association between efficient DNA repair and longevity in mice and primates (Hart & Setlow 1974). It is possible to link the genetic theories to environmental cell damage if one assumes that ageing is due to accumulated damage to macromolecules, including DNA and RNA. There is some evidence for this since age-associated cataracts, which also occur in excess in Down's syndrome, are due to cumulative protein cross-linkage, but nucleic acid damage by this route is less well documented (Davies 1993). An incidental observation is that Down's syndrome is caused by trisomy 21 and the lens protein gene is also on chromosome 21, but the relevance of this observation to natural ageing is obscure.

Waste product accumulation is another possible mechanism for ageing and we see examples of cellular and organ damage by this mechanism in amyloidosis. In amyloidosis 'active' proteins are transformed into inactive forms as beta-pleated sheets but with time the accumulation is so great that it causes pathological effects, including death. However, no similar process has been shown to underlie natural ageing. Similarly, aged cells can be recognized by their content of lipofuscin which seems to derive from free radical peroxidation of cell membranes. However, no deleterious effect from lipofuscin has ever been demonstrated and it is likely that this substance is a neutral marker of age rather than a cause of it.

Certainly the immune system can be shown to be less effective with advancing age and direct measurements of both T and B cell function have shown a progressive decline with age. This is also interesting in the light of the common view that 'you are as old as your arteries' since there is evidence to suggest that atheroma may be to some extent an immunologically determined phenomenon.

Various ageing models at the cellular level have significance for somatic ageing including the free-radical damage theory, disposable soma theory and various organelle and cell membrane theories. These are all well reviewed by Davies (1993) and although some cellular theory presumably underlies somatic ageing and death, it is too extensive to be reviewed here.

THE BIOLOGY OF DEATH

In general the concept of death is often described as irreversible loss of homeostatic control and although this definition is in a sense circular it is probably as close as we can currently get. It seems circular because the definition of life requires some factor that refers to the organism's freedom from environmental fluctuations and the ability to maintain this; even if the statements are tautologous, they are at least consistent.

It is commonly said that death is the only certainty in life, that whatever else should or should not happen, death is inevitable. But is this true? What makes death a biological inevitability? If, as most of the above-mentioned data suggest, death is an inbuilt genetic phenomenon, it must be subject to selection pressures just like any other genetic feature and must presumably have some selective advantage. Clearly the selective advantage is not for the individual and we are taught currently that we should not think of selection acting for species advantage but rather for survival of our 'selfish genes'. How could this come about? How can the death of the individual have any survival advantage for the gene pool?

If we believe that ageing is the process leading to death, then we cannot argue that the genetic advantage of death is that it removes the aged since we would simply have shifted the question back a stage to asking what is the advantage of ageing, the answer being that it produces death. It is possible to argue that ageing and death occur because they arise in the postreproductive stage and therefore escape selection processes altogether, since selection acts only on those characters that are expressed in reproduction. But if this were true it is very unlikely that such highly characteristic lifespans for species would have arisen, particularly with creatures like mayflies who live for only a day. Similarly it is difficult to argue that senescence and death occur when the risk of accumulating deleterious mutations becomes sufficiently great to present a real population risk since, again, one would expect this to be fairly uniform amongst mammals at the very least. Also it is very difficult to see why sexual reproduction should be limited to a specific period of life since the gametes are obviously viable, if they were not then there would be no next generation, and all the arguments regarding progressive genetic damage seem not to apply at the level of gametes. We must remember that sexual reproduction is not the only means of reproduction available to animals and that creatures such as many protozoa reproduce asexually. As a concomitant of this, they never die. Or at least they die only from accidents or disease: they seem to have no inbuilt, programmed death; if they had then the whole species would die.

Another possibility is that because higher animals undergo a complex developmental process ageing and death might be a direct consequence of this. Perhaps the processes that result in development in some way continue to express themselves throughout life and death is merely the final cost of these mechanisms. However, this suggestion is rather non-specific and requires more precise formulation before it can be subjected to experimental testing.

So, is death an inevitable consequence of sexuality? It is a curious thought, but our questions regarding the biological survival value of death are very similar to the questions that exercise biologists regarding the evolution of sex; it is not at all obvious why it has developed or what its value is. However, before we commit ourselves to the concept that sexuality determines death, we should remember that our somatic cells all reproduce asexually but there is good evidence that they contain their own programmes for their own death and that any coherent theory of organismal death must take account of this.

Finally, do we have to accept the tacit assumption that organismal death is the same as cellular death writ large? I am not sure that we must for the organism is not just a big cell, it is a structure that depends upon the integrity of its organs for its survival and there is no reason to believe that subcellular organelle failure is more closely related to organ failure than by simply analogy. It may be that the degree of complexity brought about by cellular, tissue and organ specialization has produced a qualitatively different type of death when we think of complex organisms; that the death of an individual is more than simply an instance of social apoptosis (Hall 1994).

ACKNOWLEDGEMENTS

I should like to thank Professor Peter Hall, Dr Simon Cross and Dr Roger Start for helpful discussions during the preparation of this article.

REFERENCES

Ashley J, Devis T 1992 Death certification from the point of view of the epidemiologist. Popul Trends 67: 2–8
Davies I 1993 Theories and general principles of aging. In: Brocklehurst JC, Tallis RC (eds) Fillit textbook of geriatric medicine and gerontology. 4th edn. Churchill Livingstone, Edinburgh, pp 26–30

Fry DE 1968 Multiple system organ failure. Surg Clin North Am 68: 107–122

Goldstein S, Murano S, Shmookler-Reis RJ 1990 Werner syndrome: a molecular genetic hypothesis. J Gerontol 45: 83–88

Goodrick CL 1975 Lifespan and inheritance of longevity of the inbred mouse. J Gerontol 30: 257–264

Gordon I 1968 The biological definition of death. J Forensic Med 15: 5–8

Hall PA 1994 Death: the cell. (personal communication)

Hart RW, Setlow RB 1974 Correlation between deoxyribonucleic acid excision repair and lifespan in a number of mammalian species. Proc Natl Acad Sci USA 71: 2169–2173

Hayflick L 1965 The limited in vitro lifetime of human diploid cell strains. Exp Cell Res 37: 614–636

Ikuta SS 1989 Dying at the right time: a critical legal theory approach to timing-of-death issues. Issues Law Med 5: 3–66

Kirk JE 1968 Premortal clinical biochemical changes. Adv Clin Chem 11: 175–212

Knight B 1991 Forensic pathology. Edward Arnold, London

Lancaster HO 1990 Expectations of life. Springer-Verlag, London

Mant AK 1984 Taylor's principles and practice of medical jurisprudence. 13th edn. Churchill Livingstone, London

Maudsley G, Williams EMI 1993 Death certification by house officers and General Practitioners—practice and performance. J Publ Health Med 15: 192–201

Modelmog D, Rahlenbeck S, Trichopoulos D 1992 Accuracy of death certificates: a population based, complete-coverage, one year autopsy study in East Germany. Cancer Causes and Control 3: 541–546

Ning Y, Weber JL, Killary AM et al 1991 Genetic analysis of indefinite division in human cells: evidence for a cell senescence-related gene(s) on human chromosome 4. Proc Natl Acad Sci USA 88: 5635–5639

Royal College of Physicians and the Royal College of Pathologists 1982 Joint report. Medical aspects of death certification. J R Coll Physicians 16: 206–217

Safar P 1988 Resuscitation from clinical death: pathophysiologic limits and therapeutic potentials. Crit Care Med 16: 923–941

Shoemaker WC 1976 Pathobiology of death: structural and functional interactions in shock syndromes. Pathobiol Ann 6: 365–407

Siegler IC 1975 The terminal drop hypothesis: fact or artifact? Exp Aging Res 1: 169–185

Underwood JCE 1993 Autopsies and clinical audit. In: Cotton DWK, Cross SS (eds) The Hospital Autopsy. Butterworth-Heinemann, London, pp 163–172

Van den Oever R 1976 A review of the literature as to the present possibilities and limitations in estimating the time of death. Med Sci Law 16: 269–276

2. Progress in gastric cancer

M. F. Dixon

Gastric cancer is the fourth commonest cause of death from cancer in the UK, the commoner causes being cancer of the bronchus, large intestine and breast. Although its incidence is gradually declining, it still accounts for about 10 000 deaths each year (Office of Population Censuses and Surveys 1989). Over 95% of malignant gastric neoplasms are adenocarcinomas. The disease frequently presents at an advanced stage and the results of surgical treatment are correspondingly poor (Thompson et al 1993). As with carcinomas at other sites, earlier detection could lead to a considerable improvement in survival but the vagueness of the symptoms, or a lack of medical awareness of their significance, usually results in delays in diagnosis and treatment. Nevertheless, the wider availability of endoscopy and improvements in surgical technique can produce a substantial increase in the proportion of patients undergoing a potentially curative operation and greatly improve survival (Sue-Ling et al 1993).

The pathologist has an important role in the diagnosis and management of gastric cancer: in the detection of premalignant changes, in the assessment of prognosis, and, increasingly, in the investigation of potential tumour markers. In addition to these practical aspects, pathologists have made a major contribution to the development of new theories regarding the aetiology of gastric cancer since the recognition of *Helicobacter pylori* as the principal cause of chronic gastritis. These aspects of gastric cancer are the subject of this review.

PREMALIGNANT CONDITIONS AND DYSPLASIA

There exists in certain quarters a degree of confusion over the concept of premalignancy. It is conventional to distinguish between a premalignant condition — a disease which on epidemiological or clinical grounds carries an increased risk of malignancy — and a premalignant change or lesion — an unequivocal neoplastic epithelial proliferation which will inevitably progress to invasion with the passage of time. The latter is almost always identified as *dysplasia* in the alimentary tract and, although the term is less than ideal from an etymological viewpoint, it has gained widespread acceptance.

13

In the stomach several conditions are recognized as having an increased risk of malignancy including gastric remnants after partial gastrectomy, autoimmune gastritis, the gastritis of hypogammaglobulinaemia and Ménétrier's disease. In these diseases, as in the majority of 'sporadic' cancers, the underlying pathology is a chronic gastritis with varying degrees of atrophy and intestinal metaplasia. However, the traditional position of intestinal metaplasia as a premalignant condition is becoming increasingly controversial. Likewise the recognition of dysplasia is highly subjective and the inevitability of progression to cancer is disputed. With these problems in mind it seems highly relevant to consider what progress and revisions have taken place in these topics.

Intestinal metaplasia

Intestinal metaplasia is a common finding in chronic gastritis of all causes and appears to increase in prevalence according to its duration. Intestinal metaplasia can be divided into three main types according to mucin content and morphology: a 'complete' type (type I) in which the epithelium resembles that of the normal small intestine; and two 'incomplete' types, type II in which goblet cells appear between normal or acid glycoprotein-containing gastric mucous cells and type III in which goblet cells and intervening diffuse mucus-containing cells stain for sulphomucins more like colonic epithelium. We have found a highly significant correlation between bile reflux and the prevalence and severity of intestinal metaplasia (Sobala et al 1993). Focal intestinal metaplasia was usually of type II, whereas extensive intestinal metaplasia was largely of type I. Type III was found in only 6% of this series of patients. The prevalence of all three types rose steadily with age. Intestinal metaplasia was only seen in 2% of individuals under 30 years and was of type II, while type III metaplasia was not seen below the age of 40 years. Each individual type of intestinal metaplasia occurred more frequently in patients with elevated intragastric bile acid concentrations than in those with bile acid concentrations within the normal limits.

These observations led us to conclude that intestinal metaplasia, usually of type II, originates by divergent differentiation during the healing of bile-induced gastric erosions, a conclusion in keeping with previous studies on the healing of gastric erosions and ulcers (Oohara et al 1983, Mukawa et al 1987, Sossai & Barbazza 1990, Silva et al 1990). Thus, other injurious agents which lead to erosions or ulceration are capable of inducing intestinal metaplasia, and this might explain why factors such as a high salt diet or non-steroidal anti-inflammatory drug use can be associated with its development. Such 'regenerative' intestinal metaplasia is likely to be transient, but repetitive injury leads to more extensive and permanent type I, or in a small minority type III, intestinal metaplasia. While the latter type, which is most closely associated with gastric cancer, might arise by the action of mutagens, we have failed to demonstrate elevated concentrations of nitroso compounds in association with intestinal metaplasia or bile reflux (Sobala et al 1991a).

Intestinal metaplasia is found more frequently in *H. pylori*-positive than -negative cases, despite the tendency for stomachs with extensive atrophy and metaplasia to become negative (Craanen et al 1992). Likewise it has been shown that *H. pylori* is an additional independent risk factor for intestinal metaplasia separate from bile reflux (Sobala et al 1993). It seems likely, therefore, that there is some synergy between *H. pylori* and bile in the production of intestinal metaplasia such that epithelium already sustaining damage from *H. pylori* is more likely to be eroded by bile reflux or other agents and be substituted by intestinal type cells during the regenerative process. In so far as *H. pylori* does not adhere to intestinal epithelium, it is possible to view intestinal metaplasia as a defence response in which gastric epithelium is substituted by an epithelium better suited to counteract two adverse factors which operate either independently or synergistically to produce chronic injury to the gastric mucosa, namely bile reflux and *H. pylori* infection. Interestingly, when well-developed intestinal metaplasia is present in *H. pylori*-associated gastritis, there is an appreciable decline in inflammatory cells in the underlying lamina propria (Wyatt & Dixon 1990), an observation which indicates that the inflammatory infiltrate is closely related to sites of bacterial adhesion and not simply a diffuse response to *H. pylori* in the stomach.

Although the epidemiological data supporting a link between intestinal metaplasia and gastric cancer is persuasive, the relationship is not sufficiently close for the finding of intestinal metaplasia to be used as a marker of 'high risk' which would indicate the need for surveillance. Because of its dilute value as a marker and its heterogeneous nature, more recent interest has focused on the relationship of individual variants to gastric cancer. In several studies involving examination of resection specimens there has been a strong association between the 'intestinal' type of gastric adenocarcinoma and the presence in adjacent mucosa of type III (sulphomucin-rich) metaplasia (Heilmann & Höpker 1979, Jass 1980, Segura & Montero 1983). However, the control material, consisting of resections for benign conditions, was not age-matched. More persuasively, this association was also present in an endoscopic biopsy study where, in all age groups, the prevalence and proportion of type III metaplasia was higher in gastric cancer patients than in other groups (Sipponen et al 1980). However, when resected stomachs from intestinal and diffuse gastric cancer cases and age-matched patients were compared, there was no special tendency for type III intestinal metaplasia to be associated with intestinal gastric cancers (Matsukuma et al 1990). The finding of type III metaplasia was a reflection of the age of the patient and the overall extent of intestinal metaplasia.

While it is generally agreed that type III intestinal metaplasia is associated with the dysplasia–carcinoma sequence, the strength of this association is disputed. Rokkas et al (1991) found it to be closely associated with the subsequent development of gastric cancer and claimed it to be a high-risk factor indicating the need for careful follow-up, while others (Ectors & Dixon 1986, Ramesar et al 1987) found the association insufficiently close in the short term to serve as a marker for surveillance purposes. Furthermore, although the type I, II, III categorization of intestinal metaplasia is widely accepted, its application in biopsy interpretation is complicated by intermediate or transitional forms and by the finding of mosaics of several intestinal metaplasia subtypes. In view of this, and its lack of clear prognostic implications, the Sydney working party suggested that typing of intestinal metaplasia is not warranted in routine practice (Misiewicz et al 1991).

Dysplasia

The cytological and architectural changes comprising dysplasia are well described in major texts on gastrointestinal pathology. However, the textbooks cannot give clear guidance on the distinction between the grades of dysplasia because no two cases are alike and no two pathologists will agree on the grade with any consistency. The problem is compounded by the difficulty in distinguishing regenerative changes from dysplasia. It would be unduly nihilistic to conclude that if the experts can't agree then there is no point in the general histopathologist attempting to grade dysplasia. A failure to recognize dysplasia and to properly assess its severity would have serious repercussions for the patient.

Until recently the natural history of dysplasia has been unclear. Areas of epithelial dysplasia can be found adjacent to some, but by no means all, gastric cancers, and it is tempting to propose a progression from dysplasia to carcinoma in the same way as colorectal cancer arises from adenomas. Follow-up studies of patients with dysplasia tend to support this hypothesis but the reports are confounded by the differing definitions and diagnostic standards employed, and by sampling errors and inadequate documentation.

The cytological atypia constituting gastric dysplasia have been divided into two main categories variously described as adenomatous and hyperplastic dysplasia (Cuello et al 1979), or types I and II (Jass 1983) which are not to be confused with types I and II intestinal metaplasia. Adenomatous dysplasia is much more frequently seen than hyperplastic dysplasia, but even the former is distinctly uncommon in Europe and the USA. Pathologists have usually graded dysplasia into mild, moderate and severe (Morson et al 1980), but the difficulties in interpretation and the wide interobserver disagreements indicate that a two-tier division into low- and high-grade has more to commend it (Tosi et al 1987, Falck et al 1990). A similar approach has been advocated for the categorization of dysplasia in ulcerative colitis (Riddell et al 1983). A major benefit of the two-grade approach is that the natural history and prognostic importance of 'low' versus 'high' can be more clearly identified, which would allow more precise guidelines for clinical management to be drawn up. Furthermore, elimination of the 'moderate' category would remove the haven of indecision towards which many histopathologists will be tempted. The use of terms such as 'intraepithelial cancer' and 'carcinoma in situ' for lesions with the cytological appearances of cancer but without evidence of invasion of the lamina propria is discouraged.

The implications of a diagnosis of high-grade dysplasia are now reasonably clear. The association with coexistent carcinoma is sufficiently close for a confirmed diagnosis of high-grade dysplasia to indicate gastrectomy. A major follow-up study of dysplasia conducted in the UK (De Dombal et al 1990) has shown that of 83 cases of high-grade dysplasia diagnosed by a panel of specialist pathologists, 65 had carcinoma subsequently diagnosed and resected, most within 6 months of the original diagnosis. Two-thirds of the resected carcinomas were found to be early gastric cancers. Eight of the patients underwent polypectomy alone, and in seven high-grade dysplasia alone was found in the specimen. Interestingly, three of the gastrectomies were 'negative', no dysplasia or cancer being found. In our own unit, 10 of 13 patients who had high-grade dysplasia in their gastric biopsies subsequently underwent radical gastrectomy: nine were found to have carcinoma and one had high-grade dysplasia (Lansdown et al 1990). Six of the resected cancers were early gastric cancer and the other three were advanced but had not invaded the serosa. None of the ten cases had lymph node metastases. Thus the prognosis for these patients is much better than for the general run of gastric cancer.

A diagnosis of low-grade dysplasia is far more problematic from a management point of view. In most series few, if any, patients have progressed to high-grade dysplasia or carcinoma; indeed, regression of low-grade dysplasia has been a frequent finding. This has been either spontaneous (Correa et al 1990) or following eradication of *H. pylori* (León-Barúa et al 1988). These findings raise the insurmountable problem of sampling error or tend to cast doubt on the original diagnosis. Reactive or regenerative epithelial changes are easily mistaken for dysplasia. In particular, foveolar hyperplasia in the postoperative stomach is frequently misdiagnosed as dysplasia (Dixon et al 1986). Several reports contain prevalence rates for dysplasia in gastric remnants which if truly premalignant would result in an incidence of carcinoma which far exceeds that observed in practice. However, when low-grade dysplasia is diagnosed by an expert panel (De Dombal et al 1990), a significant proportion will prove to have carcinoma; 14 of 69 cases of low-grade dysplasia were found to have carcinoma in a subsequent resection, half of which were early gastric cancer. A pragmatic management approach following a diagnosis of low-grade dysplasia would be to undertake immediate rebiopsy to exclude concurrent carcinoma, biopsies 6 months later and then regular (annual) surveillance. However, such an approach could put a heavy burden on endoscopy services and cause unnecessary distress to the patient if low-grade dysplasia is overdiagnosed.

Dysplasia is most commonly found in association with an ulcer. Difficulties in the diagnosis of dysplasia and carcinoma in biopsy material taken from the edge of an ulcer have been highlighted by Williams (1986), but in so far as all patients with gastric ulcers should be re-endoscoped to check healing after treatment, the second set of biopsies may well resolve the diagnostic predicament. The problem of distinguishing dysplasia from regenerative changes is particularly acute in the presence of erosions where proliferative activity in residual glands in the deep mucosa can be readily mistaken for dysplasia and even carcinoma. Pathologists should set a high threshold for the diagnosis of dysplasia in order to save the patient unnecessary endoscopies and even the possibility of receiving a 'negative' gastrectomy specimen.

STAGE, GRADE AND PROGNOSIS

The outlook for patients undergoing surgery for gastric cancer is generally poor. A recent survey of 31 000 patients with gastric cancer in the UK revealed that only 21% underwent potentially curative resection and, of these, 16% died within 1 month of surgery and only 20% were alive after 5 years (Allum et al 1989). The overall 5-year survival was just 5%. Against this background, the role of the pathologist in providing prognostic information might seem strictly limited, if not completely superfluous, but this is not the case. Histological confirmation of early gastric cancer confers an excellent prognosis, assuming that a radical operation has been performed (Sue-Ling et al 1992). Similarly, the presence of cancer that has not breached the serosa or which shows only limited lymph node spread carries a much more favourable prognosis than more advanced cancers. Thus, the pathologist has an important role in determining the stage of cancer progression. In this regard accuracy can only be achieved by meticulous attention to block-taking and lymph node dissection (Scott et al 1992).

TNM stages and prognosis

The prime responsibility of the pathologist in handling a specimen resected for gastric cancer is to determine whether or not the surgical margins are involved by carcinoma. From the point of view of the surgeon, this is best undertaken by intraoperative frozen section so that additional tissue can be resected if the original margin is found to be involved. In our recent audit of 20 years' experience in the surgical management of gastric cancer, there were no 5-year survivors among the patients in whom a potentially curative resection with clear surgical margins was not possible (Sue-Ling et al 1993).

Gastric cancers are best staged using the TNM approach as defined in the Unified 1987 TNM system (Kennedy 1987). In this system direct tumour spread through the stomach wall is categorized as: T1, tumour invades lamina propria or the submucosa; T2, spread into the muscularis propria or subserosa; T3, spread through the peritoneal aspect without invasion of adjacent structures; and T4, tumour invades adjacent structures. Lymph node spread is divided into: N0, no nodal involvement; N1, involved lymph nodes within 3 cm of the gross tumour margin; N2, involved lymph nodes greater than 3 cm from the tumour margin. The overall TNM stages (I, II and III) are made up of various combinations of the individual T and N stages; for example, stage I comprises either T1 N0, T1 N1 or T2 N0.

The value of the TNM stage in regard to prognosis is brought out by the cumulative survival figures obtained in our unit (Sue-Ling et al 1993). After excluding operative mortality, 60% of 207 patients who underwent potentially curative resection survived for 5 years after operation and 55% survived 10 years. Five-year survival was 93% in patients with stage I disease, 69% in those with stage II disease, and 28% in those with stage III disease. Metastasis to lymph nodes and depth of tumour penetration were found to be the most important predictors of outcome. To underline the detrimental influence of lymph node metastases we found that the corrected 5-year survival of patients without nodal involvement was 88% and those with lymph node metastases only 35% ($P < 0.001$). Such results emphasize the importance of harvesting the maximum number of lymph nodes from the resected specimen in order to establish as accurately as possible the extent of involvement by carcinoma.

Histological grading

Histological classification in gastric cancer has taken two main paths: the descriptive and the 'pathobiological'. The most widely used descriptive classification is that advocated by the WHO group (Oota & Sobin 1977), which recognized four variants or categories of adenocarcinoma: papillary, tubular, mucinous and signet ring cell types. Although this was not designed to have prognostic value, even as a descriptive classification, the WHO approach has certain shortcomings. The great majority of tumours fall into one category (tubular, 64% of our series). Three of the categories — papillary, mucinous and signet ring cell — are relatively infrequent (22% in all) and a proportion of poorly differentiated adenocarcinomas (15%) are unclassifiable (Martin et al 1994).

Histopathologists continue to grade gastric cancers into well, moderately and poorly differentiated adenocarcinoma despite this being of little or no value in assessing prognosis. Poorly differentiated carcinomas have usually spread more extensively than well-differentiated tumours by the time of surgery so that even amongst potentially curative resections there may be a survival advantage for the better differentiated carcinomas. When tumour stage is taken into account, however, any such advantage disappears.

The failure of the then existing histological approaches to relate to patient survival led Lauren (1965) to propose a different basis for classification in which he recognized two forms of gastric carcinoma: intestinal and diffuse. These categories take account of cytological and architectural differences, namely the tubular arrangement of cuboidal or columnar cells and more basal nuclei of the former, and the infiltrative growth pattern of single, non-cohesive cells of more polyhedral shape in the latter. The 'pathobiological' nature of this approach is reflected in the relative differences between the two patterns in terms of the stronger association between intestinal tumours and intestinal metaplasia, the higher incidence of intestinal tumours in populations at high risk of gastric cancer, and the tendency for diffuse cancers to occur at a younger age and to form a larger proportion of cancers in females, possibly reflecting a greater contribution from genetic rather than environmental factors. The Lauren classification, and its later amplification by Järvi et al (1974), has proved useful in epidemiological studies and has also been shown to be prognostic. Our study confirmed the better survival of patients with intestinal-type tumours in a univariate analysis but, as with tumour grade, the difference in behaviour became non-significant when stage was taken into account. A further failing of the Lauren approach is the high proportion of allocations to one category, intestinal-type tumours comprising 74% of our series (Martin et al 1994).

In 1977 Ming proposed an alternative classification of gastric cancer, based entirely on growth pattern. He identified 'expanding' and 'infiltrative' types and suggested that such a division was likely to reflect differences in tumour biology. In many respects this second pathobiological approach is analogous to the Lauren classification, in that a majority of expanding tumours are intestinal and, by definition, diffuse tumours are infiltrative. Therefore it is not surprising to find that several epidemiological associations are common to both classifications. Furthermore, the Ming classification is similar in its prognostic significance, patients with expanding tumours tending to have a survival advantage over those with infiltrative neoplasms in univariate analyses.

Recently Goseki and colleagues described a novel grading system based on tubular differentiation and mucin secretion which was used to categorize gastric cancers in a series of 200 patients coming to autopsy (Goseki et al 1992). We have demonstrated that the Goseki grade is significantly related to patient survival following potentially curative resection for gastric cancer, and that it was the only histological grading method which exerted an independent effect on prognosis in a multifactorial analysis (Martin et al 1994). The major contributor to the prognostic value of the Goseki grade is the intracytoplasmic mucin content, and 5-year survival of patients with mucus-rich tumours was significantly worse than that of patients with mucus-poor tumours. This was particularly evident in the more advanced tumours; for example in patients with T3 tumours (those breaching the serosa), 5-year survival was 53% for mucus-poor cases but only 18% for mucus-rich cases.

The adverse effect of a high mucin content on outcome is not a new finding. Over 20 years ago, Paile (1971) drew attention to the poorer prognosis of mucus-rich gastric carcinomas, although his categories were based on extracellular mucin content. Nevertheless, until the study of Goseki et al, little or no attention had been given to this aspect of gastric cancer.

All histological aspects of gastric cancer are heterogeneous within individual tumours and any assessment will be affected by sampling differences as well as by subjective factors. Even experienced pathologists only achieved 'moderate' agreement (kappa values 0.485–0.565) on histological grading by the WHO, Lauren, Ming and Goseki schemes (Dixon et al 1994). When agreement on the two-category situation 'mucus-rich' versus 'mucus-poor' was explored, however, a higher level of reproducibility was achieved (kappa = 0.605), suggesting that pathologists can distinguish these prognostically important categories. It seems likely, therefore, that the strength of the association between mucin content and survival will outweigh discrepancies introduced by interobserver variation.

MOLECULAR BIOLOGY AND GASTRIC CARCINOMA

Given the difficulties over the histological recognition of premalignant lesions, the assessment of cancer risk, and the determination of prognosis in established cancers, it might be predicted that recent advances in molecular biology have provided the necessary tools to overcome these problems. Unfortunately this is not the case.

The burgeoning field of molecular pathology with regard to gastric cancer has been admirably reviewed in two recent articles (Wright et al 1992, Wright & Williams 1993). The abnormalities described fall into two broad categories: allele loss or gene mutation leading to absence or inactivation of tumour suppressor genes, and amplification or overexpression of oncogenes or growth factors or their receptors. Allele loss in gastric cancers shows many similarities to colorectal cancer with losses at 5q, 18q and 17p, the latter being associated with tumour progression.

The p53 gene is thought to be an important tumour suppressor and has been referred to as 'the guardian of the genome' (Lane 1992). p53 acts as a check-point between G1 and S-phase in cells which have sustained DNA damage, and this allows for DNA repair. If repair is not possible, p53 initiates cell death by apoptosis. The gene is deleted or mutated in many human cancers. Mutations can be detected by direct DNA analysis, or inferred from the accumulation of mutant protein in cells, which can be detected by immunocytochemistry. However, such accumulation can also result from increased transcription in rapidly proliferating cells or inactivation of a factor required for degradation. p53 immunopositivity has been demonstrated in early gastric cancers and in dysplastic epithelium (Brito et al 1992), but accumulation of the mutant protein seems to be a relatively late event in the multistage process leading to malignancy which would limit its potential usefulness as a diagnostic 'marker'.

The *ras* protein p21 is thought to have a role in signal transduction, proliferation and differentiation, and mutations and overexpression of *ras* genes have been described in many forms of human neoplasia. Advanced tumours exhibit a higher prevalence of *ras* immunopositivity than early gastric cancers (Tahara et al 1986, Ohuchi et al 1987). However, *ras* overexpression does not appear to be specific for carcinoma in the stomach. High levels of *ras* expression have been found in dysplasia as well as in intestinal metaplasia, regenerative epithelium and in apparently normal epithelium adjacent to tumours (Yoshida et al 1988). It is therefore uncertain if *ras* overexpression is a cause or a consequence of neoplasia. However, it has been shown that coexpression of *ras* and TGF-α (transforming growth factor-α) in gastric cancers correlated with more advanced stage, poorer grade and worse prognosis (Yamamoto et al 1988).

The *myc* genes may also have a role in signal transduction, proliferation and control of the cell cycle. Although overexpression of c-*myc* has been demonstrated in gastric cancers (Yamamoto et al 1987), immunopositivity has also been observed in metaplasia, dysplasia and inflamed mucosa (Ciclitira et al 1987). Therefore c-*myc* may simply be a marker of increased cell proliferation.

Changes in membrane-associated óncogenes like c-*erb*-B2 and in growth factor receptors have also been studied without producing clear-cut results. Overexpression of epidermal growth factor receptor (EGF-R) (Lemoine et al 1991) and its ligand TGF-α have been found in gastric cancers, particularly of the Lauren intestinal type (Muller & Borchard 1992), but the prognostic value of this finding has yet to be determined. TGF-α can also be demonstrated in normal, metaplastic and dysplastic gastric epithelial cells (Nasim et al 1992). c-*erb*-B2 has a high level of homology with EGF-R and has been found in a small proportion of gastric cancers (Falck & Gullick 1989), more frequently of intestinal type, but not in dysplasia or non-dysplastic mucosa. The results of prognostic studies are discordant (Yonemura et al 1991, Hilton & West 1992), but overall it seems likely that c-*erb*-B2 expression, as in breast cancer, confers a poorer prognosis.

Work on other growth factors or regulatory peptides operating in the stomach, such as the trefoil peptides pS2 and hSP (Wright 1993), is still in its infancy. Likewise the role of anti-oncogenes and cell adhesion molecules like TGF-β and e-cadherin, has yet to be elucidated. Research into the molecular pathology of gastric cancer is always of interest and sometimes exciting but often appears to be a 'fishing expedition' where technology, rather than fundamental questions, drives the research. Such fishing trips have landed numerous phenomenological minnows. The 'big ones' remain elusive.

HELICOBACTER PYLORI AND GASTRIC CANCER

A commentary under this title was published in the Deutsche Medizinische Wochenschrift in 1992 (Hansen 1992). There is nothing remarkable about this; a flurry of such publications has appeared over the last 3 years. What is remarkable is that 86 years ago the same journal published an article in which a Dr Krienitz described spiral organisms associated with human gastric cancer. This article (Krienitz 1906), like other accounts of 'spirochetes' in the human stomach earlier this century, was ignored until their rediscovery by Warren & Marshall in 1983. *Helicobacter pylori*, as the bacterium was eventually named, is now accepted as the cause of the most common variety of chronic gastritis, and is credited with a major role in peptic ulceration (Tytgat et al 1993). Its role in gastric cancer is more controversial, but a strong case is emerging that the infection is also involved in gastric carcinogenesis. Could Dr Krienitz's 'Spirochäten' really be the cause of gastric cancer?

For several years the concept of a sequence of events starting with multifocal atrophic gastritis leading to intestinal metaplasia and eventually to dysplasia and carcinoma has held sway. This hypothesis, promulgated by Correa (1988), has a number of pathological and epidemiological strands to it, but the most important are dietary factors, such as a high salt intake, to explain the variable development of atrophy, and the intragastric proliferation of bacteria capable of nitrate reduction in the hypochlorhydric stomach. The latter would explain the generation of luminal nitroso compounds which could cause mutagenic events in a multistep progression towards carcinoma. There are several mechanisms whereby *H. pylori* infection can cause glandular atrophy (Dixon & Sobala 1992), and there is evidence that *H. pylori*-associated chronic gastritis progresses to atrophy in accordance with the duration of infection. It seems plausible, therefore, that infection could represent the first step in the chain of events leading to gastric cancer. It also seem likely that the speed of development of atrophy can be accelerated by other injurious agents like bile, and retarded by 'protective' dietary factors such as ascorbic acid, β-carotene and vitamin E. Thus atrophy is seen at a younger age in countries with a high prevalence of *H. pylori* infection and a low intake of fresh fruit and vegetables. Such countries also tend to have a high incidence of gastric cancer (Judd 1993).

High-incidence countries also have, or until recently have had, poor socioeconomic conditions where overcrowding in childhood leads to early and widespread acquisition of *H. pylori* infection. The geographical link between infection and gastric cancer has been elucidated in studies from China (Forman et al 1990), and more recently from the multicentre Eurogast study (Eurogast Study Group 1993). Such studies have shown a significant correlation between serological evidence of *H. pylori* infection and the gastric cancer mortality rates in the same communities. Further evidence comes from cross-sectional studies where the *H. pylori* status of patients with gastric cancer has been compared to that of controls drawn from the same overall population. Thus Sipponen et al (1992) found that 70% of 54 patients with gastric cancer were *H. pylori* positive on serological testing, whereas 49% of 35 age-matched patients with other alimentary tract neoplasms were positive ($P < 0.05$). Interestingly there was no difference in positivity rates between intestinal and diffuse gastric cancers. Similarly, Talley et al (1991), in a more comprehensive study, found that antibodies to *H. pylori* were present in 65% of patients with non-cardia gastric cancer and in only 38% of controls, giving an odds ratio for gastric cancer subjects having positive serology of 2.67 compared to non-cancer controls.

More persuasive are the results of three 'prospective' studies published in 1991 — prospective in the sense that the *H. pylori* serology was performed on serum stored many years before for other purposes (Forman et al 1991, Parsonnet et al 1991, Nomura et al 1991). This allows the investigators to compare the positivity rates in those who subsequently developed gastric cancer and age- and sex-matched controls. These were statistically powerful studies which revealed odds ratios for the development of cancer for *H. pylori* positive versus negative patients ranging from 2.8 to 6.0 and a pooled ratio of 3.8. In other words a subject who acquires *H. pylori* infection is almost four times more likely to develop gastric cancer than an uninfected individual. However, infection can only be a part of the story. The vast majority of infected individuals do not develop gastric cancer. In this connection we must not disregard the large body of evidence pointing to other risk factors, like a high salt diet, as important in the ultimate causation of neoplasia.

While the epidemiological findings are interesting and impressive, they cannot carry complete conviction until one understands how *H. pylori* infection might give rise to gastric cancer. Several factors could play a part both in the initiation and promotion of the carcinogenic process. I have already alluded to the generation of potentially mutagenic nitroso compounds in the atrophic stomach. Correa concluded that intestinal metaplasia arose by mutation and that it constituted an essential step in a metaplasia–dysplasia–carcinoma sequence. As I have argued above, it is equally valid to regard intestinal metaplasia as an adaptive or defensive response which accompanies, but is not necessarily a part of, the events leading to gastric cancer. Thus types I and II intestinal metaplasia can be considered as epiphenomena with regard to the development of cancer; only type III is likely to have significant malignant potential, but the strength of this relationship is disputed. Equally, dysplasia can arise from non-metaplastic mucosa (Ghandur-Mnaymneh et al 1988). These proposed interrelations are illustrated in Fig. 2.1. It is, of course, still possible that carcinogenic factors can act on types I and II metaplastic mucosa, but it seems somewhat ingenuous to argue, as some do, that because a cancer exhibits so-called 'intestinal' features this indicates origin from a metaplastic cell lineage.

While intragastric nitrosation offers an attractive explanation for mutagenesis, the evidence that this occurs in vivo is not totally convincing, and other mutagenic factors have been sought. In the context of *H. pylori*, other candidates readily come to mind. As a consequence of monocyte and polymorph activation in the inflammatory cell response to infection, formation of reactive oxygen metabolites and nitric oxide might lead to DNA damage via the action of free radicals or through intramucosal nitrosation. Such events might underlie the malignant potential of other long-standing chronic inflammatory conditions, of which ulcerative colitis is a prime example.

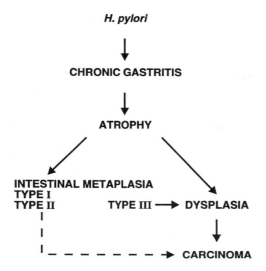

Fig. 2.1 Proposed sequence of events linking *H. pylori* infection to gastric cancer. The development of intestinal metaplasia (IM) is regarded as a parallel adaptive change which is neither an inevitable nor necessary precursor of dysplasia and carcinoma. A small subcategory of individuals having type III IM appear to carry an increased risk of malignancy but the magnitude of this risk is disputed.

Under normal circumstances there must be efficient DNA repair mechanisms which remove segments of DNA damaged by free radicals or N-nitrosation and we know little of the perturbations which permit a stable mutation. Nevertheless such damage is also minimized by antioxidants in the mucosa (Mirvish et al 1992). Interestingly, *H. pylori* infection rapidly diminishes secretion of the important antioxidant ascorbic acid into gastric juice irrespective of the plasma levels (Sobala et al 1989, 1991b). We do not know what effect infection has on intramucosal levels.

Given that there are possible mutagenic factors attributable to *H. pylori*, it is also reasonable to invoke increased cell turnover as a potentiating factor. We have demonstrated increased cell proliferation in the gastric mucosa in the presence of *H. pylori* infection which falls to normal levels after successful eradication (Lynch et al 1994). The increased proliferation is likely to be a compensatory response to increased exfoliation of surface epithelial cells, but the trophic effects of gastrin and the sustained hypergastrinaemia produced by infection cannot be disregarded.

There are thus credible explanations to add to the persuasive epidemiological evidence which point to a major role for *H. pylori* infection in gastric carcinogenesis. It would be facile to say that *H. pylori* is *the* cause of gastric cancer. Other causes of atrophy are known to be associated with an increase in cancer risk, and gastric cancer can even develop in apparently normal stomachs (Fig. 2.2). Nevertheless, it is reasonable to suggest that *H. pylori*-associated gastritis provides the background upon which carcinogenic events

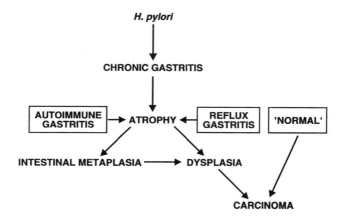

Fig. 2.2   Other routes to carcinoma. Flow chart showing how non-*H. pylori* related types of chronic gastritis can give rise to atrophy and ultimately gastric cancer. A small proportion of cancers appear to arise in normal stomachs.

are much more likely to occur. In so far as gastric cancer is the main lethal cancer in some parts of the world, the public health implications of such a conclusion will gather considerable momentum over the next few years.

REFERENCES

Allum WH, Powell DJ, McConkey CC et al 1989 Gastric cancer: a 25 year review. Br J Surg 76: 535–540

Brito MJ, Filipe MI, Lane D et al 1992 p53 overexpression in early gastric carcinoma and precancerous lesions. J Pathol 167: 95A

Ciclitira PJ, Macartney JC, Evan G 1987 Expression of c-*myc* in nonmalignant and pre-malignant gastrointestinal disorders. J Pathol 151: 293–296

Correa P 1988 A human model of gastric carcinogenesis. Cancer Res 48: 3554–3565

Correa P, Haenszel W, Cuello C et al 1990 Gastric precancerous process in a high risk population: cohort follow-up. Cancer Res 50: 4737–4740

Craanen ME, Dekker W, Blok P, Ferwerda J, Tytgat GNJ 1992 Intestinal metaplasia and *Helicobacter pylori*: an endoscopic bioptic study of the gastric antrum. Gut 33: 16–20

Cuello C, López J, Correa P et al 1979 Histopathology of gastric dysplasias. Correlations with gastric juice chemistry. Am J Surg Pathol 3: 491–500

De Dombal FT, Price AB, Thompson H et al 1990 The British Society of Gastroenterology early gastric cancer/dysplasia survey: an interim report. Gut 31: 115–120

Dixon MF, Sobala GM 1992 Gastritis and duodenitis: the histopathological spectrum. Eur J Gastroenterol Hepatol 4 (Suppl 2): 17–23

Dixon MF, O'Connor HJ, Axon ATR et al 1986 Reflux gastritis: distinct histopathological entity? J Clin Pathol 39: 524–530

Dixon MF, Martin IG, Sue-Ling HM et al 1994 Goseki grading in gastric cancer: comparison with existing systems of grading and its reproducibility (submitted for publication)

Ectors N, Dixon MF 1986 The prognostic value of sulphomucin positive intestinal metaplasia in the development of gastric cancer. Histopathology 10: 1271–1277

Eurogast Study Group 1993 An international association between *Helicobacter pylori* infection and gastric cancer. Lancet 341: 1359–1362

Falck VG, Gullick WJ 1989 c-*erb*B-2 oncogene product staining in gastric adenocarcinoma: an immunohistochemical study. J Pathol 159: 107–111

Falck VG, Novelli MR, Wright NA et al 1990 Gastric dysplasia: inter-observer variation, sulphomucin staining and nucleolar organizer region counting. Histopathology 16: 141–149

Forman D, Sitas F, Newell D et al 1990 Geographic association of *Helicobacter pylori* antibody prevalence and gastric cancer mortality in rural China. Int J Cancer 46: 608–611

Forman D, Newell DG, Fullerton F et al 1991 Association between infection with *Helicobacter pylori* and risk of gastric cancer: evidence from a prospective investigation. Br Med J 302: 1302–1305

Ghandur-Mnaymneh L, Paz J, Roldan E et al 1988 Dysplasia of nonmetaplastic gastric mucosa. A proposal for its classification and its possible relationship to diffuse-type gastric carcinoma. Am J Surg Pathol 12: 96–114

Goseki N, Takizawa T, Koike M 1992 Differences in the mode of extension of gastric cancer classified by histological type: new histological classification of gastric carcinoma. Gut 33: 606–612

Hansen WE 1992 *Helicobacter pylori* und Magenkarzinom. Dtsch Med Wochenschr 117: 1780–1781

Heilmann KL, Höpker WW 1979 Loss of differentiation in intestinal metaplasia in cancerous stomachs. A comparative morphologic study. Pathol Res Pract 164: 249–258

Hilton DA, West KP 1992 c-*erb*B-2 oncogene product expression and prognosis in gastric carcinoma. J Clin Pathol 45: 454–456

Järvi O, Nevalainen T, Ekfors T et al 1974 The classification and histogenesis of gastric tumors. Excerpta Medica International Congress Series No. 354, pp 228–234

Jass JR 1980 Role of intestinal metaplasia in the histogenesis of gastric carcinoma. J Clin Pathol 33: 801–810

Jass JR 1983 A classification of gastric dysplasia. Histopathology 7: 181–193

Judd PA 1993 Diet and precancerous lesions of the stomach. Eur J Cancer Prev 2 (Suppl 2): 65–71

Kennedy BJ 1987 The unified international gastric cancer staging classification. Scand J Gastroenterol 22 (Suppl 133): 11–13

Krienitz W 1906 Ueber das Auftreten von Spirochäten verschiedener Form im Mageninhalt bei Carcinoma Ventriculi. Dtsch Med Wochenschr 22: 872–882

Lane DP 1992 p53, guardian of the genome. Nature 358: 15–16

Lansdown M, Quirke P, Dixon MF et al 1990 High grade dysplasia of the gastric mucosa: a marker for gastric carcinoma. Gut 31: 977–983

Lauren P 1965 The two histological main types of gastric carcinoma. Acta Pathol Microbiol Scand 64: 31–49

Lemoine NR, Jain S, Silvestre F et al 1991 Amplification and overexpression of the EGF receptor and c-*erb*B2 protooncogenes in human stomach cancer. Br J Cancer 64: 79–83

León-Barúa R, Recavarren-Arce S, Ramírez-Ramos et al 1988 Reversal of gastric mucosal dysplasia associated with *Campylobacter pylori* using oral bismuth therapy. Gastroenterology 94: A256

Lynch DAF, Mapstone NP, Clarke AMT et al 1994 Cell proliferation in *Helicobacter pylori*-associated gastritis and the effect of eradication therapy. Gut (in press)

Martin IG, Dixon MF, Sue-Ling H et al 1994 Goseki histological grading of gastric cancer is an important predictor of outcome. Gut (in press)

Matsukuma A, Mori M, Enjoji M 1990 Sulphomucin-secreting intestinal metaplasia in the human gastric mucosa. Cancer 66: 689–694

Ming SC 1977 Gastric carcinoma: a pathobiological classification. Cancer 39: 2475–2485

Mirvish SS, Wallcave L, Eagen M et al 1992 Ascorbate-nitrite reaction: possible means of blocking the formation of carcinogenic N-nitroso compounds. Science 177: 65–68

Misiewicz JJ, Tytgat GNJ, Goodwin CS et al 1991 The Sydney System: a new classification of gastritis. J Hepatol Gastroenterol 6: 209–222

Morson BC, Sobin LH, Grundmann E et al 1980 Precancerous conditions and epithelial dysplasia in the stomach. J Clin Pathol 33: 711–721

Mukawa K, Nakamura T, Nakano G, Nagamachi Y 1987 Histopathogenesis of intestinal metaplasia: minute lesions of intestinal metaplasia in ulcerated stomachs. J Clin Pathol 40: 13–18

Muller W, Borchard F 1992 Expression of transforming growth factor alpha in gastric carcinoma and normal gastric mucosa cells. Cancer 69: 2871–2875

Nasim MM, Thomas DM, Alison MR et al 1992 Transforming growth factor α expression in normal gastric mucosa, intestinal metaplasia, dysplasia, and gastric carcinoma — an immunohistochemical study. Histopathology 20: 339–343

Nomura A, Stemmermann GN, Chyou P-H et al 1991 *Helicobacter pylori* infection and gastric carcinoma among Japanese Americans in Hawaii. N Engl J Med 325: 1132–1136

Office of Population Censuses and Surveys 1989 Mortality statistics by cause. HMSO, London

Ohuchi N, Hand PH, Merio G et al 1987 Enhanced expression of c-Ha-*ras* p21 in human stomach adenocarcinomas defined by immunoassays using monoclonal antibodies and in situ hybridisation. Cancer Res 47: 1413–1420

Oohara T, Tohma H, Aono G, Ukawa S, Kondo Y 1983 Intestinal metaplasia of the regenerative epithelia in 549 gastric ulcers. Hum Pathol 14: 1066–1071

Oota K, Sobin LH 1977 Histological typing of gastric and oesophageal tumours. International histological classification of tumours No. 18. World Health Organization, Geneva

Paile A 1971 Morphology and prognosis of carcinoma of the stomach. Ann Chir Gynaecol Fenn 60 (Suppl 175): 1–56

Parsonnet J, Friedman GD, Vandersteen DP et al 1991 *Helicobacter pylori* infection and the risk of gastric carcinoma. N Engl J Med 325: 1127–1131

Ramesar KCRB, Sanders DSA, Hopwood D 1987 Limited value of type III intestinal metaplasia in predicting risk of gastric carcinoma. J Clin Pathol 40: 1287–1290

Riddell RH, Goldman H, Ransohoff DF et al 1983 Dysplasia in inflammatory bowel disease: standardised classification with provisional clinical applications. Hum Pathol 14: 931–968

Rokkas T, Filipe MI, Sladen GE 1991 Detection of an increased incidence of early gastric cancer in patients with intestinal metaplasia type III who are closely followed up. Gut 32: 1110–1113

Scott N, Quirke P, Dixon MF 1992 Gross examination of the stomach: ACP Broadsheet 133. J Clin Pathol 45: 952–955

Segura DI, Montero C 1983 Histochemical characterisation of different types of intestinal metaplasia in gastric mucosa. Cancer 52: 498–503

Silva S, Filipe MI, Pinho A 1990 Variants of intestinal metaplasia in the evolution of chronic atrophic gastritis and gastric ulcer. A follow-up study. Gut 31: 1097–1104

Sipponen P, Seppälä K, Varis K et al 1980 Intestinal metaplasia with colonic type sulphomucins in the gastric mucosa; its association with gastric carcinoma. Acta Pathol Microbiol Scand Sect A 88: 217–224

Sipponen P, Kosunen TU, Valle J et al 1992 *Helicobacter pylori* infection and chronic gastritis in gastric cancer. J Clin Pathol 45: 319–323

Sobala GM, Schorah CJ, Sanderson M et al 1989 Ascorbic acid in the human stomach. Gastroenterology 97: 357–363

Sobala GM, Dixon MF, Pignatelli B et al 1991a Levels of nitrite, nitrate, N-nitrosocompounds, ascorbic acid and total bile acids in gastric juice of patients with and without pre-cancerous conditions of the stomach. Carcinogenesis 12: 193–198

Sobala GM, Crabtree J, Dixon MF et al 1991b Acute *Helicobacter pylori* infection: clinical features, local and systemic immune response, gastric mucosal histology and gastric juice ascorbic acid concentrations. Gut 32: 1415–1418

Sobala GM, O'Connor HJ, Dewar EP et al 1993 Bile reflux and intestinal metaplasia in gastric mucosa. J Clin Pathol 46: 235–240

Sossai P, Barbazza R 1990 Intestinal metaplasia and dysplasia in gastric ulcer and its tissue repair. Am J Gastroenterol 85: 829–832

Sue-Ling HM, Martin I, Griffith J et al 1992 Early gastric cancer: 46 patients treated in one surgical department. Gut 33: 1318–1322

Sue-Ling HM, Johnston D, Martin IG et al 1993 Gastric cancer: a curable disease in Britain. Br Med J 307: 591–596

Tahara E, Yasui W, Taniyama K et al 1986 Ha-*ras* oncogene product in human gastric carcinoma: correlation with invasiveness, metastasis, or prognosis. Jpn J Cancer Res 77: 517–522

Talley NJ, Zinsmeister AR, Weaver A et al 1991 Gastric adenocarcinoma and *Helicobacter pylori* infection. J Natl Cancer Inst 83: 1734–1739

Thompson GB, van Heerden JA, Starr MG 1993 Adenocarcinoma of the stomach: are we making progress? Lancet 342: 713–718

Tosi P, Luzi P, Baak JPA et al 1987 Gastric dysplasia: a stereological and morphometrical assessment. J Pathol 152: 83–94

Tytgat GNJ, Lee A, Graham DY et al 1993 The role of infectious agents in peptic ulcer disease. Gastroenterol Int 6: 76–89

Warren JR, Marshall BJ 1983 Unidentified curved bacilli on gastric epithelium in active chronic gastritis. Lancet 1: 1273–1275

Williams GT 1986 Early gastric cancer. In: Filipe MI, Jass JR (eds) Gastric carcinoma. Churchill Livingstone, Edinburgh

Wright NA 1993 Trefoil peptides and the gut. Gut 34: 577–579

Wright PA, Williams GT 1993 Molecular biology and gastric carcinoma. Gut 34: 145–147

Wright PA, Quirke P, Attanoos R et al 1992 Molecular pathology of gastric carcinoma: progress and prospects. Hum Pathol 23: 848–859

Wyatt JI, Dixon MF 1990 *Campylobacter*-associated chronic gastritis. Pathol Annu 25 (Part 1): 75

Yamamoto T, Yasui W, Ochiai A et al 1987 Immunohistochemical detection of c-*myc* oncogene product in human gastric carcinomas. Expression in tumour cells and stromal cells. Jpn J Cancer Res 78: 1169–1174

Yamamoto T, Hattori T, Tahara E 1988 Interaction between transforming growth factor alpha and c-Ha-*ras* p21 in progression of human gastric carcinoma. Pathol Res Pract 183: 663–669

Yonemura Y, Ninomiya I, Yamaguchi A et al 1991 Evaluation of immunoreactivity for c-erbB-2 protein as a marker of poor short term prognosis in gastric cancer. Cancer Res 51: 1034–1038

Yoshida K, Hamatani K, Koide H et al 1988 Analysis of *ras* gene expression in stomach cancer by anti-*ras* p21 monoclonal antibodies. Cancer Detect Prev 12: 369–376

3. Iatrogenic pathology of the gastrointestinal tract

B. F. Warren   N. A. Shepherd

This chapter is primarily concerned with pathology of the gastrointestinal tract induced by the acts of medical professionals. Gastrointestinal side-effects are the commonest to be listed on drug data sheets but such effects have, until now, received scant attention from pathologists. For instance, the effects of non-steroidal anti-inflammatory drugs have only recently been described in detail and yet these drugs, some of which are available without prescription, are a major cause of morbidity in the alimentary tract (Armstrong & Blower 1987).

Surgical procedures are also not immune from inducing gastrointestinal pathology. Novel gastrointestinal operations have brought with them a new spectrum of disease, with a need for accurate diagnosis, an understanding of their pathogenesis and a quest for appropriate treatment. In many of these newly described conditions, there are variable and confusing histological features which may lead the unwary to make an inappropriate diagnosis which may have major implications for the patient's subsequent management. In this chapter it is not intended to dwell on the early complications of investigative and therapeutic procedures such as perforation during endoscopy and we offer no apologies for any omissions, particularly rare and esoteric complications of medical management. Instead we intend to concentrate on those medical interventions which induce recently recognized and potentially confusing pathological appearances which may well mimic other pathological conditions (Haggitt 1991, Shepherd 1991). The histological features of those conditions associated with drug treatment, various surgical procedures and other therapeutic modalities will be described with an emphasis on the histopathological pitfalls in the diagnosis of these iatrogenic disorders.

DRUGS, ENEMAS AND SUPPOSITORIES

Drugs affect the gastrointestinal tract in various ways and with varied mechanisms. It should be emphasized that symptomatology, particularly nausea, vomiting, diarrhoea and constipation, is commonplace with many types of drug but this article is concerned solely with pathologically demonstrable abnormalities. Table 3.1 demonstrates the vast spectrum of pathology induced in the alimentary tract by a wide range of medicaments.

31

Table 3.1   The effects of drugs on the gastrointestinal tract

Effect	Drug	Reference
Oesophageal ulceration	Emopronium bromide doxycycline tetracycline NSAIDs	Kirkendall 1983 Heller et al 1982
Reactive gastritis	NSAIDs + others	Dixon et al 1986, Price 1991
Prepyloric ulcers	NSAIDs	Armstrong & Blower 1987
Duodenal ulcers	NSAIDs	Davies & Brightmore 1970
Jejunal ulcers and diaphragm disease	NSAIDs	Lang et al 1988
Ileal ulcers	NSAIDS Potassium chloride	Lang et al 1988 Leyonmarck & Raf 1985
Ileal inflammation	Mefenamic acid	Marks & Gleeson 1975
Colonic ulcers and diaphragms	NSAIDs	Pucius et al 1993, Hudson et al 1993
Collagenous colitis	NSAIDs	Riddell et al 1992
Lymphocytic colitis	NSAIDs	Riddell et al 1992
Pseudomembranous colitis	Various antibiotics, sulphasalazine	Price & Davies 1977
Eosinophilic colitis	Gold	Martin et al 1981
Active IBD	Methyldopa NSAIDs	Graham et al 1981 Hall et al 1983
Chronic inflammation of colonic mucosa	Penicillamine, antibiotics NSAIDs	Shepherd 1991 Sheers & Williams 1989
Crypt hyperplasia, distortion and loss	Chemotherapeutic agents especially S-fluorouracil	Floch & Hellman 1965
Exacerbation of pre-existing ulcerative colitis	NSAIDs Iron sulphate	Rampton & Sladen 1981 Kawai et al 1992
Varied effects on colonic mucosa	Enemas, bowel preparations, suppositories	Saunders et al 1977, Leriche et al 1978, Teague 1987, Shepherd 1991
Rectal inflammation ± solitary ulcer (mucosal prolapse) syndrome	NSAID suppositories Analgesics	Levy & Gaspar 1975, Fenzy & Bogomoletz 1987

The effects of non-steroidal anti-inflammatory drugs (NSAIDs) on the gastrointestinal tract represent a particularly important problem in gastroenterology because of their extensive use and availability without prescription. Lesions throughout the gastrointestinal tract have been attributed to NSAIDs whilst other drugs, particularly antibiotics, also contribute to iatrogenic gut pathology.

Oesophagus

Adverse effects of drugs on the oesophagus are limited by fast transit time but may be problematic in dysmotility disorders and in the elderly, normal oesophagus. Emopronium bromide doxycycline and tetracycline have been commonly involved. Elderly patients using these drugs are prone to large and sometimes multiple mid-oesophageal ulcers (Kirkendall et al 1983). Such ulcers are also seen with slow-release preparations of various NSAIDs (Heller et al 1982) and slow release potassium chloride (Collins et al 1979). Anticholinergic agents induce a reduction in lower oesophageal sphincter pressure, as well as reducing volume and alkalinity of saliva passing down the oesophagus. This, together with a slowing of gastric emptying, results in significant acid reflux and reflux oesophagitis (Gledhill & Hunt 1987).

Stomach

Whilst aspirin is well known for its gastric side-effects, other NSAIDs also cause gastric pathology. Reactive (chemical, type C) gastritis (Dixon et al 1986, Price 1991) is a common accompaniment of NSAID therapy (Quinn et al 1993). It is commonly misdiagnosed histologically, being frequently mistaken for normal gastric mucosa or for dysplasia (with dangers of inappropriate surgery). Its characteristic morphological features are demonstrated in Fig. 3.1. Gastric ulcers may be induced by NSAIDs: they are often multiple, characteristically prepyloric and their most useful histological hallmark on biopsy is the presence of the features of reactive gastritis in the immediately adjacent mucosa, a relative lack of inflammation and absence of *Helicobacter pylori*-associated gastritis. A major pathological pitfall is in overcalling such changes as dysplastic. NSAID-induced ulceration is thought

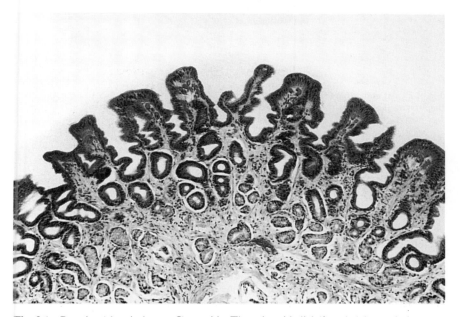

Fig. 3.1 Reactive (chemical, type C) gastritis. There is epithelial (foveolar) hyperplasia producing the typical corkscrew appearance with villiform configuration. Oedema and vascular ectasia in the lamina propria are also characteristic. The relative absence of inflammation allied to the epithelial hyperplasia may cause the unwary to diagnose dysplasia. H&E × 100.

to have two pathogenetic components (Shorrock & Rees 1992). The drugs inhibit prostaglandin synthetase activity, thus interfering with the mucosal barrier function of the gastric and small intestinal mucosa. NSAIDs also have a local chemical irritant effect. The use of NSAID suppositories does not prevent the formation of prepyloric ulcers and may also cause local complications in the rectum. Ulceration of the antrum may on occasion produce cicatrizing submucosal fibrosis and the formation of prepyloric diaphragms (Fig. 3.2) although these are much more commonly seen in the small bowel (see below).

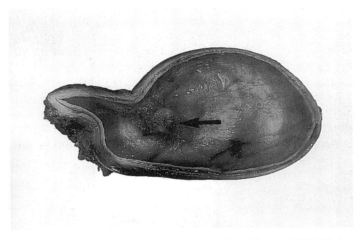

Fig. 3.2   An antrectomy from a 35-year-old man with a long history of NSAID therapy. A diaphragm-like stenosis is seen just proximal to the pylorus (arrow), with granularity of the free edge.

Small intestine

Both duodenal and ileal ulcers are seen as a consequence of therapy with many types of NSAID, whilst terminal ileal inflammation with consequent malabsorption appears to be a unique complication of mefenamic acid (Marks & Gleeson 1975). Ileal ulcers are seen with slow-release potassium chloride tablets (Davies & Brightmore 1970), probably mediated through ischaemic effect from vascular constriction caused by high concentrations of potassium ions. Histologically the changes are confined to the mucosa and submucosa, thus allowing a distinction from Crohn's disease. It may be difficult if not impossible to differentiate potassium chloride ulcers from ischaemic enteritis histologically as the pathogenic mechanisms are similar.

Diaphragm disease has received much recent attention. This striking new pathological entity was first identified in a review of small intestinal resections for recurrent subacute obstruction without a definitive diagnosis (Lang et al

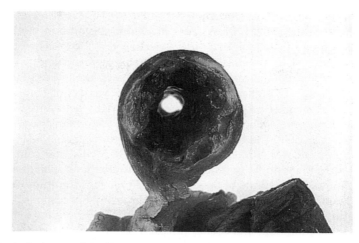

Fig. 3.3 A diaphragm of the jejunum in an elderly rheumatic lady with a long history of NSAID treatment. The gross stenosis is entirely due to the mucosal diaphragm and there is no thickening of the muscle wall.

1988). It was noted that characteristic pathological features were identifiable if the specimen was appropriately prepared (Fig. 3.3) and there was strong correlation between these features and a long history of NSAID prescription. Small intestinal diaphragms are difficult to identify at the time of surgery because the serosal surface of the bowel appears normal, but on transillumination the diaphragm-like strictures may be seen. It is important that surgeons are aware of the possible diagnosis and that the bowel is fixed by formalin insufflation. Windows cut in the wall of the bowel will then identify the diaphragms with pinhole lumina. Histologically, diaphragms consist of exaggerated mucosal folds with superficial ulceration, chronic inflammation, vascular prominence and characteristic submucosal vertical fibrosis (Lang et al 1988). The latter is probably the result of a cicatrizing healing process subsequent to circumferential ulceration. On occasion diaphragm disease may be misdiagnosed as Crohn's disease if the connective tissue changes are marked and the diaphragm is broad in outline. The absence of transmural inflammation and serosal changes are useful features against a diagnosis of Crohn's disease.

Colon and rectum

Pseudomembranous colitis is a well-known and well-understood complication of various antibiotics (Price & Davies 1977) and the disease will not be further considered here. Many other drugs cause inflammatory changes in the mucosa of the large intestine (Table 3.1) but once again NSAIDs are the most important culprits. A primary chronic inflammatory bowel disease-like pathology is described (Hall et al 1983) whilst these drugs can also induce relapse of ulcerative colitis (Rampton & Sladen 1981). It is also clear that, as in the small bowel, NSAIDs can cause ulceration (Hudson et al 1993) and colonic diaphragms (Fellows et al 1992, Pucius et al 1993). They have also been implicated as a potential cause of three enigmatic and interrelated conditions of the colon, each associated with persistent watery diarrhoea, microscopic colitis (Kingham et al 1982), lymphocytic colitis (Lazenby et al 1989) and collagenous colitis (Lindstrom 1976). Many believe that lymphocytic colitis and collagenous colitis are part of the same disease process (Giardiello et al 1989) and both have been shown to relate to NSAID therapy (Giardiello et al 1990, Riddell et al 1992). In Riddell's case-control study NSAIDs were found to be significantly related to the development of collagenous colitis and withdrawal of the drugs caused a significant improvement in symptomatology (Riddell et al 1992). Whilst probably not responsible for all cases of lymphocytic and collagenous colitis (particularly given the relationship between these conditions and coeliac disease), NSAIDs have to be considered as a potential cause. More recently these same drugs have been shown to be potent inducers of apoptosis within the crypt epithelium and this appears to be a useful pathological marker for NSAID-associated colitis (Lee 1993).

A variety of other drugs may induce colitis (Table 3.1) (Shepherd 1991). Alpha-methyldopa rarely causes a chronic inflammatory bowel disease-like acute colitis (Graham et al 1981) and gold therapy produces a florid eosinophilic infiltrate in the lamina propria associated with diarrhoea (Martin et al 1981). Several chemotherapeutic agents, particularly 5-fluorouracil, cause acute epithelial necrosis which resolves by crypt regeneration and distortion mimicking chronic ulcerative colitis in remission (Floch & Hellman 1965).

Anthraquinone laxatives are well known for inducing melanosis coli. The effects of long-term laxative abuse (particularly in some less reputable slimming clinics) on the large bowel can be very severe resulting in muscular and neural atrophy, the cathartic colon, and a sacculated malfunctioning bowel (Jass et al 1989a). Hypertonic saline and mannitol enemas, some forms of bowel preparation and bisacodyl produce crypt epithelial proliferation, goblet cell depletion and inflammatory change which may mimic various forms of colitis, especially infective and ischaemic colitis (Saunders et al 1977, Leriche et al 1978, Teague 1987). Finally, suppositories, particularly those containing NSAIDs and other analgesics, may also cause mucosal damage to the rectum (Levy & Gaspar 1975), and anterior wall ulceration with pathological features like the solitary ulcer (mucosal prolapse) syndrome are well described (Fenzy & Bogomoletz 1987).

GASTROINTESTINAL SURGERY

Oesophagus and stomach

Oesophagectomy inevitably results in the loss of antireflux mechanisms at the oesophagogastric junction and subsequent reflux-type oesophagitis in the remaining upper oesophageal segment. Possible consequences of this include stricture formation and Barrett's oesophagus with its attendant neoplastic risk. All pathologists are aware of the difficulties in the histological diagnosis of Barrett's oesophagus (particularly when no information is given by the endoscopist concerning the level of the biopsy) and this assessment may be even more difficult after oesophageal surgery. Antireflux procedures such as the Nissen fundoplication and Angelchik prosthesis have a variable effect on reflux disease of the oesophagus and bring with them an increased incidence of subsequent gastric peptic ulcer (Campbell et al 1983).

Partial gastrectomy is known to be associated with an increased neoplastic risk in the gastric stump but the magnitude of such risk remains controversial (Clark et al 1985, Caygill et al 1986). The risk appears to be greater in those patients who have had a partial gastrectomy for gastric ulcer disease than in those who have had similar surgery for duodenal ulcer disease. It has been estimated that the lifetime risk is between 1.5% and 5%, suggesting that endoscopic and histological surveillance is necessary (Sabbatini et al 1987).

The detection of dysplasia histologically would alert the pathologist to the possibility of malignant change, but the biopsy assessment of postgastrectomy gastric mucosa can be difficult. Antrectomy results in bile reflux and this (and other factors) induces the histological change of reactive gastritis (Dixon et al 1986, Price 1991). The characteristic histological features include oedema, vascular ectasia, paucity of inflammatory cells and striking foveolar hyperplasia (Dixon et al 1986) (Fig. 3.1). The latter feature may be misinterpreted by the unwary as dysplasia (particularly as there is little inflammation). Helpful histological discriminants are the preservation of epithelial cell compartments with an expanded proliferative zone which does not extend to the surface epithelium and a lack of architectural atypia (Fig. 3.1). Other rare late complications of gastric surgery include bile reflux oesophagitis (Washer et al 1984), gastric mycosis, an unusual complication of stasis and hypoacidity after antrectomy and vagotomy (Konok & Haddad 1980) and the retained antrum syndrome. In the latter, antral mucosa remains in the duodenal stump after Billroth II gastrectomy. This continues to secrete gastrin, inducing acid hypersecretion and multiple peptic ulcers at and around the gastrojejunostomy (Sabbatini et al 1987).

The small intestine

Blind loop syndrome and prestomal ileitis are well-established, if relatively rare, complications of surgery of the small intestine. The latter is characterized by a diffuse mucosal active inflammation extending proximal to an ileostomy; ulcers and even perforation are known complications (Morson et al 1990a). Malignant transformation at the site of an ileostomy has also been described (Thompson et al 1987); this is an occasional complication of surgery, particularly for familial adenomatous polyposis.

The ileal pouch operation is a cause of considerable concern and confusion amongst diagnostic pathologists. For most surgeons and patients the ileal pouch procedure is the operation of choice after colectomy for ulcerative colitis and familial adenomatous polyposis (Mortensen 1993). In this operation a pouch is constructed from terminal ileum and is anastomosed either to the abdominal wall with a continent valve (the Kock pouch) or to the anal canal (the pelvic ileal reservoir). The latter operation, restorative proctocolectomy, is now by far the more popular. It should be emphasized that the pathologist's role is not only confined to assessment of the mucosal pathological changes within the pouch mucosa. Of critical importance is the accurate selection of patients for the operation (Warren & Shepherd 1992a) and the exclusion of patients with Crohn's disease who on the whole fare badly with an ileal reservoir (Deutsch et al 1991, Grobler et al 1993).

Pelvic ileal reservoir surgery varies according to the design of reservoir and the number of stages of the procedure. The three common reservoir types are the quadruple loop (W) pouch, probably the most favoured in the UK, the triple loop (S) pouch, and the double loop (J) pouch, which was developed in Japan and is thought to bear most physiological resemblance to the rectum. Surprisingly the type of pouch has little bearing on the prevalence of subsequent pathological changes within the pouch (Warren & Shepherd 1993). Pathological involvement in pouch surgery varies according to operation sequence, either chosen by the surgeon or dictated by the disease. For example, in cases of fulminant inflammatory bowel disease, a colectomy with mucus fistula (a rectal stump) and covering ileostomy may be the operation of choice with a subsequent pouch operation when the rectal disease has ameliorated; this is the three-stage pouch procedure (Fig. 3.4). In less urgent circumstances, a pouch will be constructed at the time of proctocolectomy with a temporary covering ileostomy and subsequent connection to the faecal stream — the two-stage pouch procedure. Some surgeons have omitted the covering ileostomy — the one-stage pouch procedure. In all three operation types the reservoir is anastomosed to the anal verge, or to the distal rectum, with or without rectal mucosectomy. Preservation of distal rectal mucosa has the advantage of improved continence, outweighing, in the view of many surgeons, the potential disadvantage of leaving behind a ring of diseased and potentially neoplastic rectal mucosa (Kelly 1993). It is important for the pathologist to understand these technical procedures to ensure optimal information from subsequent pouch mucosal biopsies.

Pouch mucosal biopsies are rarely performed in the time between reservoir construction and ileostomy closure. Occasional patients develop discharge from the pouch with endoscopic evidence of inflammation (Warren et al 1990, de Silva et al 1991). Histologically, there are changes similar to those seen in late onset pouchitis (see below) and this condition has been termed preclosure pouchitis (Warren & Shepherd 1993). Its exact relationship to late onset pouchitis is uncertain since there have been few cases. Ischaemia and the

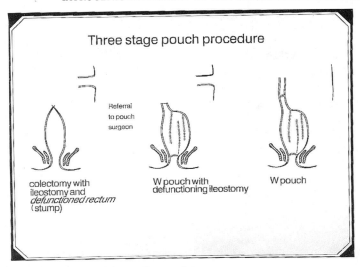

Fig. 3.4   The three-stage pelvic pouch procedure.

effects of diversion have been proposed as possible pathogenic mechanisms (Shepherd 1991), but both seem unlikely as neither preclosure pouchitis nor pouchitis are recognized in familial adenomatous polyposis and mucosal ischaemia and diversion effects would be expected as frequently in familial adenomatous polyposis pouches as in those constructed for ulcerative colitis. Although poorly understood, preclosure pouchitis does not appear to represent Crohn's disease in the pouch (Warren & Shepherd 1993).

The great majority of functioning reservoirs (i.e. after the closure of the covering ileostomy) develop chronic inflammation and villous architectural abnormality regardless of the initial indication for pouch surgery (Shepherd et al 1987, de Silva et al 1991). When villous atrophy is severe, it is associated with crypt hyperplasia (Nasmyth et al 1989, de Silva et al 1991) but does not have the intraepithelial lymphocytic infiltrate of coeliac disease (Shepherd et al 1987). These adaptive changes have been termed colonic metaplasia on account of morphological and histochemical resemblance to colonic mucosa (Fig. 3.5) (O'Connell et al 1986, Shepherd et al 1987, Corfield et al 1992). More recently this concept has been questioned by the lack of complete metaplastic change (Shepherd et al 1993) and the evidence that all pouches appear to retain small intestinal differentiation in the form of disaccharidase activity (de Silva et al 1991). The term colonic phenotypic change has been proposed for the more pronounced 'colonization' of the pouch mucosa (Shepherd et al 1993); it is likely that these changes are the result of environmental influences on the ileal mucosa, possibly instituted by changes in faecal flora (Warren & Shepherd 1993).

It is important that these commonplace pathological changes in the pouch are not equated with a diagnosis of pouchitis; this is a much abused term

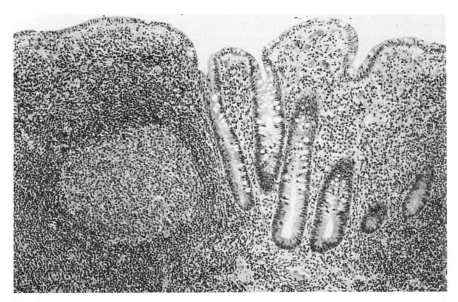

Fig. 3.5 Typical histological features of the pouch mucosa after ileostomy reversal. There is villous atrophy and diffuse chronic inflammation. Occasional polymorphs are present within the epithelium and there is striking mitotic activity. These features do not equate with pouchitis. The resemblance to colonic mucosa is striking. H&E × 100.

which should be restricted to a clinical syndrome with specific clinical, endoscopic and histopathological features (Table 3.2), occurring in 6–20% of pouch patients and representing a relapsing chronic inflammatory bowel disease of the pouch. The cause of this enigmatic condition remains uncertain and may be multifactorial: stasis, bacterial changes, mucosal ischaemia, mucosal prolapse and Crohn's disease all cause inflammatory changes in the mucosa of the pouch but it is unlikely that any are the direct cause of pouchitis. There are some interesting links between ulcerative colitis and pouchitis in terms of clinical features, response to therapy and pathological changes (Warren & Shepherd 1993). Like ulcerative colitis, pouchitis is

Table 3.2 Criteria for a diagnosis of pouchitis

Clinical	Pain, increased stool frequency, urgency, discharge, fever and other systemic effects
Endoscopic	Increased vascularity, contact bleeding and ulceration
Histological	Acute inflammation, superficial erosions and ulceration

References: Nicholls 1989, Tytgat 1989, Madden et al 1990, Warren & Shepherd 1993.

characterized histologically by a florid active inflammatory cell infiltrate including crypt abscesses, whilst erosions and ulceration are also an important feature (Shepherd et al 1987). Occasionally pseudopyloric metaplasia (ulcer-associated cell lineage (Wright et al 1990)) is observed in pouch mucosa and this appears to be a useful marker for evidence of previous ulceration and particularly pouchitis (Warren & Shepherd 1993). The theory that pouchitis represents recrudescence of ulcerative colitis in reservoirs showing a degree of colonic phenotypic change is an attractive but as yet unproven theory (Warren & Shepherd 1993). Could pouchitis represent the only available human model for ulcerative colitis (Shepherd 1990a, Kelly 1993)?

Inflammatory changes within the established pouch may be distinctly focal making the provision of multiple biopsies at endoscopy important. We recommend that biopsies are taken from both the anterior and posterior walls, avoiding suture lines, because inflammatory changes are more pronounced in the posterior wall possibly as a result of prolonged contact with static faecal matter (Shepherd et al 1993). Anterior wall biopsies may demonstrate the histological changes of mucosal prolapse in a striking analogy with the rectal changes seen in this condition (Warren & Shepherd 1993).

Crohn's disease is the strongest contraindication to pelvic ileal reservoir surgery, and pouch surgery in Crohn's disease patients results in the early development of Crohn's disease in the reservoir (Deutsch et al 1991). However, the pathologist should be aware that any of the individual histological features of Crohn's disease may be seen in pouches in patients who do not necessarily have Crohn's disease. Granulomas are occasionally seen, usually in the centre of lymphoid follicles, and can be present with or without pouchitis (Shepherd 1990b). Granulomas may also be seen in the mucosa as a response to disruptive crypt inflammation and deep in the wall, usually in relation to suture material (Warren & Shepherd 1993). Vertical fissures resembling those of Crohn's disease may also be seen in pouch mucosa in relation to ruptured deep crypt abscesses and at anastamosis lines (Warren & Shepherd 1993), a feature also seen in the defunctioned rectum in ulcerative colitis (Warren et al 1993). Fistulae may even occur soon after pouch construction, particularly at suture lines (Tytgat 1989). We believe that it is inappropriate to diagnose Crohn's disease solely on the pathological changes within the pouch mucosa; such a diagnosis should be corroborated by review of the pathology of the colectomy specimen and other clinicopathological data (Warren & Shepherd 1992a).

The first pelvic ileal reservoir was constructed in 1976 and the long-term consequences are largely unknown. The history of Kock pouches is reassuring with no evidence of increased neoplastic change and a suggestion that the ileal mucosa returns almost to normality after 20 years (Helander et al 1990). The factors influencing colonic phenotypic change, the cause of pouchitis and the neoplastic potential of the pouch mucosa are undetermined. The coexistence of colonic phenotypic change (Shepherd et al 1993) and increased epithelial proliferation (de Silva et al 1990) in the pelvic ileal pouch mucosa gives rise to some concern (Shepherd 1990a). A single case of low-grade dysplasia with associated DNA aneuploidy has been demonstrated in the phenotypically altered ileal mucosa of an ulcerative colitis pouch (Lofberg et al 1991), whilst adenomas have been described in pouches from familial adenomatous polyposis patients (Warren & Shepherd 1993). There are reports of carcinomas arising in ulcerative colitis pelvic pouches but these are considered to be derived from remaining rectal mucosa rather than altered ileal mucosa (Stern et al 1990). Surgical practice now favours the retention of a short segment of rectal mucosa to improve functional outcome (Schmitt et al 1992, Kelly 1994). All of these factors make the continuance of comprehensive endoscopic and histopathological surveillance, together with an understanding of the pathological changes seen in pouch mucosa, most important.

The large intestine

There is little doubt that diversion proctocolitis accounts for much of the pathological diagnostic confusion amongst iatrogenic pathology of the large intestine (Bosshardt & Abel 1984, Komorowski 1990, Geraghty & Talbot 1991, Shepherd 1991, Warren & Shepherd 1992b). Pathological changes are induced by diversion of the faecal stream; these are thought to be mediated by a lack of intraluminal short-chain fatty acids (Harig et al 1989, Agarwal & Schimmel 1989), particularly butyrates, which are known to be trophic to the large intestinal epithelium (Roediger 1980). Indeed, intraluminal butyrate enemas have been shown to ameliorate the inflammatory changes of diversion colitis (Harig et al 1989). Nevertheless such findings have not been supported by more recent trials (Neut et al 1989, Guillemot et al 1991) and the exact cause and mechanism remains in some doubt, although the butyrate theory undoubtedly holds sway currently. The disease was originally termed diversion colitis by Glotzer et al (1981), but it is clear that identical changes accompany defunctioning of the rectum and the term diversion proctocolitis has also been coined (Warren & Shepherd 1992b). The frequency of pathological changes within a colonic segment excluded from the faecal stream is exemplified by the demonstration of pathological abnormalities in all patients who underwent creation of a sigmoid neovagina (Toolenaar et al 1993).

Diversion colitis presents clinically with pain, discharge with blood and/or mucus and rectal discomfort from the defunctioned segment, and the inflammatory process can be observed endoscopically as nodularity, erythema, friability, oedema, erosions and ulceration (Korelitz et al 1984, Ona & Boger 1985, Roe et al 1993). There have been many and varied reports of the pathological features of diversion colitis (Korelitz et al 1984, Bosshardt et al 1984, Harig et al 1989, Komorowski 1990, Geraghty & Talbot 1991, Yeong et al 1991, Warren et al 1993). The histological features described have varied between these reports, causing much confusion. Some of this diagnostic confusion has resulted from a lack of consideration of the pre-existing disease within the colon and rectum whilst recent studies have clarified that the pre-existing state of the colon is of crucial importance in determining the histological appearances of the defunctioned colorectum (Warren & Shepherd 1992b, Warren et al 1993, Roe et al 1993). The prime indications for diversion and a summary of the pathological findings are shown in Table 3.3.

Table 3.3 Indications for diversion and pathological features according to the pre-existing disease

Pre-existing disease	Pathological features
Normal colon e.g. Hartmann's procedure for diverticular disease, colonic cancer, trauma e.g. Sigmoid neovagina	Lymphoid follicular hyperplasia Diffuse chronic inflammation, superficial erosions, seldom active inflammation, occasional granulomas
Crohn's disease Usually colon	Lymphoid follicular hyperplasia Active inflammation reduction Retention of connective tissue changes
Ulcerative colitis Usually rectal stump	Lymphoid follicular hyperplasia Often florid active inflammation with granulomas, transmural inflammation and fissures Mimicry of (1) Crohn's disease, (2) ischaemia/ pseudomembranous colitis

Faecal stream diversion from the histologically normal mucosa, performed for colonic carcinoma, diverticular disease and penetrating injury (often as Hartmann's procedure), is uncommonly symptomatic with discharge of blood and mucus (Korelitz et al 1984, Ona & Boger 1985). Nevertheless endoscopic changes of nodularity and ulceration are much more common (Fig. 3.6) and histological changes are universal. The one consistent pathological feature of diversion proctocolitis whatever the pre-existing disease is the distinctive lymphoid follicular hyperplasia (Fig. 3.7), often with small erosions overlying the hyperplastic follicles (Yeong et al 1991, Warren & Shepherd 1992b) and this accounts for the endoscopic nodularity. The histological changes are confined to the mucosa. Inflammation is diffuse throughout the lamina propria and is mainly chronic, but may include acute inflammation with cryptitis and crypt abscess formation (Fig. 3.8) and consequent mucin depletion (Komorowski 1990, Ma et al 1990). Subsequently, muciphages may be prominent in the lower half of the lamina propria (Roe et al 1993). There is usually little crypt distortion. A lack of crypt distortion can be a useful feature to differentiate diversion proctocolitis from inflammatory bowel disease (Harig et al 1989, Roe et al 1993). Intramucosal granulomas are sometimes formed in response to ruptured crypts (Anonymous 1989, Warren et al 1993).

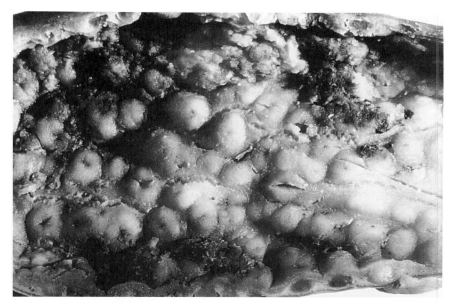

Fig. 3.6 A defunctioned colonic segment in a child after surgery for Hirschsprung's disease. There is nodularity (histologically lymphoid follicular hyperplasia) and there are small erosions overlying the hyperplastic lymphoid follicles.

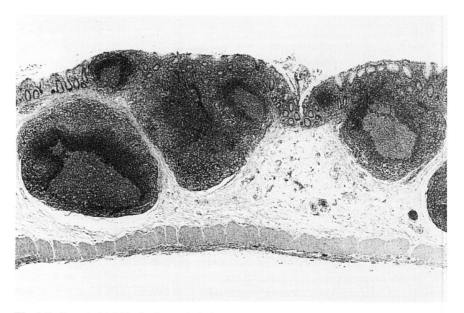

Fig. 3.7 Lymphoid follicular hyperplasia in a defunctioned segment after surgery for Hirschsprung's disease. Note the enhanced chronic inflammatory infiltrate in the mucosa. H&E × 20.

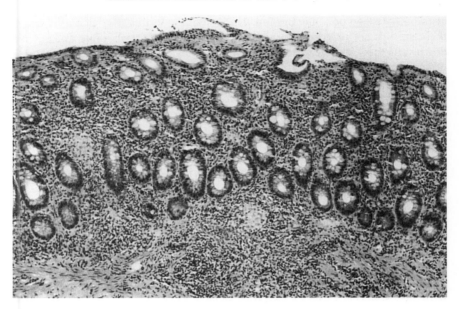

Fig. 3.8 Diversion colitis in an elderly female after a Hartmann's procedure for perforated diverticular disease. There is diffuse chronic inflammation with activity and superficial erosions. Two small granulomas (microgranulomas) are present. Although crypt distortion is slight, there is simulation of chronic inflammatory bowel disease. H&E × 100.

It is manifest that diversion of the faecal contents from the originally normal colonic mucosa can induce florid inflammatory changes which can masquerade as chronic inflammatory bowel disease. For instance, the inflammatory changes, allied to the presence of granulomas, can lead the unwary into an erroneous diagnosis of Crohn's disease whilst active inflammation with a degree of crypt architectural distortion and crypt abscesses can mimic ulcerative colitis (Geraghty & Talbot 1991, Shepherd 1991). Although the pathological changes are varied between cases, the factors underpinning such variation are largely unknown. Why there should be striking lymphoid hyperplasia when defunctioning should reduce the antigenic exposure and thus decrease the immunosurveillance activity is also unknown. It is clear that pathological changes occur relatively soon after defunctioning; one study clearly demonstrating established features of diversion colitis within 3 months of surgery (Roe et al 1993). These mucosal changes are accompanied by involution which can make surgical restoration difficult, particularly if surgery is contemplated in excess of 3 months after diversion (Korelitz et al 1984, Roe et al 1993).

Defunctioning of the rectal stump in ulcerative colitis patients can also lead to confusing histological appearances, inappropriate diagnosis and dire consequences to the patient (Warren et al 1993). Patients undergoing an emergency colectomy frequently have a closed rectal stump preserved as part of the three-stage pouch operation. Unlike defunctioning diverticular disease, these stumps are rarely defunctioned for long enough to involute and shrink down, but they are all presented for histological examination. Such defunctioned recta show the typical pronounced lymphoid follicular hyperplasia, but in addition there is frequently full thickness inflammation in the form of lymphoid aggregates, resembling Crohn's disease (Warren et al 1993). Granulomas are also seen in response to ruptured crypts in the mucosa and to sutures deep within the wall. Ruptured crypts may have overlying vertical fissures. It is not surprising that the presence of these pathological features gives rise to an erroneous diagnosis of Crohn's disease, a strong contraindication to pouch surgery (Warren & Shepherd 1992a). We strongly believe that a diagnosis of inflammatory bowel disease should be preferentially made on pathological material which has not been subject to the effects of diversion and that it is quite inappropriate to change a diagnosis of ulcerative colitis to one of Crohn's disease based on the histological features of the defunctioned rectum alone (Warren & Shepherd 1992b).

A further characteristic feature of the defunctioned rectum in ulcerative colitis is the presence of a pseudomembrane-like fibrinous exudate which lines the mucosal surface with superficial epithelial attenuation and crypt dilatation. These changes resemble pseudomembranous colitis. Whilst this pseudomembranous colitis-like picture may reflect an ischaemic element in the disease process (Warren et al 1993), it has been postulated that the florid inflammatory features seen in the defunctioned rectum of ulcerative colitis represent a combination of active ulcerative colitis and diversion proctitis (Warren & Shepherd 1992b).

Diversion of the faecal stream in Crohn's disease improves symptomatology (Burman et al 1971, Korelitz et al 1984). This contrasts with ulcerative colitis in which the changes of diversion proctitis soon supervene (Warren et al 1993). The reason for this difference in disease behaviour is not known. Diversion colitis may develop in Crohn's disease (Lohr et al 1989), although defunctioning the colon affected by Crohn's disease frequently results in reduction of histological inflammatory activity including a reduction in ulceration, fissuring and transmural inflammation (Warren & Shepherd 1992b). However, the connective tissue changes of Crohn's disease persist, including fat wrapping, neuromuscular hyperplasia and submucosal muscularization (Warren & Shepherd 1992b). A further characteristic feature is the presence of mature granulomas which develop asteroid and Schaumann bodies (Warren & Shepherd 1992b).

Urinary diversion

Ureterosigmoidostomy was a favoured surgical procedure, particularly in patients in whom abnormalities such as ectopia vesicae required removal of the bladder and urinary diversion. However, both inflammatory and neoplastic polyps are seen at the ureteric stoma in the sigmoid colon and the operation is associated with relatively high rates of adenocarcinomatous transformation (Morson et al 1990b). The operation is now less favoured compared with ileal conduit. The latter operation does have some risk of neoplastic change but this is a late and unusual occurrence. Pathological examination of the ileal conduit reveals changes akin to the colonic phenotypic change seen in pelvic ileal reservoirs and this change may contribute to the slightly increased neoplastic risk.

RADIOTHERAPY AND THE GUT

Since the mucosa of the gut is highly proliferative, it is inevitable that radiotherapy has a pronounced effect on the alimentary tract. All parts may be affected but the severity of radiation effects is proportional to the sensitivity of the part of the gut involved and the radiation dose (Fajardo 1989).

Oesophagus and stomach

Oesophagitis may be induced by local radiotherapy for bronchial carcinoma, but this is usually mild and transient. Strictures and fistulae are described as a result of radiation oesophagitis (Seaman & Ackerman 1957). Irradiation gastritis usually occurs within days or weeks of therapy and biopsy shows extensive mucosal necrosis and surface ulceration. Epithelial atypia induced by irradiation may closely mimic neoplastic change (Berthrong & Fajardo 1981). Recovery of the mucosa is accompanied by varying degrees of atrophy and underlying fibrosis with bizarre fibroblasts (Berthrong & Fajardo 1981). Acute gastric ulcers may be seen within 1–2 months after irradiation. Such ulcers are deep and penetrating, often presenting with pain and bleeding. Perforation is unusual because the ulcer is surrounded by adherent, fibrotic neighbouring structures (Berthrong & Fajardo 1981). Such ulcers may become chronic and morphologically resemble chronic peptic ulcers but with the accompanying histological stigmata of radiation (Fajardo 1989).

Small bowel and large bowel

The small and large bowel are highly sensitive to the effects of ionizing radiation, particularly because of the high mucosal cellular turnover. The most commonly damaged part of the gut are the ileum and rectosigmoid area, especially after radiotherapy for bladder, cervical and endometrial carcinoma. Acute radiation effects include ulceration with epithelial denuding, whilst more chronic features are chronic ulceration and fibrosis of the submucosa, muscularis and subserosa. The fibrosis may lead to stricture formation, which may simulate Crohn's disease. The serosa has a mottled appearance and the bowel wall is thickened and indurated. Adhesions are common and cause obstruction as often as radiation-induced strictures (Jackson 1987). The microscopic mucosal changes are many and varied (Fajardo 1989) and hence are open to misinterpretation particularly on biopsy. Villous atrophy with epithelial degenerative changes and lamina propria fibrosis are the characteristic features of mucosal radiation enteritis (Fajardo 1989), while subtle changes in the colonic mucosa may mimic forms of chronic inflammatory bowel disease. Thus crypt atrophy and distortion with fibrosis and a not insignificant chronic inflammatory cell component is seen (Novak et al 1979). Colitis cystica profunda is a rare but recognized complication of radiation colitis (Fajardo 1989).

Radiotherapy and systemic chemotherapy are known to increase the risk of subsequent neoplastic change. Leukaemia, lymphoma, bronchial carcinoma and skin cancer are amongst the more common complications of these therapies. There is controversy concerning the risk of carcinoma of the gastrointestinal tract after therapeutic radiotherapy. Increased prevalence of colorectal cancer, in particular, is described (Smith & Doll 1976, Sandler & Sandler 1983) and the risk is particularly high in those patients with a long latency period after low- to medium-dose radiation therapy (Sandler & Sandler 1983).

IMMUNOSUPPRESSION AND THE GUT

Immunosuppression particularly after whole-body irradiation and systemic chemotherapy brings an increased risk of various infections in the gut, of which pseudomembranous colitis is a characteristic example. Graft-versus-host-disease (GvHD) is now seen as the most serious complication of allogeneic bone marrow transplantation with a mortality of up to 50% (Appleton & Sviland 1993). Diarrhoea is a typical early symptom; in the gut the disease primarily affects the intestines. In acute GvHD crypt distortion and degeneration with crypt abscesses is seen (Sale et al 1979, Epstein et al 1980) and as the disease becomes chronic there is gross epithelial destruction and atrophy (Thorning & Howard 1986). The pathological mechanism of epithelial destruction is through individual cell necrosis (apoptosis) of crypt epithelial cells in both small and large intestinal mucosa, particularly in the proliferative zone (Epstein et al 1980, Appleton & Sviland 1993). This apoptosis is mediated by the intraepithelial migration of immunocompetent graft-derived lymphocytes which are often demonstrated on histological preparations adjacent to the apoptotic cell. Whilst characteristic, such apoptosis is also seen in drug-induced colitis (especially NSAIDs) (Lee et al 1993) and in primary HIV (human immunodeficiency virus) enterocolitis (Kotler et al 1986).

The crypt atrophy and destruction of GvHD may be very striking and may mimic chronic ulcerative colitis (Shepherd 1991). A characteristic morphological feature of chronic GvHD is the relative preservation of enterochromaffin cells in the colorectal mucosa and chromogranin immunohistochemistry can be a useful adjunct to diagnosis by demonstrating this feature (Lampert et al 1985).

MISCELLANEOUS IATROGENIC PATHOLOGY OF THE GUT

Radiological media

Barium sulphate is surprisingly inert even when dispersed in the tissues. Rarely barium granulomas can cause a mass effect with the potential for bowel obstruction (Jass et al 1989b). Barium is readily demonstrable on routine histological study, especially when using polarized light, and the various forms of barium have different and characteristic morphological and ultra-structural features (Levison et al 1984). Thus it is usually relatively simple to differentiate barium from other forms of granulomatous pathology. Water-soluble radiological media induce few if any pathological effects and do not usually concern the pathologist.

Laser therapy

The use of lasers for the treatment of gastrointestinal bleeding and the palliation of gastrointestinal tumours has developed exponentially in the last 10 years. In general the most important complications relate to accidental exposure of the eyes (either patient or staff) and to perforation of a hollow viscus (McKenzie 1991). Nevertheless the laser is a powerful tool which on occasion can produce unusual findings for the pathologist (Fig. 3.9). There is also a potential risk of malignant transformation induced by the laser. In general most lasers have photon energies that are too low to break molecular

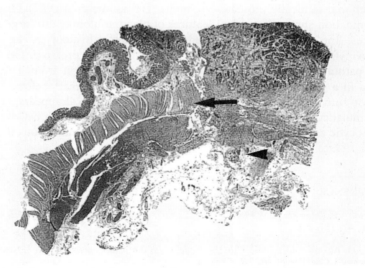

Fig. 3.9 A whole-mount section from an anterior resection in a lady with rectal carcinoma. Previous attempted laser therapy has caused a full thickness defect in the wall of the rectum (arrow) and has 'pushed' a small focus of tumour (arrowhead) through the wall, converting the tumour from a Dukes' A to a Dukes' B.

bonds and create free radicals. Nevertheless there remains a neoplastic risk with some lasers and further assessment is still needed (Boulos & Barr 1990).

Instrumentation and pneumatosis coli

Pneumatosis coli is an enigmatic condition known to be associated with emphysema. Very occasionally the condition can be induced by vigorous insufflation of the colon with carbon dioxide during colonoscopy (Eastwood & Gillon 1987).

Hot biopsy forceps artefact

Hot biopsy forceps are used to biopsy and ablate small (<1 cm) polyps. Such polyp biopsies may show considerable artefact with nuclear streaming and cytoplasmic damage (Burd et al 1992). This artefact tends to make normal mucosa resemble metaplastic polyp mucosa and metaplastic polyp mucosa resemble that of a tubular adenoma. Accurate diagnosis may not be possible but is facilitated by comparison of thermally damaged areas of the biopsy with relatively undamaged areas (Burd et al 1992).

Oleogranuloma and Ivalon tumour

Injection sclerotherapy with almond oil/phenol for haemorrhoids and pro-lapse may cause a fibrotic oily mass in the anorectal area, the oleogranuloma, which may clinically simulate carcinoma (Hernandez et al 1967). Histological examination shows the typical features of oleogranuloma with large rounded spaces lined by uninucleate and multinucleate histiocytes. Ivalon is a polyvinyl sponge used in rectopexy surgery for rectal prolapse. On occasion the pathologist may be confronted by a biopsy/excision from a retrorectal mass in a patient who had undergone this operation years before. So-called Ivalon tumour shows highly distinctive histopathological appearances with a resemblance to a bone tumour, the material itself resembling osteoid and the histiocytic and fibrotic reaction mimicking osteoclasts and fibrous tissue (Jass et al 1989c).

REFERENCES

Agarwal VP, Schimmel EM 1989 Diversion colitis: a nutritional deficiency syndrome? Nutr Rev 47: 257–261
Anonymous 1989 NSAIDs and gut damage. Lancet 2: 600
Appleton AL, Sviland L 1993 Current thoughts on the pathogenesis of graft versus host disease. J Clin Pathol 46: 785–789
Armstrong CP, Blower AL 1987 Non-steroidal anti-inflammatory drugs and life-threatening complications of peptic ulceration. Gut 28: 527–531
Berthrong M, Fajardo LF 1981 Radiation injury in surgical pathology. Am J Surg Pathol 5: 153–178

Bosshardt RT, Abel ME 1984 Proctitis following fecal diversion. Dis Colon Rectum 27: 605–607

Boulos PB, Barr H 1990 Lasers and their application to surgery. In: Hadfield J, Hobsley M, Treasure T (eds) Current surgical practice. Edward Arnold, London, vol 5: 21–37

Burd E, Warren BF, Mountford RA et al 1992 Hot biopsy forceps artefact in the colon — a cause of diagnostic confusion. J Pathol 167 (Suppl): 110A

Burman JH, Thompson H, Cooke WT et al 1971 The effects of diversion of intestinal contents on the progress of Crohn's disease of the large bowel. Gut 12: 11–15

Campbell R, Kennedy T, Johnson GW 1983 Gastric ulceration after Nissen fundoplication. Br J Surg 70: 406–407

Caygill C, Hill MJ, Kirkham JS et al 1986 Mortality from gastric cancer following gastric surgery for peptic ulcer. Lancet 1: 929–931

Clark CG, Fresini A, Gledhill T 1985 Cancer following gastric surgery. Br J Surg 72: 591–594

Collins FJ, Mathews HR, Baker SE, Strakova JM 1979 Drug induced oesophageal injury. Br Med J i: 1673–1676

Corfield AP, Warren BF, Bartolo DCC et al 1992 Colonic metaplasia following restorative proctocolectomy monitored using a new metabolic labelling technique for mucin. Br J Surg 79: 1209–1212

Davies DR, Brightmore T 1970 Idiopathic and drug-induced ulceration of the small intestine. Br J Surg 57: 134–139

de Silva HJ, Gatter KC, Millard PR et al 1990 Crypt cell proliferation and HLA-DR expression in pelvic ileal pouches. J Clin Pathol 43: 824–829

de Silva HJ, Millard PR, Kettlewell M et al 1991 Mucosal characteristics of pelvic ileal pouches. Gut 32: 61–65

Deutsch AA, McLeod RS, Cullen J et al 1991 Results of the pelvic pouch procedure in patients with Crohn's disease. Dis Colon Rectum 34: 160–163

Dixon MF, O' Connor HJ, Axon ATR et al 1986 Reflux gastritis: a distinct histopathological entity? J Clin Pathol 39: 524–530

Eastwood M, Gillon J 1987 Pneumatosis cystoides intestinalis. In: Misiewicz JJ, Pounder RE, Venables CW (eds) Diseases of the gut and pancreas. Blackwell Scientific, Oxford, pp 1092–1096

Epstein RJ, McDonald GB, Sale GE et al 1980 The diagnostic accuracy of the rectal biopsy in acute graft-versus-host disease: a prospective study of thirteen patients. Gastroenterology 78: 764–771

Fajardo LF 1989 Radiation-induced pathology of the alimentary tract. In: Whitehead R (ed) Gastrointestinal and oesophageal pathology. Churchill Livingstone, Edinburgh, pp 813–822

Fellows IW, Clarke JM, Roberts PF 1992 Non-steroidal anti-inflammatory drug induced jejunal and colonic diaphragm disease; a report of two cases. Gut 33: 1424–1426

Fenzy A, Bogomoletz WV 1987 Anorectal ulceration due to abuse of dextropropoxyphene and paracetamol suppositories. J R Soc Med 80: 62

Floch MH, Hellman L 1965 The effect of 5-fluorouracil on rectal mucosa. Gastroenterology 48: 430–437

Geraghty JM, Talbot IC 1991 Diversion colitis: histological features in the colon and rectum after defunctioning colostomy. Gut 32: 1020–1023

Giardiello FM, Lazenby AJ, Bayless TM et al 1989 Lymphocytic (microscopic) colitis. Clinicopathologic study of 18 patients and comparison to collagenous colitis. Dig Dis Sci 34: 1730–1738

Giardiello FM, Hansen III FC, Lazenby AJ et al 1990 Collagenous colitis in setting of nonsteroidal antiinflammatory drugs and antibiotics. Dig Dis Sci 35: 257–260

Gledhill T, Hunt RH 1987 Oesophagitis and hiatus hernia. In: Misiewicz JJ, Pounder RE, Venables CW (eds) Diseases of the gut and pancreas. Blackwell Scientific, Oxford, pp 139–140

Glotzer DJ, Glick ME, Goldman H 1981 Proctitis and colitis following diversion of the faecal stream. Gastroenterology 80: 438–441

Graham CF, Gallagher K, Jones JK 1981 Acute colitis with methyldopa. N Engl J Med 304: 1044–1045

Grobler SP, Hosie KB, Affie E et al 1993 The outcome of restorative proctocolectomy when the diagnosis is suggestive of Crohn's disease. Gut 34: 1384–1388

Guillemot F, Colombel JF, Neut C et al 1991 Treatment of diversion by short-chain fatty acids. Prospective and double-blind study. Dis Colon Rectum 35: 511–512

Hall RI, Pelty AH, Cobden I et al 1983 Enteritis and colitis associated with mefenamic acid. Br Med J 287: 1182

Haggitt RC 1991 The differential diagnosis of idiopathic inflammatory bowel disease. In: Norris HT (ed) Pathology of the colon, small intestine and anus. 2nd edn. Churchill Livingstone, New York, pp 23–60

Harig JM, Soergel KH, Komorowski RA et al 1989 Treatment of diversion colitis with short chain fatty acid irrigation. N Engl J Med 320: 23–28

Helander KG, Ahren C, Philipson BM et al 1990 Structure of mucosa in continent ileal reservoirs 15 to 19 years after construction. Hum Pathol 21: 1235–1238

Heller SR, Fellows IW, Ogilvie AL et al 1982 Non-steroidal anti-inflammatory drugs and benign oesophageal stricture. Br Med J 285: 167–168

Hernandez V, Hernandez IA, Berthrong M 1967 Oleogranuloma simulating carcinoma of the rectum. Dis Colon Rectum 10: 205–207

Hudson N, Wilkinson MJ, Swannell AJ et al 1993 Ileo-caecal ulceration associated with the use of diclofenac slow release. Aliment Pharmacol Ther 7: 197–200

Jackson BT 1987 Radiation damage to the gut. In: Misiewicz JJ, Pounder RE, Venables CW (eds) Diseases of the gut and pancreas. Blackwell Scientific, Oxford, pp 1045–1055

Jass JR, Shepherd NA, Maybee JD 1989a Miscellaneous conditions. In: Atlas of surgical pathology of the colon, rectum and anus. Churchill Livingstone, Edinburgh, p 170

Jass JR, Shepherd NA, Maybee JD 1989b Miscellaneous conditions. In: Atlas of surgical pathology of the colon, rectum and anus. Churchill Livingstone, Edinburgh, p 174

Jass JR, Shepherd NA, Maybee JD 1989c Tumours of the retrorectal space. In: Atlas of surgical pathology of the colon, rectum and anus. Churchill Livingstone, Edinburgh, p 220

Kawai M, Sumimito S, Kasajima Y et al 1992 A case of ulcerative colitis induced by oral ferrous sulphate. Acta Paediatr Jpn 34: 476–478

Kelly K 1994 Ileoanal anastamosis. In: Rachmilewitz D, (ed) Falk Symposium No. 72, IVth International Symposium on Inflammatory Bowel Diseases. Kluwer, Lancaster, pp 264–275

Kirkendall JW, Friedman AC, Oyewole MA 1983 Pill induced oesophageal injury: case reports and review of the medical literature. Dig Dis Sci 28: 174–182

Kingham JGC, Levison DA, Ball JA et al 1982 Microscopic colitis — a cause of chronic watery diarrhoea. Br Med J 285: 1601–1604

Komorowski RA 1990 Histologic spectrum of diversion colitis. Am J Surg Pathol 14: 548–554

Konok G, Haddad H 1980 Postoperative gastric mycosis. Surg Gynecol Obstet 150: 337–341

Korelitz BI, Cheskin LJ, Sohn N et al 1984 Proctitis after faecal diversion in Crohn's disease and its elimination with reanastomosis: implications for surgical management. Gastroenterology 87: 1171–1173

Kotler DP, Weaver SC, Terzakis JA 1986 Ultrastructural features of epithelial cell destruction in rectal crypts of patients with AIDS. Am J Surg Pathol 10: 531–538

Lampert IA, Thorpe P, van Noorden S et al 1985 Selective sparing of enterochromaffin cells in graft-versus-host-disease affecting the colonic mucosa. Histopathology 9: 875–886

Lang J, Price AB, Levi AJ et al 1988 Diaphragm disease: pathology of disease of the small intestine induced by non-steroidal anti-inflammatory drugs. J Clin Pathol 41: 516–526

Lazenby A, Yardley J, Giardello F et al 1989 Lymphocytic ('microscopic') colitis. A comparative histopathologic study with particular reference to collagenous colitis. Hum Pathol 20: 18–28

Lee FD 1993 The importance of apoptosis in the histopathology of drug-related lesions of the large intestine. J Clin Pathol 46: 118–122

Leriche M, Devroede G, Sanchez G et al 1978 Changes in the rectal mucosa induced by hypertonic enemas. Dis Colon Rectum 21: 227–236

Levison DA, Crocker PR, Smith A et al 1984 Varied light and scanning electron microscopic appearances of barium sulphate in smears and histological sections. J Clin Pathol 37: 481–487

Levy N, Gaspar E 1975 Rectal bleeding and indomethacin suppositories. Lancet 1: 577

Leyonmarck CE, Raf L 1985 Ulceration of the small intestine due to slow-release potassium tablets. Acta Chir Scand 151: 273–278

Lindstrom CG 1976 'Collagenous colitis' with watery diarrhoea — a new entity? Pathol Eur 11: 87–92

Lofberg R, Liljequist L, Lindquist K et al 1991 Dysplasia and DNA aneuploidy in a pelvic pouch. Dis Colon Rectum 34: 280–284

Lohr HF, Mayet WJ, Singe CC et al 1989 Diversion colitis in Crohn's disease. A case report and review of the literature. Gastroenterology 27: 221–224

Ma CK, Gottlieb C, Haas PA 1990 Diversion colitis: a clinicopathological study of 21 cases. Hum Pathol 21: 429–436

McKenzie AL 1991 Laser safety in gastroenterology. In: Krasner N (ed) Lasers in gastroenterology. Chapman & Hall, London, pp 51–72

Madden MV, Farthing MJG, Nicholls RJ 1990 Inflammation in the ileal reservoir: pouchitis. Gut 31: 247–249

Marks JS, Gleeson MH 1975 Steatorrhoea complicating therapy with mefenamic acid. Br Med J 4: 442

Martin DM, Goldman JA, Gilliam J et al 1981 Gold-induced eosinophilic enterocolitis: response to oral chromolyn sodium. Gastroenterology 80: 1567–1570

Morson BC, Dawson IMP, Day DW et al 1990a Inflammatory disorders. In: Morson & Dawson's gastrointestinal pathology. 3rd edn. Blackwell Scientific, Oxford, p 498

Morson BC, Dawson, IMP, Day DW et al 1990b Benign epithelial tumours and polyps. In: Morson & Dawson's gastrointestinal pathology. 3rd edn. Blackwell Scientific, Oxford, p 591

Mortensen NJ 1993 Patient selection for restorative proctocolectomy. In: Nicholls J, Bartolo D, Mortensen N (eds) Restorative proctocolectomy. Blackwell Scientific, Oxford, pp 7–17

Nasmyth DG, Godwin PGR, Dixon MF et al 1989 Ileal ecology after pouch–anal anastamosis or ileostomy. A study of mucosal morphology, fecal bacteriology, fecal volatile fatty acids and their interrelationship. Gastroenterology 96: 817–824

Neut C, Colombel JF, Guillemot F et al 1989 Impaired bacterial flora in human excluded bowel. Gut 30: 1094–1098

Nicholls RJ 1989 Clinical diagnosis. In: Pouchitis Workshop. Int J Colorectal Dis 4: 213–216

Novak JM, Collins JT, Donowitz M et al 1979 Effects of radiation on the human gastrointestinal tract. J Clin Gastroenterol 1: 9–39

O'Connell PR, Rankin DR, Weiland LH et al 1986 Enteric bacteriology, absorption, morphology and emptying after ileal pouch–anal anastamosis. Br J Surg 73: 909–914

Ona FV, Boger JN 1985 Rectal bleeding due to diversion colitis. Am J Gastroenterol 80: 40–41

Price AB 1991 The Sydney system: histological division. J Gastroenterol Hepatol 6: 209–222

Price AB, Davies DR 1977 Pseudomembranous colitis. J Clin Pathol 30: 1–12

Pucius RJ, Charles AK, Adair HM et al 1993 Diaphragm-like strictures of the colon induced by non-steroidal anti-inflammatory drugs. Br J Surg 80: 395–396

Quinn CM, Bjarnason I, Price AB 1993 Gastritis in patients on non-steroidal anti-inflammatory drugs. Histopathology 23: 341–348

Rampton DS, Sladen GE 1981 Relapse of chronic proctocolitis after treatment with non-steroidal inflammatory drugs. Postgrad Med J 57: 297–299

Riddell RH, Tanaka M, Mazzoleni G 1992 Non-steroidal anti-inflammatory drugs as a possible cause of collagenous colitis: a case-control study. Gut 33: 683–686

Roe AM, Warren BF, Brodribb AJM et al 1993 Diversion colitis and the involution of the defunctioned rectum. Gut 34: 382–385

Roediger WE 1980 Role of anaerobic bacteria in the metabolic welfare of the colonic mucosa in man. Gut 21: 793–798

Sabbatini F, Siewert JR, Blum AL 1987 Sequelae of gastric surgery. In: Misiewicz JJ, Pounder RE, Venables CW (eds) Diseases of the gut and pancreas. Blackwell Scientific, Oxford, pp 344–360

Sale GE, McDonald GB, Shulman HM et al 1979 Gastrointestinal graft-versus-host disease in man. A clinicopathological study of rectal biopsy. Am J Surg Pathol 3: 291–299

Sandler RS, Sandler DP 1983 Radiation-induced cancers of the colon and rectum: assessing the risk. Gastroenterology 84: 51–57

Saunders DR, Sillery J, Rachmilewitz D et al 1977 Effect of bisacodyl on the structure and function of rodent and human intestine. Gastroenterology 72: 849–856

Schmitt SL, Wexner SD, Lucas FV et al 1992 Retained mucosa after double stapled ileal reservoir and ileoanal anastomosis. Dis Colon Rectum 35: 1051–1060

Seaman WB, Ackerman LV 1957 The effect of radiation on the esophagus. Radiology 68: 534–541

Sheers R, Williams WR 1989 NSAIDs and gut damage. Lancet 2: 1154

Shepherd NA 1990a The pelvic ileal reservoir: apocalypse later? Br Med J 301: 886–887

Shepherd NA 1990b The pelvic ileal reservoir: pathology and pouchitis. Neth J Med 37: S57–S64

Shepherd NA 1991 Pathological mimics of chronic inflammatory bowel disease. J Clin Pathol 44: 726–733

Shepherd NA, Jass JR, Duval I et al 1987 Restorative proctocolectomy with ileal reservoir: pathological and histochemical study of mucosal biopsy specimens. J Clin Pathol 40: 601–607

Shepherd NA, Healey CJ, Warren BF et al 1993 Distribution of mucosal pathology and an assessment of colonic phenotypic change in the pelvic ileal reservoir. Gut 34: 101–105

Shorrock CJ, Rees WDW 1992 Mucosal adaptation to indomethacin induced gastric damage in man — studies on morphology, blood flow and prostaglandin E_2 metabolism. Gut 33: 164–169

Smith PG, Doll R 1976 Late effects of X-radiation in patients treated for metropathia haemorrhagica. Br J Radiol 49: 224–232

Stern H, Walfisch S, Mullen B et al 1990 Cancer in an ileoanal reservoir: a new late complication? Gut 31: 473–475

Teague RH 1987 Investigation of the colon. In: Misiewicz JJ, Pounder RE, Venables CW (eds) Diseases of the gut and pancreas. Blackwell Scientific, Oxford, pp 869–883

Thompson H, Alexander-Williams J, Suarez V et al 1987 Carcinoma of the ileostomy stoma — an increasing problem. J Pathol 152: 233A

Thorning D, Howard JD 1986 Epithelial denudation in the gastrointestinal tract of two bone marrow transplant recipients. Hum Pathol 17: 560–566

Toolenaar TAM, Freundt I, Huikeshoven FJM et al 1993 The occurrence of diversion colitis in patients with a sigmoid neovagina. Hum Pathol 24: 846–849

Tytgat GNJ 1989 The role of endoscopy in pouch monitoring and pouchitis. In: Pouchitis Workshop. Int J Colorectal Dis 4: 210–213

Warren BF, Shepherd NA 1992a The role of pathology in pelvic ileal reservoir surgery. Int J Colorectal Dis 7: 68–75

Warren BF, Shepherd NA 1992b Diversion proctocolitis. Histopathology 21: 91–93

Warren BF, Shepherd NA 1993 Pouch pathology. In: Nicholls J, Bartolo D, Mortensen N (eds) Restorative proctocolectomy. Blackwell Scientific, Oxford, pp 147–162

Warren BF, Bartolo DCC, Collins CMP 1990 Preclosure pouchitis. J Pathol 160: 170A

Warren BF, Shepherd NA, Bartolo DCC et al 1993 The pathology of the defunctioned rectum in ulcerative colitis. Gut 34: 514–516

Washer GF, Gear MWL, Dowling BL et al 1984 Randomised prospective trial of Roux en Y duodenal diversion versus fundoplication for severe reflux oesophagitis. Br J Surg 71: 181–184

Wright NA, Pike C, Elia G 1990 Induction of a novel epidermal growth factor-secreting cell lineage by mucosal ulceration in human gastrointestinal stem cells. Nature 343: 82–85

Yeong ML, Bethwaite PB, Prasad J et al 1991 Lymphoid follicular hyperplasia — a distinctive feature of diversion colitis. Histopathology 19: 55–61

4. Progress in Hodgkin's disease

A. S. Krajewski   R. F. Jarrett

The histopathological criteria for the diagnosis and the classification of Hodgkin's disease (HD) appear to be well established (Lukes & Butler 1966, Lukes 1971, Colby et al 1981, Bennett et al 1991). The diagnosis of HD remains largely dependent on histological findings and is usually made by lymph node biopsy, extranodal presentation being extremely rare. Neck and mediastinal nodes are the most common sites of presentation and less commonly axillary, inguinal and intra-abdominal nodes (Colby et al 1981, Mauch et al 1993). Diagnosis is conventionally considered to require the identification of classical Reed–Sternberg (RS) cells, with or without variants, in an appropriate cellular background (Figs 4.1–4.3) (Lukes 1971). The

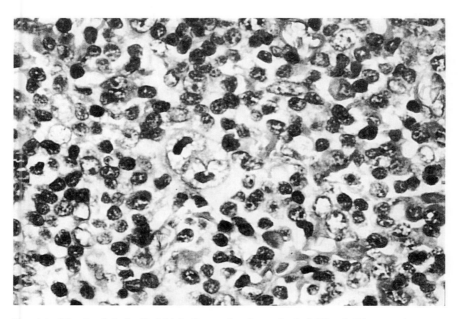

Fig. 4.1 Mixed cellularity·Hodgkin's disease showing a classical RS cell. These are large (> 30 μm), multinucleated cells with moderate to abundant, usually eosinophilic, cytoplasm in which there are large vesicular nuclei, containing prominent nucleoli. H&E × 400.

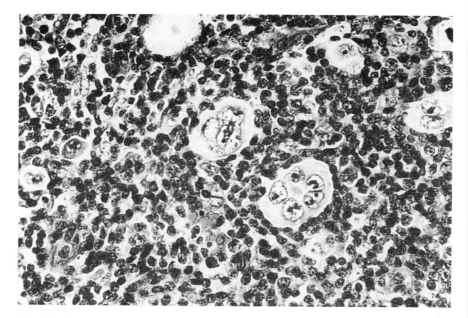

Fig. 4.2 Nodular sclerosing Hodgkin's disease showing pleomorphic multinucleated RS cells. H&E × 250.

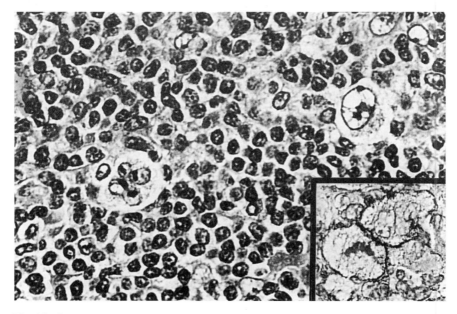

Fig. 4.3 Lymphocyte predominant Hodgkin's disease showing the L&H variant RS cell with a polylobated nucleus. H&E × 400. The inset shows CD20 (L26) membrane staining of L&H cells.

nature of the cellular background in which RS cells are found forms the basis of the Rye classification of Hodgkin's disease (Lukes & Butler 1966, Butler 1992) which divides HD into four main subgroups: lymphocyte predominant (LP), nodular sclerosis (NS), mixed cellularity (MC), lymphocyte depleted (LD).

The Rye classification of Hodgkin's disease, unlike classifications of non-Hodgkin's lymphomas (NHL), has remained stable over 25 years and remains generally accepted as clinically and pathologically relevant (Bennett et al 1991). However, certain problems exist with this classification as the accurate distinction of histological subtypes can be difficult (Bernhards et al 1992). This difficulty has been compounded by the recently proposed histological subdivision of NSHD, which accounts for around 70% of cases in most series, into good (NS-1) and poor (NS-2) prognosis categories (MacLennan et al 1989). Another problem is the concept, implicit in the Rye classification, that the four subtypes are interrelated with possible progression from good to poor prognosis subtypes, i.e. transition from lymphocyte predominant to mixed cellularity to lymphocyte depleted. It is now clear that LPHD is a biologically distinct entity that does not progress to other types but may rarely transform to a high grade B cell lymphoma (Poppema 1992).

A further difficulty for the histopathologist is that it is now apparent that there is considerably more morphological overlap between HD and NHL than was previously recognized and it is necessary to be aware that certain types of NHL may closely resemble and be misdiagnosed as HD (Harris 1992). T cell rich B cell lymphomas (Chittal et al 1991) and peripheral T cell lymphomas (Patsouris et al 1989) may be confused histologically with the diffuse lymphocyte predominant or mixed cellularity Hodgkin's disease. High grade large cell lymphomas, especially Ki-1 positive anaplastic lymphomas, may show considerable morphological and immunophenotypic overlap with LDHD and lymphocyte depleted variants of NSHD (Frizzera 1992).

The introduction of sophisticated immunohistochemical and immuno-genotypic analyses have contributed less to the diagnosis of HD than to NHL, and a major unresolved problem in the study of HD is the failure to determine the histogenesis of the RS cell. The current consensus is that the RS cell is an activated lymphoid cell with an aberrant phenotype. There is, however, no consensus as to whether the RS cell is of T or B cell origin. The detection of Epstein–Barr virus (EBV) in RS cells in up to 50% of cases of HD has led to a renewal of interest in a possible viral aetiology for HD (Armstrong et al 1992b) and to the suggestion that HD may be a histogenetically hetero-geneous group of diseases in which viral transformation of an immature lymphoid cell plays a major role in the induction of the aberrant lymphoid cell phenotype of the RS cell (Herbst et al 1989, Stein et al 1991).

In the first part of this article we review the histopathological criteria for the diagnosis and classification of HD and its distinction from other lymphomas, including where appropriate details of the contribution of immunophenotyp-ing and genotyping to diagnosis and classification. In the second part of this article we will review some of the progress that has been made in defining the histogenesis of HD and review the evidence for a viral aetiology in the pathogenesis of HD.

HISTOPATHOLOGY OF HODGKIN'S DISEASE

Lymphocyte predominant Hodgkin's disease (LPHD)

Lymphocyte predominant Hodgkin's disease (LPHD) accounts for around 5–10% of cases of HD, shows a marked male predominance and usually occurs in younger patients, LPHD most commonly presents with involvement of neck nodes and less commonly with other peripheral nodes. Mediastinal involvement is uncommon (Mauch et al 1993). LPHD includes two subtypes originally defined by Lukes and Butler: nodular lymphocytic and histiocytic predominance (NLPHD) and diffuse lymphocytic and histiocytic predominance (DLPHD).

Histological and immunophenotypic features

NLPHD is characterized histologically by loss of normal lymph node architecture and replacement by poorly defined, often large nodules, best identified by reticulin staining, consisting predominantly of small lymphocytes between which L&H type RS cells can be found (Fig. 4.3). Identification of the L&H cell is essential for the diagnosis of NLPHD. These cells are larger than centroblasts and contain large polylobated nuclei ('popcorn cells') with medium sized nucleoli and have moderate surrounding cytoplasm. L&H cells may be present in only small numbers or may form obvious large aggregates. Epithelioid histiocytes may be found and may form small aggregates or large sarcoid-like granulomas. In some cases residual follicles can be seen compressed at the periphery of the node. Other enlarged follicles showing features of progressive transformation of germinal centres with or without L&H cells may sometimes be seen (Hansmann et al 1990). It is now generally accepted that classical RS cells are rarely found in NLPHD and are not required for diagnosis (Wright 1989, Butler 1992). If classical RS cells are easily found it is more likely that the correct diagnosis is either cellular phase NSHD or MCHD. It should be stressed that positive identification of L&H RS cells is essential for diagnosis of LPHD and to prevent misdiagnosis of progressive transformation of germinal centres.

NLPHD has a distinct phenotype allowing differentiation from other types of HD in most cases (Poppema 1992). In paraffin sections the L&H cells stain with antibodies to CD20 (L26) in over 90% of cases and with antibodies to CD45 and EMA in around 50% of cases. Very variable results have been reported using antibodies to CD30 (Ki-1, Ber-H2) staining. Although most cases show CD30 (Ki-1) staining of L&H cells in frozen sections, Ber-H2 stains less than 50% of cases in paraffin sections. CD15 (Leu-M1, Dako-M1) staining of L&H cells is unusual in NLPHD (Nicholas et al 1990, Bishop et al 1991).

These findings suggest that L&H cells are of B cell origin, a hypothesis that is supported by the finding of J chains in L&H cells (Stein et al 1986). It should be noted that in most cases L&H cells show polytypic (presumably endocytosed) immunoglobulin light chain expression. However it has been reported that in some cases L&H cells express monotypic kappa or lambda light chains (Schmid et al 1991b, Momose et al 1992). This has recently been confirmed by in situ hybridization for light chain mRNA (Hell et al 1993). Most studies have failed to demonstrate immunoglobulin gene rearrangements (Algara et al 1991, Said et al 1991).

The background lymphocyte population within the nodules of NLPHD differs from that of other types of HD with the majority of lymphocytes marking as B cells, rather than T cells, and expressing polyclonal immunoglobulin kappa and lambda chains. Within the nodules containing these B cells there is a prominent dendritic cell network which can be demostrated by antibodies to CD21 or DRCs (Alavaikko et al 1991, Poppema 1992). A further distinguishing feature in NLPHD is that the T cells within the nodules and clustered around L&H cells have a unique follicle centre T cell phenotype, expressing the Leu-7 (CD57) which is absent from T cells in other subtypes (Poppema 1989, Kamel et al 1993).

Diffuse lymphocyte predominant HD (DLPHD) may coexist with NLPHD or present with a purely diffuse growth pattern often associated with large numbers of histiocytes (Hansmann et al 1991). Most cases contain polylobated L&H RS cells which usually show an identical B cell phenotype to those of NLPHD (i.e. CD20$^+$ CD15$^-$). In contrast to NLPHD the reactive background population shows loss of Dentritic Reticular Cells (DRCs) with fewer B cells and more T cells. A major problem in the diagnosis of DLPHD is that this condition shows morphological and some immunophenotypic overlap with other subgroups of HD, especially MCHD (Bishop et al 1991), and with NHL including T cell rich or histiocyte rich B cell lymphoma and peripheral T cell lymphomas, especially Lennert's lymphoma. The differential dignosis of these conditions from HD is discussed in the section on MCHD. If classical RS cells, with a CD20$^-$ CD15$^+$ phenotype, are present cases should probably be classified as MCHD or NSHD. Classification of cases which lack typical RS cells but show L&H cells with an atypical CD15$^+$ CD20$^{+/-}$ phenotype is more controversial with some authors advocating classification as mixed cellularity (Wright 1989, Nicholas et al 1990). Most authors, however, believe that the morphology, immunophenotypic overlap and similar clinical behaviour to NLPHD supports retention of such cases in the LPHD group (Borg-Grech et al 1989, Hansmann et al 1991, Tefferi et al 1990).

Nodular sclerosing Hodgkin's disease (NSHD)

Nodular sclerosing Hodgkin's disease (NSHD) is the most common type of HD and accounts for around 70% of cases. It occurs mainly in young adults and in contrast to other histological subtypes does not show male predominance. The mediastinum and neck nodes are the most commonly involved sites (Colby et al 1981, Mauch et al 1993).

Histological and immunophenotypic features

The diagnosis of NSHD requires identification of classical RS cells together with nodule formation, lacunar cells and at least some evidence of intranodal fibrosis with organized birefringent collagen bands (Bennett et al 1991). Lacunar cells show abundant clear cytoplasm within which there is an ovoid or polylobated nucleus showing fine chromatin and smaller nucleoli than in classical RS cells. Lacunar cells may be found singly or in aggregates, sometimes forming large 'syncytial' sheets within which there are areas of necrosis (Fig. 4.3). The number and morphology of RS and lacunar cells and the composition of the cellular background in NSHD are widely variable, ranging from lymphocyte predominant to lymphocyte depleted (Figs 4.4, 4.5) with variable numbers of eosinophils, plasma cells and histiocytes as well as widely varying amounts of banding sclerosis and intranodular sclerosis.

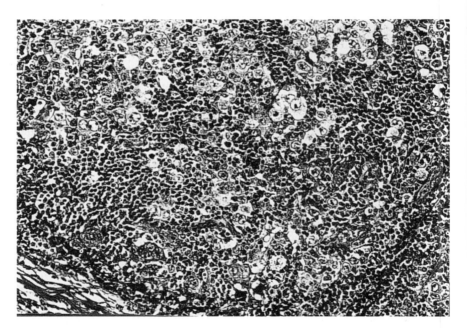

Fig. 4.4 Nodular sclerosing Hodgkin's disease showing a nodule in which clusters of lacunar cells are present in a background of small lymphocytes. H&E × 100.

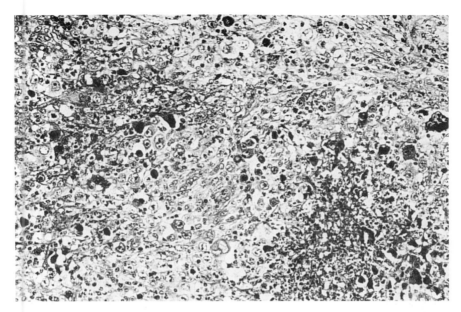

Fig. 4.5   Nodular sclerosing Hodgkin's disease showing lymphocyte depletion (NS-2). The infiltrate consists almost entirely of abnormal large mononuclear cells with occasional RS cells. Two areas of necrosis are also present. H&E × 100.

Although bands of fibrosis are usually a prominent feature, distinction of cellular phase NSHD with minimal sclerosis from other subtypes may sometimes only be possible after careful examination of sections from several areas. Subdivision of NSHD into good (NS-1) and poor (NS-2) prognostic categories has been proposed with classification of NS-2 defined as follows (MacLennan et al 1989): > 25% of nodules show lymphocyte depletion resembling reticular lymphocyte depleted HD, or > 80% show fibrohistiocytic lymphocyte depletion, or > 25% of nodules show bizarre and highly anaplastic Hodgkin's cells without lymphocyte depletion. Although some reports have supported the value of this subdivision (Ferry et al 1993, Wijlhuizen et al 1989) other groups have failed to substantiate its reproducibility and prognostic significance (Bernhards et al 1992, D'Amore et al 1992, Masih et al 1992). It is important to be aware of the existence of lymphocyte depleted and fibrohistiocytic variants of NSHD, including the syncytial variant of NSHD (Ben-Yehuda-Salz et al 1990), as they may be misclassified as lymphocyte depleted HD or misdiagnosed as high grade NHL, especially sclerosing mediastinal NHL (Perrone et al 1986, Al-Sharabati et al 1991).

Immunophenotyping using paraffin sections in NSHD shows that RS cells and lacunar cells express CD15 and CD30 in over 80% of cases but only rarely express CD20 (L26) or T cell markers such as CD3 or CD45RO (UCHL1) (Figs 4.6, 4.7) (reviewed by Hugh & Poppema 1992, Drexler 1992). Using frozen sections, several groups have reported that over 50% of cases

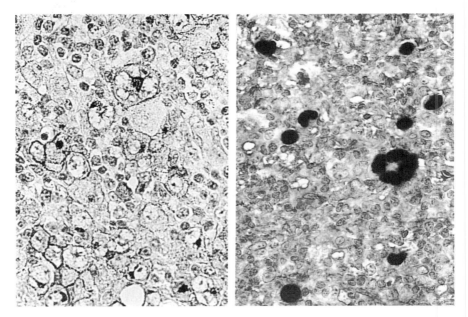

Fig. 4.6   Nodular sclerosing Hodgkin's disease. Left panel: CD30 (Ber-H2) showing membrane and cytoplasmic staining of multinucleated RS and uninucleated Hodgkin's cells. ABC peroxidase staining × 250. Right panel: EBER in situ hybridization showing staining of multinucleated RS and uni-nucleated Hodgkin's cells. × 250.

express T cell antigens such as CD2, CD3 or T cell receptor (TCR) β chains (Agnarsson & Kadin 1989, Dallenbach & Stein 1989). Accurate interpretation of staining of RS cells, which are surrounded by reactive T lymphocytes, with T cell markers is, however, extremely difficult and frozen section studies are not generally helpful in the diagnosis of HD. The background lymphocyte population in NSHD consists predominantly of T lymphocytes with a mature T helper phenotype (CD3$^+$ CD4$^+$ CD45RO$^+$).

Although immunophenotyping is probably unnecessary in most cases of NSHD, it is essential in some cases showing lymphocyte depletion in order to exclude high grade B cell or T cell NHL. Immunogenotyping may be helpful in excluding T cell lymphoma as TCR rearrangements, although reported, are rare in HD. Detection of immunoglobulin (Ig) rearrangements are of limited value as these are present in around 20% of cases of NSHD as well in B cell lymphomas (Gledhill et al 1990).

Mixed cellularity Hodgkin's disease (MCHD)

Mixed cellularity Hodgkin's disease (MCHD) is the second most common type of HD and accounts for between 20% and 40% of cases. It occurs mainly in young adults but is also more common than other subtypes in older patients. It is more common in males. The neck nodes are the most

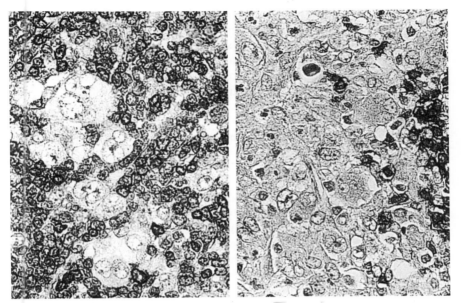

Fig. 4.7 Nodular sclerosing Hodgkin's disease. Left panel: CD3 (poly CD3) showing staining of small lymphocytes between and around RS cells but with no staining of RS cells. ABC peroxidase staining × 250. Right panel: CD20 (L26) showing a small aggregate of normal B cells but no staining of RS or mononuclear Hodgkin's cells. ABC peroxidase staining × 250.

commonly involved site and mediastinal involvement is less common than in NSHD (Colby et al 1981, Mauch et al 1993).

Histological and immunophenotypic features

The diagnosis of MCHD requires identification of classical RS cells. The number and morphology of RS cells and the composition of the cellular background in cases of MCHD are widely variable. The latter ranges from lymphocyte predominant to areas of lymphocyte depletion but usually includes eosinophils, plasma cells and histiocytes and may also show irregular sclerosis. Both lacunar cells and pleomorphic variants of RS cells may be present. The distinction of MCHD from other subtypes of HD is not always clear since MCHD represents a dumping ground where cases are placed if they do not fulfil all the criteria for NSHD or LPHD. The presence of classical RS cells that express CD15 and CD30 usually allows distinction from LPHD. Distinction from cellular phase NSHD can, however, often be difficult but the identification of at least minimal organized sclerosis with birefringent collagen within the lymph node and the presence of lacunar cells and nodularity should be seen before cellular phase NSHD is diagnosed (Bennett et al 1991). Areas of lymphocyte depletion may also be identified but these cases show similar clinical behaviour to typical MCHD and should therefore be retained in the MCHD group (Bennett et al 1991).

Immunophenotyping using paraffin sections gives similar results to NSHD (see above) with expression of CD15 and CD30 in around 80% of cases. As with NSHD, in occasional cases RS cells may express B or T cell markers. The background lymphocyte population in MCHD as in NSHD consists predominantly of T lymphocytes with a mature T helper phenotype.

The distinction of MCHD from NHL may present difficulty. Cases of peripheral T-cell lymphoma (Lennert's lymphoma, T zone lymphoma, AIL-like lymphoma) and T cell rich and histiocyte rich B cell lymphoma (Patsouris et al 1989, Chittal et al 1991, Delabie et al 1992) may show considerable morphological overlap with MCHD. In peripheral T cell lymphomas there may be a similar polymorphous infiltrate including eosinophils, plasma cells and histiocytes. However, classical RS cells are absent or present in only very small numbers and there is usually clear expression of T cell markers by neoplastic blast cells as well as small and intermediate lymphocytes. The lymphocyte population in peripheral T cell lymphomas also tends to show more pleomorphism, frequent presence of clear cells and a high mitotic rate compared to MCHD (Harris 1992, Krajewski et al 1988, Osborne et al 1990b). In T cell lymphoma, although CD30 expression by large blasts is common, CD15 expression, particularly strong membrane and/or golgi area staining, is rare and favours a diagnosis of HD (Krajewski et al 1988, Patsouris et al 1989, Tosi et al 1992).

Demonstration of clonal TCR rearrangements may help in the distinction of MCHD from peripheral T cell lymphomas in some cases. Absence of TCR rearrangements would support the diagnosis of MCHD (Gledhill et al 1990, Harris 1992) although it should be noted that some groups have reported that up to 20% of cases HD show TCR β chain rearrangements (Griesser et al 1987) and conversely rearrangements may not be detectable in some T cell lymphomas (Weiss et al 1988).

In T cell rich B cell lymphoma only rare RS cells can be identified together with more numerous large blast cells in a background of small lymphocytes which may show nuclear irregularity. Although histiocytes may occasionally be numerous, other accompanying cells such as eosinophils and plasma cells are not present. Immunophenotyping shows that the large cells, including RS-like cells, express B cell antigens such as CD20, and also express EMA but do not express the RS-associated antigens CD15 and CD30. The B cells show monotypic Ig expression in some cases (Ramsay et al 1988) and most cases show clonal Ig gene rearrangements (Osborne et al 1990a).

Lymphocyte depleted Hodgkin's disease (LDHD)

Lymphocyte depleted Hodgkin's disease (LDHD) is the least common type of HD and in most recent series accounts for less than 5% of cases, although in an earlier series from Lukes' group it represented 18% of cases (Lukes et al

1966). Two histological subtypes of LDHD are recognized: diffuse fibrosis and reticular (Lukes & Butler 1966).

Histological and immunophenotypic features

In the diffuse fibrosis subtype there is disorganized sclerosis with a hypocellular background containing few classical RS cells and numerous abnormal large mononuclear Hodgkin's cells. In the reticular subtype, cellular sheets of pleomorphic RS cells, with bizarre multilobated nuclei and large nucleoli, as well as large mononuclear cells are present together with small numbers of lymphocytes, neutrophils and eosinophils. Features of both subtypes commonly coexist within the same biopsy and both subtypes often show foci of necrosis.

The rarity of LDHD in recent series is largely a result of the recognition that some cases previously diagnosed as LDHD show organized birefringent collagen band formation and therefore should be classified as NSHD. These cases include fibrohistiocytic variants of NSHD resembling the diffuse fibrosis subtype of LDHD and cases of reticular, pleomorphic or syncytial lymphocyte depleted variants of NSHD (Bennett et al 1991) resembling reticular LDHD. Following the introduction of immunophenotyping many other cases previously diagnosed as reticular LDHD are now diagnosed as NHL, usually of Ki-1 positive large cell anaplastic type.

The distinction of reticular LDHD from large cell anaplastic lymphoma (LCAL) can be extremely difficult and depends on careful assessment of both cytological and architectural features of the tumour cell infiltrate and immunophenotypic investigation (Agnarsson & Kadin 1988). Cytologically LCALs show marked pleomorphism and include both mononuclear immunoblast-like cells and multinucleated tumour giant cells with large vesicular nuclei containing large nucleoli which may resemble RS cells. In most cases tumour cells have abundant eosinophilic cytoplasm. There is a high mitotic and apoptotic rate and necrosis may be seen. Architecturally, tumour cells tend to show cohesive growth, with preferential sinusoidal and paracortical node infiltration. Some cases may show capsular and intranodal sclerosis. Immunophenotypic studies have shown considerable overlap between RS cells and the cells in LCAL. Definite distinction between the two tumours is not possible on the basis of immunohistochemistry alone. There are, however, certain antigens that are more commonly expressed in LCAL than HD. About 80–90% cases of LCAL express CD45 and 50% express EMA, both of which are only expressed in 10–20% of cases of HD. About 50% express T cell markers such as CD43, CD45RO and CD3 and 20% express B cell markers such as MB1, CD20 (L26), which are only occasionally expressed by RS cells in a small number of cases of HD (Herbst et al 1989, Carbone et al 1992). CD15 expression is common in HD (80–90%) but uncommon in LCAL (Carbone et al 1992, Leoncini et al 1990). Genotypic analyses have shown a higher incidence of TCR and Ig gene rearrangements in LCAL than HD with around 60% of cases showing TCR rearrangements and 20% of cases showing Ig gene rearrangements (Herbst et al 1989).

HISTOGENESIS OF HODGKIN'S DISEASE

Immunophenotype and genotype of Hodgkin's and RS cells

A large number of studies have investigated the immunophenotype of RS cells using frozen or more recently paraffin sections and less commonly using imprint preparations or cytospins (reviewed by Hugh & Poppema 1992, Drexler 1992). There is now a general consensus that classical RS cells and their mononuclear variants (H/RS cells) have a phenotype consistent with derivation from an activated lymphoid cell. RS cells consistently express activation-associated antigens such as CD71 (transferrin receptor), CD25 (interleukin 2 receptor, IL-2R), MHC II (Hugh & Poppema 1992), adhesion molecules such as CD54 (ICAM-1), CD58 (LFA-3), CD44 and CD15 (Paietta 1992), and growth factor receptors such as CD30 and CD40 (members of the nerve growth factor receptor family) (Durkop et al 1992, O'Grady et al 1994).

In LPHD the L&H variant RS cells consistently express B cell antigens such as CD20, and LPHD is now regarded as a distinct subgroup of HD of B cell derivation (Poppema 1992). The histogenesis of the other subtypes of HD remains much more controversial. Using routine diagnostic panels, limited to a few T or B cell specific antibodies on paraffin sections, inconsistent and usually negative results are obtained with T and B cell markers (Hall et al 1988, Hugh & Poppema 1992). In detailed phenotypic studies using extended antibody panels some authors have claimed that B cell antigens are expressed by H/RS cells in a majority of cases of NSHD and MCHD (Schmid et al 1991a), although others have claimed that few cases express B cell markers while in many cases of NSHD and MCHD the RS cells express T cell markers (Agnarrson & Kadin 1989, Dallenbach & Stein 1989).

Recently, attempts to resolve the identity of the RS cell have been made using the novel technique of single cell polymerase chain reaction (PCR) to study gene expression by RS cells isolated from biopsy specimens by micromanipulation (Trumper et al 1993). In this study RS cells were found to coexpress genes characteristic of several haematopoietic lineages and therefore could not be unequivocally identified as macrophage, B, or T cell derived. A group of genes was expressed by the large majority of RS cells examined; this included c-*myc*, the c-*fes/fps* oncogene, the *fyn* tyrosine kinase, the IL-2R β chain, tumour necrosis factor-β and CD4. Overall, the expression pattern was consistent with that of an activated haematopoietic cell.

The analysis of Ig and TCR genes has been used to investigate the histogenesis of RS cells and as a potential diagnostic tool. The proportion of cases with detectable rearrangement of Ig genes varies from 0% to 25% between studies (Knowles et al 1986, Griesser et al 1987, Herbst et al 1989, Gledhill et al 1991). In studies which have selected cases on the basis of high RS cell numbers or enriched for RS cells, a higher proportion of rearrangements has been found (Sundeen et al 1987, Weiss et al 1986). It is clear that Ig gene rearrangements are not present in all cases since some cases with high percentages of abnormal cells have Ig genes in the germline configuration (Gledhill et al 1991, Knowles et al 1986). Although there are two reports describing a high incidence of TCR β chain gene rearrangement (4/22 and 6/39 respectively) (Griesser et al 1987, Herbst et al 1989), many other studies have failed to confirm these findings and TCR β chain rearrangements are probably rare even in cases that show expression of T cell markers on H/RS cells (Gledhill et al 1991, Schmid et al 1991a). Evidence that the rearrangements are present in RS cells is only indirect but results following RS cell enrichment, and comparison of the percentage of abnormal cells with intensity of rearranged bands, lend some support to the interpretation that rearrangements are present in RS cells rather than the reactive lymphocytic infiltrate (Gledhill et al 1987, Sundeen et al 1987, Weiss et al 1986).

The conflicting results obtained from immunophenotypic and genotypic studies outlined above have not yet clearly defined whether RS cells are of T or B cell origin. There is a strong possibility that while HD appears to be a clinically and histopathologically well-defined entity it would be better regarded as a syndrome that includes related but histogenetically distinct tumours. It has been suggested that RS cells may be derived from immature T or B cell precursors which differentiate abnormally to show dissociation between lineage specific and genotypic markers (Herbst et al 1989) and that the abnormal phenotype and expression of activation antigens may be a consequence of viral infection (Stein et al 1991). It is thought likely that the common histopathological pattern with the characteristic polymorphous cellular infiltrate associated with tumour cells in Hodgkin's disease is consequent upon the secretion of cytokines by H/RS cells and T cells interacting with H/RS cells (Merz et al 1991).

Oncogenes

Studies of oncogene involvement in HD have been hindered by the relative paucity of RS cells within tumour infiltrates and have largely been restricted to analyses of HD derived cell lines (Jucker et al 1990). These studies have shown a number of different oncogenes and are expressed by cell lines in vitro but the in vivo relevance of these findings is uncertain. A further problem in identifying oncogenes involved in HD is the lack of any consistent chromosomal abnormality detectable by cytogenetics (Sandberg 1990). Recent results on bcl-2 and p53 are, however, worthy of mention.

The proto-oncogene bcl-2 was first identified because of its involvement in the chromosomal translocation t(14;18), which is found in the majority of follicular lymphomas and around 30% of diffuse large cell lymphomas. *bcl*-2 inhibits apoptosis and therefore increases cell survival. In 1990 it was reported that t(14;18) could be detected in 17/53 (32%) of HD cases using PCR (Stetler-Stevenson et al 1990). This finding stimulated a number of similar studies which gave rise to conflicting results. Some workers failed to detect any *bcl*-2 rearrangements (Schmid et al 1991a, Said et al 1991) whereas others detected rearrangement in a minority of cases (Lorenzen et al 1992, Reid et al 1993). Since t(14;18) has been detected in benign lymphoid tissue using PCR, the key issue is whether this translocation is present in the RS cells. Reid et al (1993) addressed this question in one case by separating nuclei into large and small populations and showing that the rearrangement was present in large nuclei. Poppema analysed 28 cases using both PCR and cytogenetics coupled with in situ hybridization; *bcl*-2 rearrangements were found in almost 40% of the cases using PCR but their detection did not correlate with the presence of t(14;18) detected cytogenetically (Poppema et al 1992). Thus, they concluded that this translocation was most probably present within cells in the reactive infiltrate. Studies which have examined the expression of *bcl*-2 by RS cells have also given varying results but overall it would appear that RS cells in many cases express low to moderate levels of *bcl*-2 protein. There is, however, no correlation between the presence of *bcl*-2 protein in RS cells and t(14;18) detectable by PCR (Schmid et al 1991a, Lorenzen et al 1992). It therefore seems unlikely that the *bcl*-2 proto-oncogene plays a major role in the pathogenesis of HD.

Mutation of the p53 tumour suppressor gene is thought to be the most frequent abnormality detectable in human tumours. This protein has a short half-life and levels in non-transformed cells are low, but stabilization by mutation or binding to cellular or viral proteins renders it detectable using immunohistological techniques. Studies investigating p53 expression in HD have detected p53, restricted to the RS cells, in 32–74% of cases (Doglioni et al 1991, Gupta et al 1992, Niedobitek et al 1993); p53 expression has been detected in all subtypes with the exception of LPHD (Doglioni et al 1991, Gupta et al 1992, Niedobitek et al 1993). Using single cell PCR techniques Trumper et al (1993) detected a mutation in exon 7 of the p53 gene in five out of seven RS cells from the one case they examined. These results suggest that p53 may play a role in the pathogenesis of some cases of HD.

Viruses and Hodgkin's disease

Many features of the epidemiology and pathology of HD suggest that an infectious agent is involved in its causation. Early seroepidemiological studies linked the EBV with HD, but it was not until 1987 that Weiss and colleagues demonstrated the presence of EBV genomes within HD biopsies (Levine et al 1971, Weiss et al 1987).

Although most healthy adults are infected with EBV, the virus remains latent in B cells at a level of infection of about 1 in 10^5–10^6 peripheral blood mononuclear cells. This level of infection is not sufficient to enable detection by conventional Southern blot analysis. Using Southern blot analysis EBV genomes are, however, detected in biopsy samples from 19–41% of cases of HD (Weiss et al 1987, Boiocchi et al 1989, Gledhill et al 1991, Jarrett et al 1991). Analysis of the terminal repeats of the EBV genome, which is present in a plasmid form and not integrated in infected cells, has shown that the infected cells in HD biopsies are clonal with respect to EBV, consistent with the expansion of a single infected cell (Weiss et al 1987, Boiocchi et al 1989, Gledhill et al 1991, Jarrett et al 1991).

Demonstration that the virus is present in the RS cells in HD has been accomplished using immunohistochemical and in situ hybridization techniques (Fig. 4.6) (Pallesen et al 1991a, Armstrong et al 1992b, Weiss et al 1991). Comparison of immunohistochemical staining, using antibodies to EBV latent membrane protein (LMP-1), and in situ hybridization, using probes to the EBV EBER RNA molecules, has shown that the latter technique is more reliable in the detection of latent EBV infection (Armstrong et al 1992b). The EBER transcripts are two small, abundantly transcribed RNA molecules which are present in the nuclei of all cells latently infected with EBV (Howe & Mei-Di Shu 1989). Many studies have now been performed using this assay on HD samples and the results are remarkably consistent: EBV can be detected in the RS cells of 28–48% of cases (Armstrong et al 1992b, Weiss et al 1991, Niedobitek et al 1993); within a positive case the vast majority of abnormal cells are positively stained; consistent results are obtained following examination of samples removed at different time points; scattered EBV positive lymphocytes are detectable within the reactive infiltrate (Armstrong et al 1992b, Ambinder et al 1993, Chang et al 1993).

EBV has the capacity to encode around 80 proteins but in latent infection only a restricted group of proteins is expressed. These include six nuclear proteins (the EBNAs), and three membrane proteins (LMP-1, -2a and -2b) (reviewed by Kieff & Liebowitz 1990). The EBNA-1 protein is a DNA binding protein which plays a crucial role in maintaining the viral genome in a plasmid form. Expression of EBNA-2 and LMP-1 appears to be essential for the immortalization of B cells and the LMP-1 protein is the only EBV latent protein which, in isolation, has been shown to have transforming properties. In B cells three patterns of expression of these latent proteins have been described: in type I latency only the EBNA-1 protein is expressed; in type II EBNA-1 is expressed along with the LMPs; and in type III all nine proteins are expressed (Rowe et al 1992). The different patterns of latent gene expression have been associated with the various malignancies associated with EBV. In Burkitt's lymphoma only the EBNA-1 protein is expressed whereas in lymphomas in immunosuppressed persons type III latency is seen. Immunohistochemical studies provide convincing evidence that the LMP-1 protein is expressed by RS cells in EBV positive cases whereas EBNA-2 expression has not been detected (Pallesen et al 1991a, Armstrong et al

1992b). A study on EBV latent gene expression at the RNA level showed the presence of EBNA-1 and LMP-1 and -2 transcripts but absence of EBNA-2 mRNA (Deacon et al 1993). This conforms to the type II pattern of latency described above. EBV lytic cycle proteins have been detected in only occasional RS cells in a minority of cases of HD (Pallesen et al 1991b).

The expression of LMP-1 by RS cells suggests that the EBV is likely to be playing some role in the pathogenesis of HD. LMP-1 is known to induce a number of cellular genes including CD23, CD30, CD40 and bcl-2. There is, however, no clear correlation between the detection of these proteins and LMP-1 expression in RS cells (Armstrong et al 1992a, O'Grady et al 1994). Further studies are required to determine the role of LMP-1 in HD.

It is clear that EBV is involved in only a proportion (33–50%) of cases of HD. Epidemiological studies have consistently suggested, however, that HD is a heterogeneous condition which is likely to have more than one aetiology (Correa & O'Conor 1971, MacMahon 1966). HD has a bimodal age/incidence curve: in developed countries the first peak occurs in young adults, there is a decline in incidence in the fourth decade and in older age groups the incidence increases or plateaus. In contrast, in developing countries the first age incidence peak is seen in childhood, the young adult peak is absent and the second peak is again seen in older adults (Correa & O'Conor 1971, MacMahon 1966, McKinney et al 1989). NSHD largely accounts for the young adult age incidence peak whereas MCHD is relatively more common in childhood and older adults (McKinney et al 1989, Correa & O'Conor 1971, MacMahon 1966). Risk factors for the development of HD vary in the different age groups with young adult HD being associated with factors which suggest a high standard of living in early childhood (Gutensohn & Cole 1977, MacMahon 1966, Alexander et al 1991). These features lead to two hypotheses regarding the aetiology of HD: first that HD is a group of conditions with different aetiologies in different age groups and secondly that HD in young adults in developed countries is related to delayed exposure to a common infectious agent (MacMahon 1966, Gutensohn & Cole 1977).

EBV has been detected within the RS cells of all subtypes of HD. However, many studies have shown a significant excess of EBV positive cases within the MCHD subtype (Pallesen et al 1991a, Weiss et al 1991). The number of LDHD cases examined has been smaller but it is likely that EBV is also associated with this subtype. We have also shown a significant association between age at diagnosis and EBV positivity, with paediatric and older adult cases being more likely to be EBV-associated than young adult cases (Jarrett et al 1991). Some, but not all, other studies have confirmed this age distribution; different results can in part be explained by different age and subtype distributions within individual case series (Khan et al 1993).

A high incidence of EBV-associated cases has been noted in Peru and the proportion of EBV positive cases was found to be higher in children from Honduras than in those from the USA (Ambinder et al 1993, Chang et al 1993). We compared the incidence of EBV positivity in children from Brazil with children from the UK; although samples from Brazilian children were more likely to be EBV positive, differences were not apparent when adjustment for age and subtype were included in the analysis (Armstrong et al 1993). A striking feature of the above study was that almost all children under the age of 10 years, from any of the locales tested, had EBV-associated disease. The above results are consistent with a model which suggests that EBV is associated with paediatric cases < 10 years, the majority of older adult cases and most cases of mixed cellularity disease, and that EBV-associated disease is relatively more common in countries in which the young adult age incidence peak is not present. Despite the association between EBV and subtypes with a less favourable clinical outcome there is no evidence that EBV status is a useful prognostic marker (Vestlev et al 1992).

We believe that another virus may be involved in the pathogenesis of HD in young adults in developed countries. Candidate viruses are the recently identified herpesviruses HHV-6 and HHV-7. Infection with both agents is common and widespread and the majority of healthy adults are persistently infected. HD patients, particularly those in the young adult age group, have elevated antibody titres to HHV-6 antigens (Clark et al 1990). Using Southern blot analysis we have not detected HHV-6 genomes in any of > 50 biopsy specimens analysed and Khan et al did not detect HHV-6 in 77 cases examined using DNA in situ hybridization (Gledhill et al 1991, Jarrett et al 1991, Khan et al 1993). Torelli et al (1991) detected HHV-6 using PCR in tumour samples from three cases and in two of these Southern blot analysis indicated a relatively high viral load in the specimens. In one HD case they further showed that HHV-6 sequences were integrated into cellular DNA in peripheral blood mononuclear cells (Luppi et al 1993). Viral sequences have not been localized to RS cells and a sensitive in situ hybridization assay is needed to confirm or refute the direct involvement of this virus in HD. Studies on HHV-7 are more limited at present, but we have not detected HHV-7 sequences in over 50 samples examined to date (our unpublished results with Zwi Berneman). Studies on cytomegalovirus have also given negative results (Weiss et al 1987, Khan et al 1993).

CONCLUSIONS

The diagnosis of HD is primarily dependent on histological findings and requires the identification of classical Reed–Sternberg (RS) cells, or variants, in an appropriate cellular background.

The nature of the cellular background in which RS cells are found forms the basis of the Rye classification of Hodgkin's disease which divides HD into four main subgroups: lymphocyte predominant (LP), nodular sclerosis (NS), mixed cellularity (MC), lymphocyte depleted (LD). It has been proposed that NSHD should be further subclassified into good (NS-1) and poor (NS-2) prognosis categories.

Immunophenotypic studies have shown that LPHD is a biologically distinct entity, of B cell origin, in which B cell antigens are consistently expressed by L&H type RS cells. In other subtypes the detection of RS-associated antigens, such as CD15 and CD30, in the absence of T or B cell markers on tumour cells may be useful diagnostically, especially in the differential diagnosis of HD and certain types of NHL which show morphological overlap with HD.

Despite intensive effort there is still uncertainty regarding the histogenesis of the RS cell. Conventional immunophenotyping and immunogenotyping studies have given conflicting results. It is likely that future progress will depend on the introduction of new methods to the study of HD. These include the use of single cell techniques to generate cDNA libraries from RS cells and the development of improved in situ hybridization methodologies on tissue sections.

Since the first description of HD it has been suggested that there may be an infectious aetiology. However, it has only been in the last 7 years that an infectious agent, EBV, has been definitively linked with HD. At present the role of the virus is not clear and further studies, on EBV and the host immune response to EBV, are needed to resolve this question. It is clear that EBV is involved in only around 40% of cases. Epidemiological studies suggest that another infectious agent is present in the remaining cases.

REFERENCES

Agnarsson BA, Kadin ME 1988 Ki-1 Positive large cell lymphoma. A morphologic and immunologic study of 19 cases. Am J Surg Pathol 12: 264–274

Agnarsson BA, Kadin ME 1989 The immunophenotype of Reed–Sternberg cells. A study of 50 cases of Hodgkin's disease using fixed frozen tissues. Cancer 63: 2083–2087

Alavaikko MJ, Hansmann ML, Nebendahl C et al 1991 Follicular dendritic cells in Hodgkin's disease. Am J Clin Pathol 95: 194–200

Alexander FE, McKinney PA, Williams J et al 1991 Epidemiological evidence for the 'Two-disease hypothesis' in Hodgkin's disease. Int J Epidemiol 202: 354–361

Algara P, Martinez P, Sanchez L et al 1991 Lymphocyte predominance Hodgkin's disease (nodular paragranuloma) — a bcl-2 negative germinal centre lymphoma. Histopathology 19: 69–75

Al-Sharabati M, Chittal S, Duga-Neulat I et al 1991 Primary anterior mediastinal B-cell lymphoma. A clinicopathologic and immunohistochemical study of 16 cases. Cancer 67: 2579–2587

Ambinder RF, Browning PJ, Lorenzana I et al 1993 Epstein–Barr virus and childhood Hodgkin's disease in Honduras and the United States. Blood 81: 462–467

Armstrong AA, Gallagher A, Krajewski AS et al 1992a The expression of the EBV latent membrane protein (LMP-1) is independent of CD23 and bcl-2 in Reed–Sternberg cells in Hodgkin's disease. Histopathology 21: 72–73

Armstrong AA, Weiss LM, Gallagher A et al 1992b Criteria for the definition of Epstein–Barr virus association in Hodgkin's disease. Leukemia 6: 869–874

Armstrong, AA, Alexander FE, Pinto Paes R et al 1993 Association of Epstein Barr virus with paediatric Hodgkin's disease. Am J Pathol 142: 1683–1688

Bennett MH, MacLennan KA, Vaughan Hudson B et al 1991 The clinical and prognostic relevance of histopathologic classification in Hodgkin's disease. Prog Surg Pathol 10: 127–151

Ben-Yehuda-Salz D, Ben-Yehuda A, Polliack A et al 1990 Syncytial variant of nodular sclerosing Hodgkin's disease. A new clinicopathologic entity. Cancer 65: 1167–1172

Bernhards J, Fischer R, Hubner K et al 1992 Histopathological classification of Hodgkin's lymphomas. Results from the reference pathology of the German Hodgkin Trial. Annals of Oncology 3 (Suppl 4): 31–33

Bishop PW, Harris M, Smith AP et al 1991 Immunophenotypic study of lymphocyte predominance Hodgkin's disease. Histopathology 18: 19–24

Boiocchi M, Carbone A, De Re V et al 1989 Is the Epstein–Barr virus involved in Hodgkin's disease? Tumori 75: 345–350

Borg-Grech A, Radford JA, Crowther D et al 1989 A comparative study of the nodular and diffuse variants of lymphocyte-predominant Hodgkin's disease. J Clin Oncol 7: 1303–1309

Butler JJ 1992 The histologic diagnosis of Hodgkin's disease. Semin Diagn Pathol 9: 252–256

Carbone A, Gloghini A, Volpe R 1992 Paraffin section immunohistochemistry in the diagnosis of Hodgkin's disease and anaplastic large cell (CD30 +) lymphomas. Virchows Arch A Pathol Anat 420: 527–532

Chang KL, Albujar PF, Chen YY et al 1993 High prevalence of Epstein–Barr virus in the Reed–Sternberg cells of Hodgkin's disease occurring in Peru. Blood 81: 496–501

Chittal SM, Brousset P, Voigt J-J, Delsol G 1991 Large B-cell lymphoma rich in T-cells and simulating Hodgkin's disease. Histopathology 19: 211–220

Clark DA, Alexander FE, McKinney P et al 1990 The seroepidemiology of human herpesvirus-6 (HHV-6) from a case control study of leukaemia and lymphoma. Int J Cancer 45: 829–833

Colby TV, Hoppe RT, Warnke RA 1981 Hodgkin's disease: a clinicopathologic study of 659 cases. Cancer 49: 1848–1858

Correa P, O'Conor GT 1971 Epidemiologic patterns of Hodgkin's disease. Int J Cancer 8: 192–201

Dallenbach FE, Stein H 1989 Expression of T-cell receptor β chain in Reed–Sternberg cells. Lancet 2: 828–830

Deacon EM, Pallesen G, Niedobitek G et al 1993 Epstein–Barr virus and Hodgkin's disease: transcriptional analysis of virus latency in the malignant cells. J Exp Med 177: 339–349

Delabie J, Vandenberghe E, Kennes C et al 1992 Histiocyte-rich B-cell lymphoma: a distinct clinicopathologic entity possibly related to lymphocyte predominant Hodgkin's disease, paragranuloma subtype. Am J Surg Pathol 16: 37–48

D'Amore ESG, Lee CKK, Aeppli DM et al 1992 Lack of prognostic value of histopathologic parameters in Hodgkin's disease, nodular sclerosis type: a study of 123 patients with limited stage disease who had undergone laparotomy and were treated with radiation therapy. Arch Pathol Lab Med 116: 856–861

Doglioni C, Pelosio P, Mombello A et al 1991 Immunohistochemical evidence for abnormal expression of the antioncogene-encoded phosphoprotein in Hodgkin's disease and CD30 + anaplastic lymphomas. Hematol Pathol 5: 67–73

Drexler HG 1992 Recent results on the biology of Hodgkin and Reed–Sternberg cells. I. Biopsy material. Leukemia Lymphoma 8: 283–313

Durkop H, Latza U, Hummel M et al 1992 Molecular cloning and expression of a new member of the nerve growth factor receptor family that is characteristic for Hodgkin's disease. Cell 68: 421–427

Ferry JA, Linggood RM, Convery KM et al 1993 Hodgkin disease, nodular sclerosis type. Implications of histologic subclassification. Cancer 71: 457–463

Frizzera G 1992 The distinction of Hodgkin's disease from anaplastic large cell lymphoma. Semin Diagn Pathol 9: 291–296

Gledhill S, Krajewski AS, Dewar AE et al 1990 Analysis of T-cell receptor and immunoglobulin gene rearrangements in the diagnosis of Hodgkin's and non-Hodgkin's lymphoma. J Pathol 161: 245–254

Gledhill S, Gallagher A, Jones DB et al 1991 Viral involvement in Hodgkin's disease: detection of clonal type A Epstein–Barr genomes in tumour samples. Br J Cancer 64: 227–232

Griesser H, Feller A, Mak TW et al 1987 Clonal rearrangements of T-cell receptor and immunoglobulin genes and immunophenotypic antigen expression in different subclasses of Hodgkin's disease. Int J Cancer 40: 157–160

Gupta RK, Norton AJ, Thompson IW et al 1992 p53 expression in Reed–Sternberg cells of Hodgkin's disease. Br J Cancer 66: 649–652

Gutensohn N, Cole P 1977 Epidemiology of Hodgkin's disease in the young. Int J Cancer 19: 595–604

Hall PA, D'Ardenne AJ, Stansfeld AG 1988 Paraffin section immunohistochemistry. II. Hodgkin's disease and large cell anaplastic (Ki1) lymphoma. Histopathology 13: 161–169

Hansmann ML, Fellbaum C, Hui PK et al 1990 Progressive transformation of germinal centers with and without association to Hodgkin's disease. Am J Clin Pathol 93: 219–226

Hansmann ML, Stein H, Dallenbach F et al 1991 Diffuse lymphocyte predominant Hodgkin's disease (diffuse paragranuloma). A variant of the B-cell-derived nodular type. Am J Pathol 138: 29–36

Harris NL 1992 Differential diagnosis between Hodgkin's disease and non-Hodgkin's lymphoma. Int Rev Exp Pathol 33: 1–25

Hell K, Pringle JH, Hansmann ML et al 1993 Demonstration of light chain mRNA in Hodgkin's disease. J Pathol 171: 137–143

Herbst H, Tippelman G, Anagnostopoulos et al 1989 Immunoglobulin and T-cell receptor gene rearrangements in Hodgkin's disease and Ki-1 positive anaplastic large cell lymphoma: dissociation between phenotype and genotype. Leukemia Res 13: 103–116

Howe JG, Mei-Di Shu 1989 Epstein–Barr virus small RNA (EBER) genes: unique transcription units that combine RNA polymerase II and III promoter elements. Cell 57: 825–834

Hugh J, Poppema S 1992 Immunophenotype of Reed–Sternberg cells. Int Rev Exp Pathol 33: 81–114

Jarrett RF, Gallagher A, Jones DB et al 1991 Detection of Epstein–Barr virus genomes in Hodgkin's disease: relation to age. J Clin Pathol 44: 844–848

Jucker M, Schaadt M, Diehl V et al 1990 Heterogeneous expression of proto-oncogenes in Hodgkin's disease derived cell lines. Hematol Oncol 8: 191–204

Kamel OW, Gelb AB, Shibuya RB et al 1993 Leu 7 (CD57) reactivity distinguishes nodular lymphocyte predominance Hodgkin's disease from nodular sclerosing Hodgkin's disease, T-cell-rich B-cell lymphoma and follicular lymphoma. Am J Pathol 142: 541–546

Khan G, Norton AJ, Slavin G 1993 Epstein–Barr virus in Hodgkin disease. Relation to age and subtype. Cancer 71: 3124–3129

Kieff E, Liebowitz D 1990 Epstein–Barr virus and its replication. In: Fields BN, Knipe DM (eds) Virology. 2nd edn. Raven Press, New York, pp 1889–1920

Knowles DM, Neri A, Pelicci PG et al 1986 Immunoglobulin and T-cell receptor B-chain gene rearrangement analysis of Hodgkin's disease: implications for lineage determination and differential diagnosis. Proc Natl Acad Sci USA 83: 7942–7946

Krajewski AS, Myskow MW, Cachia PG et al 1988 T-cell lymphoma: morphology, immunophenotype and clinical features. Histopathology 13: 19–41

Leoncini L, Del Vecchio MT, Kraft R et al 1990 Hodgkin's disease and CD30-positive anaplastic large cell lymphomas — a continuous spectrum of malignant disorders. A quantitative morphometric and immunohistologic study. Am J Pathol 137: 1047–1057

Levine PH, Ablashi DV, Berard CW et al 1971 Elevated antibody titers to Epstein–Barr virus in Hodgkin's disease. Cancer 27: 416–421

Lorenzen J, Hansmann M, Pezzella F et al 1992 Expression of the bcl-2 oncogene product and chromosomal translocation t(14;18) in Hodgkin's disease. Hum Pathol 23: 1205–1209

Lukes RJ 1971 Criteria for involvement of lymph node, bone marrow, spleen and liver in Hodgkin's disease. Cancer Res 31: 1755–1767

Lukes RJ, Butler JJ 1993 The pathology and nomenclature of Hodgkin's disease. Cancer Res 26: 1063–1081

Lukes RJ, Butler JJ, Hicks EB 1966 Natural history of Hodgkin's disease as related to its pathologic picture. Cancer 19: 317–344

Luppi M, Marasca R, Barozzi P et al 1993 Three cases of human herpesvirus-6 latent infection: integration of viral genome in peripheral blood mononuclear cell DNA. J Med Virol 40: 44–52

McKinney PA, Alexander FE, Ricketts TJ et al 1989 A specialist leukaemia/lymphoma registry in the UK. Part 1: incidence and geographical distribution of Hodgkin's disease. Br J Cancer 60: 942–947

MacLennan KA, Bennett MH, Tu A et al 1989 Relationship of histopathologic features to survival and relapse in nodular sclerosing Hodgkin's disease: a study of 1659 patients. Cancer 64: 1686–1693

MacMahon B 1966 Epidemiology of Hodgkin's disease. Cancer Res 26: 1189–1200

Masih AS, Weisenburger DD, Vose JM et al 1992 Histologic grade does not predict prognosis in optimally treated advanced-stage nodular sclerosing Hodgkin's disease. Cancer 69: 228–232

Mauch PM, Kalish La, Kadin M et al 1993 Patterns of presentation of Hodgkin's disease: implications for etiology and pathogenesis. Cancer 71: 2062–2071

Merz H, Fliedner A, Orscheschek K et al 1991 Cytokine expression in T cell lymphomas and Hodgkin's disease: its possible implication in autocrine or paracrine production as a potential basis for neoplastic growth. Am J Pathol 139: 1173–1180

Momose H, Chen YY, Ben-Ezra J et al 1992 Nodular lymphocyte-predominant Hodgkin's disease: study of immunoglobulin light chain protein and mRNA expression. Hum Pathol 23: 1115–1119

Nicholas DS, Harris S, Wright DH 1990 Lymphocyte predominance Hodgkin's disease — an immunohistochemical study. Histopathology 16: 157–165

Niedobitek G, Rowlands DC, Young LS et al 1993 Overexpression of p53 in Hodgkin's disease: lack of correlation with Epstein–Barr virus infection. J Pathol 169: 207–212

O'Grady JT, Stewart S, Lowrey J et al 1994 CD40 expression in Hodgkin's disease. Am J Pathol 144: 21–26

Osborne BM, Butler JJ, Pugh WC 1990a The value of immunophenotyping on paraffin sections in the identification of T-cell rich B-cell large-cell lymphomas: lineage confirmed by J(H) rearrangement. Am J Surg Pathol 14: 933–938

Osborne BM, Uthman MO, Butler JJ et al 1990b Differentiation of T-cell lymphoma from Hodgkin's disease. Mitotic rate and S-phase analysis. Am J Clin Pathol 93: 227–232

Paietta E 1992 Cell adhesion molecules in Hodgkin's disease. Ann Oncol 3 (Suppl 4): 17–19

Pallesen G, Hamilton-Dutoit SJ, Rowe M et al 1991a Expression of Epstein–Barr virus latent gene products in tumour cells of Hodgkin's disease. Lancet 337: 320–322

Pallesen G, Sandvej K, Hamilton-Dutoit SJ et al 1991b Activation of Epstein–Barr virus replication in Hodgkin and Reed–Sternberg cells. Blood 78: 1162–1165

Patsouris E, Noel H, Lennert K 1989 Cytohistologic and immunohistochemical findings in Hodgkin's disease, mixed cellularity type, with a high content of epithelioid cells. Am J Surg Pathol 13: 1014–1022

Perrone T, Frizzera G, Rosai J 1986 Mediastinal diffuse large-cell lymphoma with sclerosis. A clinicopathologic study of 60 cases. Am J Surg Pathol 10: 176–191

Poppema S 1989 The nature of the lymphocytes surrounding Reed–Sternberg cells in nodular lymphocyte predominance and in other types of Hodgkin's disease. Am J Pathol 135: 351–357

Poppema S 1992 Lymphocyte-predominance Hodgkin's disease. Semin Diagn Pathol 9: 257–264

Poppema S, Kaleta J, Hepperle B 1992 Chromosomal abnormalities in patients with Hodgkin's disease: evidence for frequent involvement of the 14q chromosomal region but infrequent bcl-2 gene rearrangement in Reed–Sternberg cells. J Natl Cancer Inst 84: 1789–1793

Ramsay AD, Smith WJ, Isaacson PG 1988 T-cell-rich B-cell lymphoma. Am J Surg Pathol 12: 433–443

Reid AH, Cunningham RE, Frizzera G et al 1993 bcl-2 rearrangement in Hodgkin's disease. Results of polymerase chain reaction, cytometry, and sequencing on formalin-fixed, paraffin-embedded tissue. Am J Pathol 142: 395–402

Rowe M, Lear AL, Croom-Carter D et al 1992 Three pathways of Epstein–Barr virus gene activation from EBNA1-positive latency in B lymphocytes. J Virol 66: 122–131

Said JW, Sassoon AF, Shintaku IP et al 1991 Absence of bcl-2 major breakpoint region and JH gene rearrangement in lymphocyte predominance Hodgkin's disease. Am J Pathol 138: 261–264

Sandberg AA 1990 Lymphoproliferative disorders. In: Sandberg AA (ed) The chromosomes in human cancer and leukemia. 2nd edn. Elsevier, New York, pp 625–751

Schmid C, Pan L, Diss T et al 1991a Expression of B-cell antigens by Hodgkin's and Reed–Sternberg cells. Am J Pathol 139: 701–707

Schmid C, Sargent C, Isaacson PG 1991b L and H cells of nodular lymphocyte predominant Hodgkin's disease show immunoglobulin light-chain restriction. Am J Pathol 139: 1281–1289

Stein H, Hansmann ML, Lennert K et al 1986 Reed–Sternberg and Hodgkin cells in lymphocyte predominant Hodgkin's disease of nodular subtype contain J chain. Am J Clin Pathol 86: 292–297

Stein H, Herbst H, Anagnostopoulos I et al 1991 The nature of Hodgkin and Reed–Sternberg cells, their association with EBV, and their relationship to anaplastic large-cell lymphoma. Ann Oncol 2 (Suppl 2): 33–38

Stetler-Stevenson M, Crush-Stanton S, Cossman J 1990 Involvement of the *bcl-2* gene in Hodgkin's disease. J Natl Cancer Inst 82: 855–858

Sundeen J, Lipford E, Uppenkamp M et al 1987 Rearranged antigen receptor genes in Hodgkin's disease. Blood 70: 96–103

Tefferi A, Zellers RA, Banks PM et al 1990 Clinical correlates of distinct immunophenotypic and histologic subcategories of lymphocyte-predominance Hodgkin's disease. J Clin Oncol 8: 1959–1965

Torelli G, Marasca R, Luppi M et al 1991 Human herpesvirus-6 in human lymphomas: identification of specific sequences in Hodgkin's lymphomas by polymerase chain reaction. Blood 77: 2251–2258

Tosi P, Leoncini L, Del Vecchio MT et al 1992 Phenotypic overlaps between pleomorphic malignant T-cell lymphomas and mixed-cellularity Hodgkin's disease. Int J Cancer 52: 202–207

Trumper LH, Brady G, Bagg A et al 1993 Single-cell analysis of Hodgkin and Reed Sternberg cells: molecular heterogeneity of gene expression and p53 mutations. Blood 81: 3097–3115

Vestlev PM, Pallesen G, Sandvej K et al 1992 Prognosis of Hodgkin's disease is not influenced by Epstein–Barr virus latent membrane protein. Int J Cancer 51: 1–2

Weiss LM, Strickler JG, Hu E et al 1986 Immunoglobulin gene rearrangements in Hodgkin's disease. Hum Pathol 17: 1009–1014

Weiss LM, Strickler JG, Warnke RA et al 1987 Epstein–Barr viral DNA in tissues of Hodgkin's disease. Am J Pathol 129: 86–91

Weiss LM, Picker LJ, Grogan TM et al 1988 Absence of clonal beta and gamma T-cell receptor gene rearrangements in a subset of peripheral T-cell lymphomas. Am J Pathol 130: 436–442

Weiss LM, Chen Y, Liu XF et al 1991 Epstein–Barr virus and Hodgkin's disease. A correlative in situ hybridization and polymerase chain reaction study. Am J Pathol 139: 1259–1265

Wijlhuizen TJ, Vrints LW, Jairam R et al 1989 Grades of nodular sclerosis (NSI-NSII) in Hodgkin's disease. Are they of independent prognostic value? Cancer 15; 63: 1150–1153

Wright DH 1989 Pathology of Hodgkin's disease: anything new? Recent Res Cancer Res 117: 3–13

5. The bone marrow trephine biopsy: recent progress and current issues

B. S. Wilkins

Bone marrow trephine biopsies (BMTs) have been subject to less systematic scientific study over recent years than biopsies of other commonly sampled tissues. This relates largely to their bone content, which makes frozen section studies difficult and creates a requirement for decalcification or resin embedding prior to processing for routine histological examination.

The aim of this article is firstly to highlight areas where recent studies have advanced our understanding of bone marrow structure and secondly to describe areas of active current research employing BMTs.

WHAT IS AN ADEQUATE BIOPSY?

Needles most commonly used for obtaining BMTs in the UK are those of the Jamshidi or Islam types, yielding cores of 1–4 mm diameter (Jamshidi et al 1971, Islam 1982). The length of sample obtained and its integrity are highly operator-dependent. Frisch et al (1985), who employ a myelotomy drill giving cores of 8 mm diameter, have proposed that 15 mm or five intertrabecular spaces is a minimum adequate biopsy length. This figure appears somewhat arbitrary and cannot readily be converted into a value applicable to Jamshidi or Islam cores. Additional length may not be directly equivalent to an equal area of additional width, particularly if the sample contains marrow from the immediate subcortical region, which may be unrepresentative of the marrow elsewhere. Also, the useful area for interpretation in sections from BMTs is diminished by inclusion in the sample of cartilage, tendon, cortical bone, crushed trabecular bone and blood clot. Bishop et al (1992) recently reviewed more than 700 BMTs taken within the Christie Hospital, Manchester, during a 12-month period. They evaluated the contribution of cortex, crushed tissue, etc., to each biopsy and attempted to define minimum adequate biopsy lengths appropriate for a range of suspected disorders. This is of great importance, as a small core may be adequate for detection of diffuse bone marrow disease such as leukaemia, while focal lesions such as metastatic or lymphomatous deposits may be missed by even quite large biopsies. Their results also emphasize that operators performing few or infrequent BMTs collect significantly less satisfactory biopsies than do individuals who frequently take BMTs.

The problem of detection of focal lesions, particularly in the sphere of lymphoma diagnosis, has prompted several approaches to improve the volume of tissue sampled. One group has recommended the collection of particularly long BMTs to enhance sample size and quality (Islam & Henderson 1988). Other authors favour bilateral BMTs, arguing that sampling two sites (usually the two posterior iliac crests) is superior to sampling an equivalent volume of tissue from one site (Kuneja et al 1990).

HOW SHOULD BONE MARROW TREPHINE BIOPSIES BE PROCESSED?

This issue continues to generate controversy. Traditional methods of processing for embedding in paraffin wax require that BMTs undergo decalcification during or after fixation, by exposure to acids (e.g. formic or trichloroacetic acid) or chelating agents (e.g. EDTA). Both methods extend the time required for processing relative to other tissues handled routinely by a histopathology laboratory and alter the morphology of the tissue. Acid decalcification impairs demonstration of neutrophil granules and haemosiderin deposits, in addition to causing shrinkage artefacts. EDTA also produces shrinkage artefacts, although granules are better preserved. One major advantage of EDTA over acid decalcification is that chloroacetate esterase activity (Leder's stain) is more readily demonstrable following the former.

Resins have been developed over the past 15–20 years that are suitable for embedding, sectioning and staining of routinely fixed tissues. Use of such resins now permits avoidance of decalcification and is claimed by some authors to offer improvements in the preservation of morphology compared with wax embedding after decalcification (Islam & Frisch 1985). Shrinkage artefacts are minimal, granules and iron deposits are well preserved and sections of 1–2 μm thickness can be cut with relative ease, allowing better appreciation of cytological detail. Other authors argue that carefully prepared sections from decalcified, wax-embedded BMTs are not inferior to resin-embedded sections for diagnostic evaluation (Gatter et al 1987, Vincic et al 1989). Production of wax-embedded sections is also less expensive and requires less technical specialization than is needed for resin embedding and sectioning.

Currently, the most persuasive argument in favour of decalcification and wax embedding for BMTs is that this methodology permits good preservation of antigens within the tissue and demonstration of these by standard immunohistochemical techniques. Frozen section immunohistochemistry is technically difficult to perform with BMTs. Because of their mixed composition of bone, fat and haemopoietic tissue, high quality frozen sections are difficult to obtain and morphology is much less well preserved than in fixed tissue sections. Consequently, although immunostaining can be performed as for frozen sections of other tissues (White et al 1989, Shin et al 1992, Dilly et al 1993), interpretation of the results is difficult and small or focal lesions may not be recognizable. Immunostaining methods for use with resin-embedded biopsies are still undergoing development. Epoxy resins such as Araldite require etching with sodium ethoxide to permit penetration of antibodies to antigenic sites within the tissue, and this process is detrimental to the preservation of some antigens. Acrylic resins such as methyl methacrylate and glycol methacrylate do not require etching prior to staining. Some success has been achieved with immunostaining of BMTs embedded in such resins (Islam et al 1988). Care is necessary to avoid the generation of excessive heat during setting of the resin, which may destroy epitopes, and the conditions for immunostaining may vary with time for any particular block as the resin continues to harden progressively over a long period. To date, the range of antigens that have been demonstrated successfully in resin-embedded sections of bone marrow is much smaller than that applicable to wax-embedded sections.

In summary, resin embedding of BMTs has advantages and disadvantages when compared with wax embedding. Both methods are generally satisfactory for diagnostic purposes and the choice of method depends on individual preference. For some purposes, one or other method is superior. For instance, morphometric studies should undoubtedly be performed using resin-embedded BMTs wherever possible, to avoid distortions caused by shrinkage. By contrast, until more reliable immunostaining methods for use with resin sections have been developed, immunohistochemical studies are better performed using decalcified, wax-embedded BMTs.

It should not be forgotten that modifications of wax embedding exist which reduce the need for decalcification and facilitate preparation of high quality thin sections. Waxes which set to a harder consistency than paraffin wax have been used successfully to embed BMTs for sectioning at 2–3 μm. Further modifications involve the addition of plasticizers such as piccolytes to wax, giving products that have properties intermediate between those of wax and resin (Bogomoletz & Potet 1987). Little attention has been given to these techniques in recent years, but they seem worthy of further investigation. In particular, it will be important to demonstrate whether good immunohistochemical staining can be achieved after embedding in such compounds.

THE SPATIAL ORGANIZATION OF HAEMOPOIESIS WITHIN BONE MARROW

The production of red and white blood cells by bone marrow is an orderly and highly regulated process. Within a BMT, haemopoietic cells show spatial orientation with respect to bone trabeculae and larger blood vessels (Wilkins 1992, Brown & Gatter 1993). This reflects the existence of cell–stroma interactions which vary between the different haemopoietic lineages and also between cells at different stages of maturation. Precise recognition of individual cell types within BMT sections is a source of difficulty to many pathologists and has limited the appreciation of spatial disturbances in pathological haemopoiesis. Chloroacetate esterase staining can demonstrate clearly the organization of promyelocytes and myelocytes around trabeculae, small veins and arteries. Metamyelocytes and neutrophil polymorphs occupy the central areas of intertrabecular spaces. Erythroid cells, recognizable in wax-embedded sections by their clear perinuclear haloes and the dense nuclei of maturing normoblasts, occur as rounded clusters in the central intertrabecular areas. In resin sections, perinuclear haloes are not formed and erythroid cell clusters have a syncytial appearance because the margins of individual cells are indistinct. Megakaryocytes occur singly, usually centrally, and occasionally can be seen closely applied to the wall of a sinusoid, into which proplatelets are shed from their cytoplasm. Recognition of developing monocytes and their distinction from granulocytes is difficult. Basophil precursors can rarely be visualized, because their granule contents are soluble in aqueous fixatives and, although eosinophil granules are often well preserved, little is known about the organization of developing eosinophils within bone marrow. They usually appear randomly dispersed.

Immunohistochemistry is a useful tool for the demonstration of cells of different haemopoietic lineages and maturation stages (Van der Valk et al 1989, Wilkins & Jones 1989). The antibodies listed in Table 5.1 have differential reactivity with developing precursors of the main haemopoietic lineages and have been used to study spatial disturbances in such pathological states as myelodysplastic syndromes, myeloproliferative disorders and chemotherapy-induced dysplasia (Van der Valk et al 1989, Wilkins et al 1993). Using such antibodies, it has been shown that developing monocytes can be distinguished from granulocytes and that they have a non-zonal distribution within marrow spaces (Wilkins & Jones 1992).

Table 5.2 lists other commonly used antibodies which are used primarily for immunohistochemical demonstration of lymphoid and non-haematological cells, but which have additional reactivity with marrow cells in formalin-fixed, wax-embedded BMTs. These antibodies are nonetheless of considerable value for the diagnosis of lymphomas or metastases, as long as their staining patterns are interpreted with care to take into account the background of normal marrow tissue staining.

BONE MARROW STROMA

To date, few studies of the marrow stroma in BMTs have been reported. Stroma contains alkaline phosphatase positive cells (loosely termed 'reticulum cells'), fat cells, endothelium and macrophages. It is unclear at present how these cells influence the differentiation of haemopoietic cells. On the basis of bone marrow culture studies, stromal cells are believed to present growth factors to haemopoietic precursors in association with heparan sulphate proteoglycan in the extracellular matrix (Quesenberry et al 1989).

Dilly & Jagger (1990) have investigated changes in marrow stromal macrophages, reticulum cells and endothelium in patients with a variety of

Table 5.1 Antibodies of use for the demonstration of haemopoietic cells of different lineages and other components of bone marrow

Antibody	Antigen	Granulocytes	Monocytes	Erythrocytes	Megakaryocytes	Other
Anti-α_1-antitrypsin	α_1-antitrypsin	+	+	–	–	–
Anti-muramidase	Muramidase	+	+	–	–	–
KP1	CD68	+	+	–	±	Osteoclasts Mast cells
PG-M1	CD68	–	+	–	±	Osteoclasts Mast cells
NP57	Neutrophil elastase	+	–	–	–	–
LeuM1	CD15	+	+ some	–	–	–
MAC 387	Calgranulin	+	+	–	–	–
1B5	MHC class II	+	+	–	–	Lymphocytes Some stromal cells
Hermes 3	CD44	+	±	–	–	Lymphocytes Osteocytes
JC70A	CD31	–	+	–	±	Endothelium Stem cells
QBEnd10	CD34	–	–	–	–	Endothelium
Ret40f	β-Sialoglycoprotein	–	–	+	–	–
BRIC101	α-Sialoglycoprotein	–	–	+	–	–
BNH9	Not characterized	–	–	+	+	ALCL
Anti-FVIII	von Willebrand factor	–	–	–	+	Endothelium
Y2/51	CD61	–	–	–	+	–
Anti-tryptase	Most cell tryptase	–	–	–	–	Mast cells
CBL-419	Major basic protein	+*	–	–	–	–

*Only cells of the eosinophil lineage. ALCL = anaplastic large cell lymphoma.

Table 5.2 Bone marrow reactivities with commonly used antibodies whose usual use in diagnosis is to demonstrate unrelated cell types

Antibody	Antigen	'Usual' reactivity sought	Reactivity with haemopoietic and other cells in BMT
LCA	CD45	Lymphocytes	Granulocytes and monocytes[a]
MTI	CD43	T lymphocytes	Granulocytes and monocytes. Early erythroid precursors
UCHLI	CD45RO	T lymphocytes	Granulocytes and monocytes
MB2	Unclustered	B lymphocytes	Granulocytes and monocytes. Endothelium
LNI	CDw75	B lymphocytes	Erythroid cells, particularly non-nucleated erythrocytes
Anti-CEA	CEA	Epithelium	Granulocytes
Anti-S100	S100	Melanocytes	Granulocytes. Occasional dendritic cells
BerH2	CD30	RS cells, ALCL	Erythroid cells, particularly early forms.[b] Plasma cells and osteoblasts[b]
Anti-PGP9.5	PGP9.5	Neuroendocrine cells neuroblastoma	Granulocytes. New collagen at growth plate. Chondrocytes

[a]Myeloid CD45 reactivity can be at least partly abolished by trypsin digestion of sections prior to immunostaining.
[b]These CD30 reactivities can be abolished by microwave irradiation of sections in citrate buffer (pH 6.0) prior to immunostaining.
RS cell = Reed–Sternberg cell; ALCL = anaplastic large cell lymphoma.

haematological neoplasms, using frozen section enzyme histochemistry and immunostaining. They found that, in contrast to myeloid leukaemias, lymphoid neoplasms were associated with reduction in reticulum cell numbers, suggesting that stromal damage results from marrow infiltration. These authors have also studied marrow stroma of patients who died following bone marrow transplantation (Dilly et al 1993). In this group of patients, a reduced number of reticulum cells and altered proportions of macrophage subpopulations were found in association with depressed haemopoiesis, suggesting that stromal injury may have contributed to poor engraftment.

Other recent studies in fixed, wax-embedded BMTs have demonstrated increased numbers of macrophages and altered vascular architecture in patients with chronic myeloproliferative disorders compared with normal marrow (Thiele et al 1992a,b). Tenascin, a matrix protein normally present only at the endosteal surfaces of bone trabeculae in BMTs, has been shown to be increased in myelofibrosis and a variety of other haemopoietic conditions associated with megakaryocyte hyperplasia (Soini et al 1993). The significance of this observation with regard to the pathogenesis of such disorders is uncertain at present.

NORMAL AND NEOPLASTIC LYMPHOID TISSUE WITHIN BONE MARROW

Published studies are contradictory concerning the composition of normal lymphoid tissue within bone marrow. Small numbers of diffusely scattered lymphocytes and occasional discrete lymphoid nodules are normal marrow constituents (Rywlin et al 1974), but reports vary as to the proportions of T and B lymphocytes present (Sangster et al 1986, Nash et al 1988, Farhi 1989, Pich et al 1991, Horny et al 1993). With increasing numbers of studies and harmonization of immunohistochemical methods, a concensus is emerging; approximately three quarters of dispersed lymphocytes are T cells while nodules and aggregates consist predominantly of B cells. The proportion of B cells in lymphoid nodules is highest in those that appear most reactive, with prominent germinal centre formation.

Distinguishing normal and reactive lymphoid tissue from infiltrates of neoplastic lymphocytes is of great importance in the diagnosis and staging of lymphoid malignancies. Rywlin et al (1974) defined morphological criteria for the differentiation of benign from malignant lymphoid infiltrates in bone marrow. They described two main forms of physiological lymphoid tissue: small, discrete lymphoid infiltrates and larger lymphoid follicles, both characterized by rounded shape, well-defined margins and non-paratrabecular distribution. Lymphoid follicles might be seen to contain a central arteriole and/or a germinal centre and they represent the bone marrow equivalent of lymph node follicles (Fig. 5.1). In fact, a spectrum of appearances exists between the two extreme variants described by Rywlin and his colleagues. Subsequently, one study has shown that patients with morphologically benign lymphoid aggregates and nodules have a higher than expected incidence of

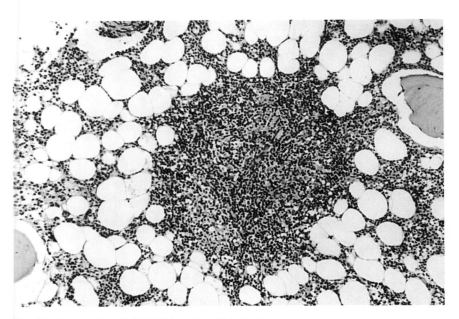

Fig. 5.1 Reactive lymphoid follicle with well-defined margin occupying the centre of an intertrabecular space. H&E.

subsequent lymphoma, sometimes after many years of follow-up (Faulkner-Jones et al 1988). This may partly reflect inaccuracies in the initial diagnosis of benign lymphoid nodules. However, the long timespan over which tumours developed in some patients suggests that benign lymphoid nodules (possibly indicating persistent antigenic stimulation and hence proliferation of marrow lymphoid tissue) may allow the development of neoplasia.

Malignant lymphoid infiltrates vary in appearance, reflecting the nature of the neoplastic process (Schmidt & Isaacson 1992). Marrow involvement by low grade lymphomas is generally more problematic to discriminate from reactive changes than is high grade lymphoid neoplasia. Lymphocytic lymphoma/leukaemia is characterized by nodules composed of monotonous small lymphocytes, lacking germinal centre formation but with occasional proliferation centres present. Accompanying these nodules there is usually, but not always, a diffuse interstitial infiltrate of small lymphocytes. Sometimes the pattern is entirely diffuse, and infiltration may be sufficiently heavy as to obscure any residual normal haemopoiesis. Lymphoplasmacytic lymphoma (LPL) shows essentially similar patterns of bone marrow involvement. Plasmacytic differentiation may be inapparent in BMT sections, but the infiltrates of LPL are characteristically accompanied by large numbers of mast cells (Fig. 5.2).

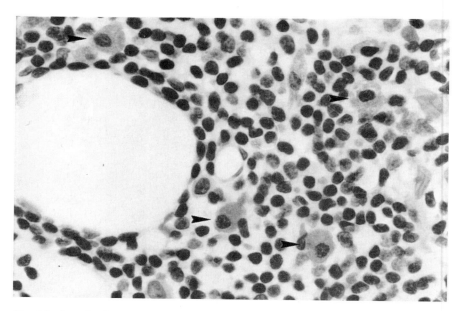

Fig. 5.2 Lymphoplasmacytic lymphoma infiltrate within a BMT. The neoplasm consists of a diffuse infiltrate of small lymphocytes with no obvious plasmacytic features. The presence of abundant mast cells (arrows) is helpful in distinguishing this from chronic lymphocytic leukaemia. H&E.

Follicle centre cell (FCC) lymphomas typically infiltrate paratrabecular areas. Marrow involvement is common in low grade FCC lymphoma, being present in up to approximately 60% of cases. It is important to be aware that FCC infiltrates may be very subtle and that they do not always occupy paratrabecular sites. Also, much of the infiltrate which is visible may be composed of reactive lymphocytes accompanying the tumour, so that classical centrocytes and centroblasts may be inapparent amongst a predominant population of small lymphocytes. Giemsa stain is very helpful in aiding visualization of small infiltrates, which in a well-stained preparation will have a bright blue appearance against the general lilac/pink hue of haemopoietic tissue. In doubtful cases, immunohistochemistry for B cell-associated antigens such as CD20 can be helpful in confirming the presence of small infiltrates at abnormal sites in marrow. Demonstration of light chain restriction, to confirm clonality, is difficult in BMTs because the presence of abundant immunoglobulin in the background stroma and the contribution of reactive cells to infiltrates make interpretation problematical.

Relatively few data exist concerning patterns of marrow infiltration exhibited by other low and intermediate grade B cell lymphomas such as centrocytic lymphoma, monocytoid B cell lymphoma and lymphomas derived from mucosa-associated lymphoid tissue (MALT). Centrocytic lymphoma has been described as having a strong propensity for marrow involvement and a paratrabecular distribution (Schmidt & Isaacson 1992). MALT lymphomas spread to bone marrow late in their evolution, tending to remain localized to their primary site of origin and adjacent lymph nodes. It is to be hoped that marrow involvement by these entities will become better characterized over the next few years.

Two unrelated entities, hairy cell leukaemia (HCL) and myeloma, usually cause little problem in diagnosis unless the quantity of disease is so small that recognition of tumour cells is difficult. Clonality of plasma cell infiltrates can usually be demonstrated easily by immunostaining for cytoplasmic light chains, although the threshold for minimal disease involvement has not yet been established. Identification of minimal marrow involvement by HCL (e.g. in assessment of residual disease following interferon therapy) has been aided recently by the development of monoclonal antibodies such as DBA.44, which are relatively specific for HCL amongst low grade lymphomas (Hounieu et al 1992). In normal lymphoid tissue, DBA.44 reacts preferentially with mantle zone B cells. However, a relationship between HCL and monocytoid B cells, which are probably related to marginal zone cells, has been claimed (Traweek et al 1989).

High grade B cell lymphomas (centroblastic, immunoblastic, lymphoblastic, etc.) are usually easy to recognize in bone marrow by virtue of their cytological features. Marrow involvement is proportionately less frequent than with low grade lymphomas (15% in the series of Schmidt & Isaacson 1992), and they show variable infiltration patterns. Frequently, there is massive marrow involvement by the time of diagnosis or staging. Where infiltration is focal or slight, differential diagnoses of melanoma, early leukaemia or epithelial neoplasia should be considered.

Hodgkin's disease and peripheral T cell lymphomas remain difficult to distinguish in bone marrow, as both usually provoke a marked stromal reaction with sclerosis and infiltration by reactive plasma cells, eosinophils and macrophages (Hanson et al 1986, Myers et al 1974). Immunostaining for CD30, CD15 and a variety of T cell markers can be performed successfully on BMT sections to assist in making this distinction. A high grade B cell lymphoma mimicking T cell lymphoma (the pattern of so-called 'T cell rich B cell lymphoma') can have a primary presentation in bone marrow (Provan et al 1993) and should be included in the differential diagnosis of infiltrates suggestive of Hodgkin's disease or T cell lymphoma.

It is important in diagnostic practice to accept the limitations of BMT morphology for the classification of lymphomas. It is often only possible to decide that an infiltrate is either low or high grade, because cytological and architectural features used for categorization within the Kiel classification are absent or difficult to appreciate in BMTs. Similarly, in the diagnosis of Hodgkin's disease, bone marrow does not show the range of morphological subtypes described by the Rye classification. It is important to recognize the manifestations of different types of lymphoma in BMT in order to provide a diagnosis when disease presents primarily at this site. However, BMT is usually performed during the staging of non-Hodgkin's lymphoma or Hodgkin's disease, following diagnosis of the disease by biopsy of lymph node or other tissue. In these circumstances, confirmation of involvement rather than precise classification is required by the clinician.

NON-LYMPHOID METASTATIC TUMOURS IN BONE MARROW

BMT is frequently performed in the investigation of suspected metastatic disease of unknown primary origin and it has an important place in the staging of paediatric solid tumours, particularly neuroblastoma.

In adult malignancies, traditional teaching is that carcinomas of breast, bronchus, kidney, thyroid and prostate are the most likely to involve bone and bone marrow. This, however, does not translate accurately into a list of carcinomas most likely to be the source of metastatic deposits found in a BMT. The discrepancy reflects (1) the circumstances under which BMT is performed, usually in the context of an occult primary tumour, and (2) the distance, or the unfavourable circulatory route, of the iliac crests from the primary tumour. Thus, thyroid carcinoma is a very rare diagnosis in a BMT. Prostatic carcinoma, in men, and breast carcinoma, in women, are the most frequent sources of tumours diagnosed from marrow metastases, followed by bronchogenic carcinomas (particularly oat cell carcinoma) and carcinomas of the gastrointestinal tract. Immunohistochemistry as yet offers only limited assistance in determining the tissue of origin of metastatic carcinoma in BMTs, as in other tissues.

Bone marrow examination for the evaluation of metastatic neuroblastoma in children has been a focus of specific study in the last few years (Carey et al 1990, Reid et al 1990, 1991). Recognition of marrow involvement at the time of diagnosis and during follow-up after therapy is of prognostic importance. Detection of minimal marrow involvement, or of residual disease after treatment, can be extremely difficult and immunohistochemistry has a useful role in this process. Markers of neuronal (neuron-specific enolase, neurofilament protein) or glial (glial fibrillary acidic protein) differentiation have been used to aid recognition of involvement of marrow by neuroblastoma, but one of the most reliable antibodies available at present is PGP9.5 (Wirnsberger et al 1992). Studies of bone marrow aspirate and trephine samples from patients with neuroblastoma have shown that metastases can be detected significantly more often using immunostaining in addition to routine stains than by histology alone (Reid et al 1991). Using immunohistochemistry, very low levels of marrow involvement can be detected (Fig. 5.3). However, the clinical significance of such minimal involvement remains uncertain at present.

Another focus of interest in the study of neuroblastoma in BMT has been the tendency of the tumour to cause stromal fibrosis, often marked following therapy (Turner & Reid 1993). Sometimes sclerosis is demonstrable in the absence of any evidence of residual neuroblastoma cells and is a source of

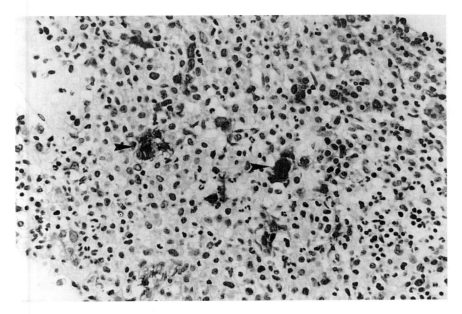

Fig. 5.3 BMT performed during the staging of neuroblastoma in a young child. PGP9.5 positive cells are present (arrows), scattered in small numbers amongst reactive haemopoietic cells. Streptavidin–biotin complex method with monoclonal antibody PGP9.5.

diagnostic difficulty. It is believed that such stromal fibrosis is evidence of persistent tumour and should at least prompt a detailed search of multiple sections for malignant cells. The cause of the fibrosis is not known. Stromal fibrosis is seen at other sites of involvement in some cases of neuroblastoma. Although neurofilament protein and/or glial fibrillary acidic protein are sometimes expressed by the fibrous tissue, suggesting that it may be neurophil produced by tumour cells, it is more usual for the tissue in BMT to resemble loose, new collagen and there is frequently associated osteoblastic activity at the margins of adjacent trabeculae, suggesting a marrow stromal reaction to tumour cells (unpublished observations).

THE ROLE OF TREPHINE BIOPSY MORPHOLOGY IN ASSESSMENT OF MYELODYSPLASIA, MYELOPROLIFERATIVE SYNDROMES AND LEUKAEMIAS

The diagnosis of these conditions is principally based upon a combination of clinical features, peripheral blood findings and bone marrow aspirate appearances. However, BMT morphology can provide additional information of assistance in diagnosis and assessment of prognosis (Winfield & Polacarz 1992).

In myelodysplasia (MDS), attempts have been made to correlate histological appearances with the subtypes of the French–American–British (FAB) Group classification (Van der Weide et al 1988, Kitigawa et al 1989). Morphological patterns in BMTs cannot be matched precisely to the FAB categories of MDS, but cytological features of dysplasia can be appreciated in biopsy sections. The general trend of an increasing proportion of blast cells from refractory anaemia (RA, with or without ringed sideroblasts) to RA with excess blasts (RAEB) to RAEB in transformation (RAEBt) can be seen (Rios et al 1990). Chronic myelomonocytic leukaemia is difficult to recognize in BMT sections, unless the proportion of blasts and promonocytes is high. A useful aid to diagnosis is loss of the normal zonal pattern of granulopoiesis (Fig. 5.4) (Wilkins & Jones 1992).

The most valuable information provided by BMT in MDS which cannot be obtained by aspirate examination is that relating to the spatial disturbances of haemopoietic cells which are present. Megakaryocytes and erythroid cell clusters may be found adjacent to trabeculae and granulocyte precursors may be displaced from their normal location there. This abnormal localization of immature myeloid precursors (ALIP) is typically apparent as clusters of blast cells and promyelocytes in the central areas of intertrabecular spaces (Tricot et al 1984a,b). The presence of such clusters has been shown to carry an adverse prognosis in patients with less than 5% of blast cells in their aspirate. Patients with higher blast cell counts almost always have at least some ALIP present in BMT sections and these are not independently associated with poor outcome (Mufti 1992). Immunohistochemistry has been used to show that myeloid ALIP can be distinguished from clusters showing an erythroid or

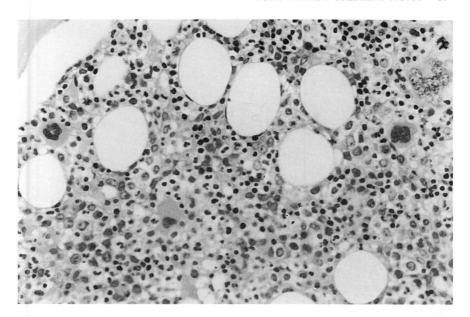

Fig. 5.4 Chronic myelomonocytic leukaemia. Cells of the various haemopoietic lineages show little evidence of spatial organization. In particular, no zone of early granulopoietic cells adjacent to the trabecular margin (top left).

megakaryocytic phenotype (which they term 'pseudo-ALIP') and that only the former are of prognostic significance (Mangi et al 1991, Mangi & Mufti 1992). Some ALIP clusters have a monocytic rather than a granulocytic phenotype (Wilkins & Jones 1992), but the prognostic significance of this difference is not known.

BMT examination has also contributed to appreciation of the extent to which overlap exists between MDS and the chronic myeloproliferative disorders (CMPD). Profound cytological and spatial atypia resembling MDS is commonly present in CMPD. In the absence of the grossly exaggerated zonal granulopoiesis around trabeculae and blood vessels seen in some forms of chronic granulocytic leukaemia (Fig. 5.5), BMT examination alone may not be able to distinguish CMPD from MDS. Usually, however, clinical features and the peripheral blood picture help to confirm the diagnosis. Megakaryocyte morphology in BMT sections can be a helpful guide in difficult cases (Fig. 5.6).

Burkhardt et al (1986) have proposed a morphological classification of CMPD based on the predominance of each major haemopoietic lineage and patterns of cell distribution within the marrow. This has been shown to be of some prognostic importance (Burkhardt et al 1990). Assignment of patients to subtypes involves assessment of numerous morphological parameters, however, and interobserver variation may limit the usefulness of this classification in routine application.

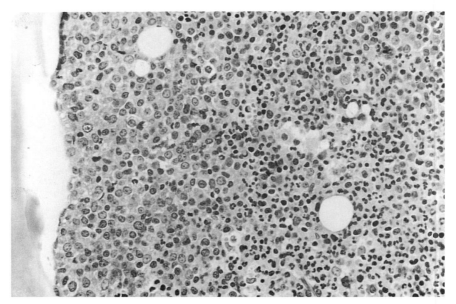

Fig. 5.5 Chronic granulocytic leukaemia. There is expansion of the normal paratrabecular zone of early granulocytes (left side of photograph) with metamyelocytes and neutrophils confined to the central area of the intertrabecular space (right side of photograph).

BMT has been regarded historically as having relatively little to contribute to the diagnosis of acute leukaemias. The FAB classification of acute leukaemias is based on bone marrow aspirate cytology and cytochemistry. FAB subtypes of acute myeloid and lymphoid leukaemia do not correlate precisely with prognosis, although several clinically distinct entities (e.g. acute promyelocytic leukaemia, AML-M3, with a strong tendency for disseminated intravascular coagulation and responsiveness to retinoic acid treatment) are highlighted. FAB subtypes also do not correlate closely with the chromosomal abnormalities which have been shown in recent years to be associated with acute leukaemias (Fenaux et al 1989). Morphological assessment of leukaemic blast cell infiltrates in BMTs is not a sensitive means of subclassifying these diseases, as there is extensive overlap, even between myeloid and lymphoid neoplasms. However, BMT is of value in the quantification of response of leukaemia to therapy, for which a pretreatment 'baseline' sample is desirable. BMT can also indicate whether or not acute leukaemia has developed from a background of myelodysplasia. This is of importance as there is evidence that AML secondary to MDS differs cytogenetically from de novo AML and may carry a worse prognosis (Berger & Flandrin 1992).

In recent years, there has been increasing interest in the use of immuno-histochemistry as an aid to classifying acute leukaemias in BMTs (Horny et al 1990, Wilkins et al 1993a). Expression of antigens such as neutrophil elastase (AML-M3), calgranulin and the monocyte-restricted form of CD68 (AML-M4 and AML-M5) and CD61 (AML-M7) correlates well with FAB subtyping.

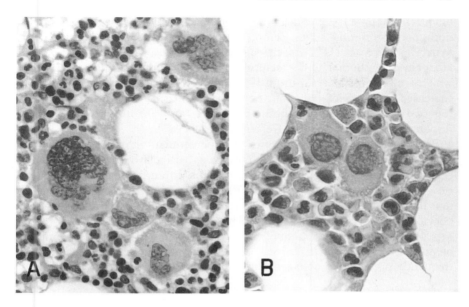

Fig. 5.6 **A** Large megakaryocytes with high nuclear lobulation/high ploidy from a case of polycythaemia rubra vera. **B** Small, mononuclear megakaryocytes from a case of MDS-RA.

Antibodies such as Ret40f, directed against β-sialoglycoprotein, are of value in estimating the proportion of erythroid blast cells in suspected cases of AML-M6. It remains to be shown whether immunohistochemical demonstration of myelomonocytic antigens in leukaemic blasts can assist in the diagnosis of less-differentiated variants of AML (AML-M0 to AML-M2). AML-M0 and AML-M1 blast cells express the form of CD68 recognized by KP1 and can thus be distinguished from blasts of acute lymphoblastic leukaemia (ALL), which lack expression of such myelomonocytic antigens (Wilkins et al 1993).

ALL blast cells have been less intensively studied in routinely fixed BMTs because of the limited range of primitive lymphoid, B and T cell antigens which has been available for use with fixed tissue until recently. It is to be hoped that, with the advent of microwave-based techniques for antigen retrieval from fixed tissue sections (Shi et al 1991), better immunohistochemical characterization of ALL will be achieved. It is not known whether BMT immunophenotype in acute leukaemia correlates with the presence of cytogenetic or molecular genetic abnormalities.

BONE MARROW BIOPSY APPEARANCES IN HUMAN IMMUNODEFICIENCY VIRUS INFECTION AND AUTOIMMUNE DEFICIENCY SYNDROME

BMT may be performed in HIV positive patients for investigation of cytopenias or pyrexia of unknown origin. Morphological features present often reflect opportunistic infections (granulomas and perivascular inflammation), poor nutritional status (serous atrophy or gelatinous transformation of marrow stroma) or HIV-associated malignancy (usually high grade non-Hodgkin's lymphoma). Other features represent disturbances of haemopoiesis which are believed to result from HIV infection of haemopoietic precursors. Increased numbers of lymphoid nodules and plasma cells have also been reported in BMTs from HIV positive patients, but these may be non-specific responses to occult infection (Delacretaz et al 1987).

BMT sections are usually normo- or hypercellular, although they may be hypocellular in up to 30% of cases. Dysplasia, particularly affecting erythroid cells and megakaryocytes, is marked in patients with cytopenias. Morphometric assessment of megakaryocytes in BMTs from AIDS patients has shown that they differ from megakaryocytes in primary MDS or idiopathic thrombocytopenia (Thiele et al 1992c). They are generally larger than MDS megakaryocytes, with few mononuclear variants, but they have lower numbers of nuclear segments than normal. A mild increase in reticulin staining is frequently present, but collagen fibrosis is rare (Ricci et al 1993).

APPLICATION OF NEW TECHNIQUES TO TREPHINE BIOPSIES

The application of immunohistochemistry to BMTs has been discussed extensively in preceding sections. Methodology for use with decalcified, wax-embedded samples is well established. Some progress has been made in recent years with development of methods for use with resin-embedded BMT and this is an area in which advances are likely to continue. Meanwhile, microwave irradiation as a means of improving antigen demonstration in fixed tissues (Shi et al 1991) has opened a new chapter in BMT immunohistochemistry, particularly with regard to study of stromal cells and extracellular matrix.

In situ hybridization for mRNA demonstration has been shown to be possible in EDTA or formic acid decalcified BMTs. The first report of application of such techniques to BMTs came from Akhtar et al (1989), who demonstrated total mRNA and mRNA for kappa and lambda light chains in cases of multiple myeloma. Subsequently, *in situ* hybridization for monocyte colony stimulating factor mRNA in BMTs has been performed (Wilkins & Jones 1993). *In situ* hybridization with mRNA species will provide a valuable tool over the next few years for investigation of the roles of growth factors and cytokines in haemopoiesis.

In situ hybridization methods using chromosome-specific probes are also being developed currently. They offer a useful addition to traditional cytogenetic studies in a variety of pathological conditions. Although methods for application to cytological preparations are more advanced than those for use with tissue sections at present, abnormalities involving loss or gain of whole chromosomes or large parts of chromosomes (e.g. trisomy of chromosome 8 or loss of the long arm of chromosomes 5 or 7) have been demonstrated successfully in MDS (Kibbelaar et al 1992a,b). With refinements in methodology and increasing availability of probes for chromosome regions of interest, DNA *in situ* hybridization is becoming a field of intense investigation in bone marrow research.

SUMMARY

BMT is a valuable adjunct to marrow aspirate in diagnosis. High quality sections can be achieved with either wax or resin embedding. It is important to be familiar with the differences in BMT morphology which result from processing for either wax or resin embedding.

Diagnosis and staging of lymphomas are important areas of practice in bone marrow pathology. Patterns of marrow infiltration by different types of lymphoma are of assistance in distinguishing benign from malignant lymphoid tissue and in typing lymphomatous infiltrates.

Disturbances of the spatial organization of haemopoietic cells in BMTs, in addition to cytological abnormalities, are seen in conditions such as myeloproliferative disorders and myelodysplastic syndromes.

Immunohistochemistry has aided our understanding of the normal structure of bone marrow and has wide-ranging applications to diagnosis. The availability of new antibodies and improved methods for antigen retrieval make this an area of continuing interest.

Techniques are currently being developed for *in situ* hybridization with RNA and DNA in BMTs. These methods promise to add to our knowledge of mechanisms underlying normal and abnormal haemopoiesis during the next few years.

SOURCES FOR ANTIBODIES REFERRED TO IN THE TABLES AND TEXT

These can be found in the Appendix at the end of the chapter on p. 97.

REFERENCES

Akhtar N, Ruprai A, Pringle J et al 1989 *In situ* hybridisation detection of light chain mRNA in routine bone marrow trephines from patients with suspected myeloma. Br J Haematol 73: 296–301

Berger R, Flandrin G 1992 Chromosomal abnormalities in secondary acute myeloid leukaemia and the myelodysplastic syndromes. In: Mufti G, Galton D (eds) The myelodysplastic syndromes. Churchill Livingstone, London, pp 129–139

Bishop P, McNally K, Harris M 1992 Audit of bone marrow trephines. J Clin Pathol 45: 1105–1108

Bogomoletz W, Potet F 1987 Paraplast–Piccolyte double embedding of bone marrow biopsies in routine histopathology. Histopathology 11: 989

Brown D, Gatter K 1993 The bone marrow trephine biopsy: a review of normal histology. Histopathology 22: 411–422

Burkhardt R, Bartl R, Jäger K et al 1986 Working classification of chronic myeloproliferative disorders based on histological, haematological and clinical findings. J Clin Pathol 39: 237–252

Burkhardt R, Jaeger K, Kettner G et al 1990 Chronic myeloproliferative disorders: prognostic importance of new working classification. J Clin Pathol 43: 357–364

Carey P, Thomas L, Buckle G et al 1990 Immunocytochemical examination of bone marrow in disseminated neuroblastoma. J Clin Pathol 43: 9–12

Delacretaz F, Perey L, Schmidt P et al 1987 Histopathology of bone marrow in human immunodeficiency virus infection. Virchows Arch A Pathol Anat 411: 543–551

Dilly S, Jagger C 1990 Bone marrow stromal cell changes in haematological malignancies. J Clin Pathol 43: 942–946

Dilly S, Jagger C, Sloane J 1993 Stromal cell populations in necropsy bone marrow sections from allogeneic marrow recipients and non-transplant patients. J Clin Pathol 46: 611–616

Farhi D 1989 Germinal centers in the bone marrow. Hematol Pathol 3: 133–136

Faulkner-Jones B, Howie A, Boughton B et al 1988 Lymphoid aggregates in bone marrow: study of eventual outcome. J Clin Pathol 41: 768–775

Fenaux P, Preudhomme C, Lai J et al 1989 Cytogenetics and their prognostic value in de novo acute myeloid leukaemia: a report on 283 cases. Br J Haematol 73: 61–67

Frisch B, Lewis S, Burkhardt R et al 1985 Introduction. In: Biopsy pathology of bone and bone marrow. Chapman and Hall, London, p 10

Gatter K, Heryet A, Brown D et al 1987 Is it necessary to embed bone marrow biopsies in plastic for haematological diagnosis? Histopathology 11: 1–7

Hanson C, Brunning R, Gajl-Peczalska K et al 1986 Bone marrow manifestations of peripheral T-cell lymphoma. A study of 30 cases. Am J Clin Pathol 86: 449–460

Horny H-P, Campbell M, Steinke B et al 1990 Acute myeloid leukaemia: immunohistological findings in paraffin-embedded bone marrow biopsy specimens. Hum Pathol 21: 648–655

Horny H-P, Wehrmann M, Griesser H et al 1993 Investigation of bone marrow lymphocyte subsets in normal, reactive and neoplastic states using paraffin-embedded biopsy specimens. Am J Clin Pathol 99: 142–149

Hounieu H, Chittal S, Al Saati T et al 1992 Hairy cell leukaemia. Diagnosis of bone marrow involvement in paraffin-embedded sections with monoclonal antibody DBA.44. Am J Clin Pathol 98: 26–33

Islam A 1982 A new bone marrow biopsy needle with core securing device. J Clin Pathol 35: 359–364

Islam A, Frisch B 1985 Plastic embedding in routine histology I: Preparation of semi-thin sections of undecalcified marrow cores. Histopathology 9: 1263–1274

Islam A, Henderson E 1988 Value of long-core biopsy in the detection of discrete bone marrow lesions. Histopathology 12: 641–648

Islam A, Archimbaud E, Henderson E et al 1988 Glycol methacrylate (GMA) embedding for light microscopy. II. Immunohistochemical analysis of semithin sections of undecalcified marrow cores. J Clin Pathol 41: 892–896

Jamshidi K, Windschitl H, Swaim W 1971 A new biopsy needle for bone marrow. Scand J Haematol 8: 69–71

Kibbelaar R, van Kamp H, Dreef E, et al 1992a Combined immunophenotyping and DNA in situ hybridisation to study lineage involvement in patients with myelodysplastic syndromes. Blood 79: 1823–1828

Kibbelaar R, Mulder J, van Kamp H et al 1992b Nonradioactive in situ hybridisation of the translocation t(1;7) in myeloid malignancies. Genes Chromosom Cancer 4: 128–134

Kitagawa M, Kamiyama R, Takemura T et al 1989 Bone marrow analysis of the myelodysplastic syndromes: histological and immunohistochemical features related to the evolution of overt leukemia. Virchows Arch B Cell Pathol 57: 47–53

Kuneja S, Wolf M, Cooper I 1990 Value of bilateral bone marrow biopsy specimens in non-Hodgkin's lymphoma. J Clin Pathol 43: 630–632

Mangi M, Mufti G 1992 Primary myelodysplastic syndromes: diagnostic and prognostic significance of immunohistochemical assessment of bone marrow biopsies. Blood 79: 198–205

Mangi M, Salisbury J, Mufti G 1991 Abnormal localization of immature precursors (ALIP) in the bone marrow of myelodysplastic syndromes: current state of knowledge and future directions. Leukaemia Res 15: 627–639

Mufti G 1992 Primary myelodysplastic syndrome: prognostic value of FAB classification, scoring systems, bone marrow histology and karyotypic analysis. In: Mufti G, Galton D (eds) The myelodysplastic syndromes. Churchill Livingstone, London, pp 207–223

Myers C, Chabner B, DeVita V et al 1974 Bone marrow involvement in Hodgkin's disease — pathology and response to MOPP chemotherapy. Blood 44: 197–204

Nash J, Smith S, Mackie M 1988 An immunocytochemical study of lymphocyte and macrophage populations in the bone marrow of patients with non-Hodgkin's lymphoma. J Pathol 154: 141–149

Pich A, Gastaldi M, Tragni G et al 1991 Lymphocyte subsets in bone marrow lymphoid nodules and malignant lymphoma nodular involvement. Basic Appl Histochem 35: 81–89

Provan A, Wilkins B, Hodges E et al 1993 Immunohistochemical and molecular genetic analysis of a case of T cell-rich B cell lymphoma presenting in bone marrow. Clin Exp Haematol 15: 211–217

Quesenberry P, McNiece I, McGrath H et al 1989 Stromal regulation of hematopoiesis. Ann NY Acad Sci 554: 116–124

Reid M, Malcolm A, McGuckin A 1990 Immunohistochemical detection of neuroblastoma in frozen sections of bone marrow trephine biopsy specimens. J Clin Pathol 43: 334–336

Reid M, Wallis J, McGuckin A et al 1991 Routine histological compared with immunohistological examination of bone marrow trephine biopsy specimens in disseminated neuroblastoma. J Clin Pathol 44: 483–486

Ricci D, Ponzoni M, Zoldan M et al 1993 Bone marrow morphology in 50 AIDS patients. Pathol Res Pract 189: 793

Rios A, Casizo M, Sanz M et al 1990 Bone marrow biopsy in myelodysplastic syndromes: morphological characteristics and contribution to the study of prognostic factors. Br J Haematol 75: 26–33

Rywlin A, Ortega R, Dominguez C 1974 Lymphoid nodules of bone marrow: normal and abnormal. Blood 43: 389–400

Sangster G, Crocker J, Nar P et al 1986 Benign and malignant (B cell) focal lymphoid aggregates in bone marrow trephines shown by means of an immunogold–silver technique. J Clin Pathol 39: 453–457

Schmidt C, Isaacson P 1992 Bone marrow trephine biopsy in lymphoproliferative disease. J Clin Pathol 45: 745–750

Shi S, Key M, Kalra K 1991 Antigen retrieval in formalin-fixed, paraffin-embedded tissues: an enhancement method for immunohistochemical staining based on microwave oven heating of tissue sections. J Histochem Cytochem 38: 741–748

Shin SS, Sheibani K, Kezirian J et al 1992 Immunoarchitecture of normal human bone marrow: a study of frozen and fixed tissue sections. Hum Pathol 23: 686–694

Soini Y, Kamel D, Apaja-Sarkkinen M et al 1993 Tenascin immunoreactivity in normal and pathological bone marrow. J Clin Pathol 46: 218–221

Thiele J, Braeckel C, Wagner S et al 1992a Macrophages in normal human bone marrow and in chronic myeloproliferative disorders: an immunohistochemical and morphometric study by a new monoclonal antibody (PG-M1) on trephine biopsies. Virchows Arch A Pathol Anat 421: 33–39

Thiele J, Rompcik V, Wagner S et al 1992b Vascular architecture and collagen type IV in primary myelofibrosis and polycythaemia vera: an immunomorphometric study on trephine biopsies of the bone marrow. Br J Haematol 80: 227–234

Thiele J, Titius B, Quitman H et al 1992c Megakaryocytopoiesis in bone marrow biopsies of patients with acquired immunodeficiency syndrome (AIDS). Pathol Res Pract 188: 722–728

Traweek S, Sheibani K, Winberg C et al 1989 Monocytoid B-cell lymphoma: its evolution and relationship to other low-grade B cell neoplasms. Blood 73: 573–578

Tricot G, De Wolf-Peeters C, Hendricks B et al 1984a Bone marrow histology in the myelodysplastic syndromes I. Histological findings in the myelodysplastic syndromes and comparison with bone marrow smears. Br J Haematol 57: 423–430

Tricot G, De Wolf-Peeters C, Hendricks B et al 1984b Bone marrow histology in the myelodysplastic syndromes II. Prognostic value of abnormal localisation of immature precursors in MDS. Br J Haematol 58: 217–225

Turner G, Reid M 1993 What is marrow fibrosis after treatment of neuroblastoma? J Clin Pathol 46: 61–63

Van der Valk P, Mullink H,.Huijgens P et al 1989 Immunohistochemistry in bone marrow diagnosis; value of a panel of monoclonal antibodies on routinely processed bone marrow biopsies. Am J Surg Pathol 13: 97–106

Van der Weide M, Sizoo W, Krefft J et al 1988 Myelodysplastic syndromes: analysis of morphological features related to the FAB classification. Eur J Haematol 41: 58–61

Vincic L, Weston S, Riddell R 1989 Bone core biopsies. Plastic or paraffin? Am J Surg Pathol 13: 329–334

White D, Smith A, Whitehouse J et al 1989 Peripheral T cell lymphoma: value of bone marrow trephine immunophenotyping. J Clin Pathol 42: 402–408

Wilkins B 1992 Histology of normal haemopoiesis: bone marrow histology I. J Clin Pathol 45: 645–649

Wilkins B, Jones D 1989 The use of immunohistochemical techniques with formalin-fixed, decalcified, wax-embedded bone marrow trephine biopsies. Haematol Rev 3: 149–163

Wilkins B, Jones D 1992 Cell–stroma interactions in monocytopoiesis. FEMS Microbiol Immunol 105: 347–354

Wilkins B, Jones D 1993 Non-isotopic in situ hybridisation with M-CSF mRNA in routinely processed, formic acid decalcified bone marrow trephine biopsies. J Pathol 170 (Suppl): 36

Wilkins B, Bostanci A, Ryan M et al 1993 Haemopoietic regrowth following chemotherapy for acute leukaemia: an immunohistochemical study of bone marrow trephine biopsy specimens. J Clin Pathol 46: 915–921

Winfield D, Polacarz S 1992 Bone marrow histology. 3: Value of bone marrow core biopsy in acute leukaemia, myelodysplastic syndromes and chronic myeloid leukaemia. J Clin Pathol 45: 855–859

Wirnsberger S, Becker H, Ziervogel K et al 1992 Diagnostic immunohistochemistry of neuroblastic tumors. Am J Surg Pathol 16: 49–57

APPENDIX

Antibody	Antigen	Source
Anti-A1AT	Alpha-1-antitrypsin	DAKO
Antimuramidase	Muramidase (lysozyme)	DAKO
KP1	CD68	DAKO
PG-M1	CD68	DAKO
NP57	Neutrophil elastase	DAKO
LeuM1	CD15	Miles, UK
MAC 387	Calgranulin	DAKO
1B5	MHC Class II	ICRF, London
Hermes 3	CD44	S Jalkanen, Turku, Finland
JC/70A	CD31	DAKO
QBEnd10	CD34	Novocastra, UK
Ret40f	β-Sialoglycoprotein	DAKO
BRIC101	α-Sialoglycoprotein	D Anstee, IBGRL, Bristol
BNH9	Uncharacterized	DAKO
Anti-FVIII	von Willebrand Factor	DAKO
Y2/51	CD61	DAKO
Antitryptase	Mast cell tryptase	DAKO
CBL 419	Major basic protein	Cymbus Bioscience, Southampton
L26	CD20	DAKO
LCA	CD45	DAKO
MT1	CD43	Euro-Path Ltd
UCHL1	CD45R0	DAKO
MB2	Unclustered	Euro-Path Ltd
LN1	CDw75	Biotest UK, Ltd
Anti-CEA	Carcinoembryonic antigen	DAKO
Anti-S100	S100 protein	DAKO
BerH2	CD30	DAKO
Anti-PGP9.5	PGP9.5	Ultraclone, Isle of Wight
Anti-HCL	DBA.44	DAKO

6. Current trends in immunocytochemistry

K. D. Miller   N. Singh   A. C. Wotherspoon

Many advances have taken place over the last 50 years to enable histopathologists to exploit the interaction between antibodies and their specific antigens. With numerous cell types possessing either highly selective or specific epitopes, identification of components in routinely processed paraffin sections and cytological preparations using immunocytochemical techniques has become an essential task of the diagnostic cellular pathology laboratory. Among the technological innovations that established immunocytochemistry as a diagnostic tool, monoclonal antibody technology developed by Kohler & Milstein (1975), proteolytic digestion by Huang et al (1976) and advances in labelling systems (Heggeness & Ash 1977) must be considered major contributions. More recently, synthetic peptide technology (Mason et al 1989) has allowed the production of specific antibodies for diagnostic purposes.

This chapter will concern itself essentially with technical progress, including recent developments, external quality assessment and current advances in immunocytochemistry.

HISTORY

The first significant routine diagnostic application was the identification of immunoglobulin and complement deposits in renal and skin diseases using fluorescent labelling as devised by Coons et al (1941).

As morphological characteristics were not easily seen with fluorescent labelling, enzyme immunocytochemical marking gained popularity. The enzyme horseradish peroxidase (Nakane & Pierce 1966) combined with the chromogen diaminobenzidine (DAB) (Graham & Karnovsky 1966), which gives a golden brown reaction product, became the most prevalent. Morphological detail provided by haematoxylin counterstain enabled the diagnostic pathologist to identify cells expressing particular antigens. The popularity of the DAB–peroxidase reaction product remains, even today, because of its resistance to processing through to resinous mounting and hence giving excellent resolution and prolonged storage qualities. The brown colour can be enhanced using imidazole (Straus 1982), or altered using heavy metal salts such as copper or cobalt (Hsu & Soban 1982), osmication or treatment with gold chloride.

The most popular detection systems for routine diagnostic work, especially in the early 1980s, were the indirect peroxidase and peroxidase antiperoxidase methods (Sternberger et al 1970). Cordell et al (1984) devised the alkaline phosphatase–anti-alkaline phosphatase (APAAP) method which later became accepted as the technique of choice for demonstrating antigens in bone marrow smears as it overcame the difficulties with endogenous peroxidase. The combination of an appealing red reaction product and enhancement, by repeating the bridge and tertiary layers, has enabled APAAP methodology to establish a role in antigen detection on cytological preparations and frozen sections.

As research and development of immunocytochemistry took place, so commercial interest increased and eventually a number of suppliers entered the field. Not only did this enable many research reagents to be more widely available, but the competition ensured reasonable prices. The quality of most products and data sheets have improved to what today is a very high standard from the majority of suppliers. However, the quality of some reagents for immunocytochemistry fail to meet an acceptable standard.

EXTERNAL QUALITY ASSESSMENT OF IMMUNOCYTOCHEMISTRY

The United Kingdom National External Quality Assessment Scheme (UK NEQAS) for Immunocytochemistry (Department of Histopathology, University College London Medical School), begun in 1984, received official recognition in 1988 from the Department of Health Histopathology Steering Committee for External Quality Assessment.

The scheme currently requests the demonstration of two antigens on sections provided by the UK NEQAS centre. The participants are requested to return the best stained section for each antigen together with their own 'in-house' controls. Data are also collected on the methods and reagents employed by each participating laboratory. All slides are coded so as to ensure the participants remain anonymous to the assessors. Anti-kappa light chain immunoglobulin staining is always requested with mantle zone demonstration being the gold standard. It allows monitoring of progress of performance on the same antigen. As kappa light chain immunoglobulin demonstration is one of the most complex immunocytochemical tests, it is considered that good performance with this antibody implies that the participating laboratory is able to perform well with most antibodies. However, the demonstration of a second antigen is requested for confirmation. In-house controls ensure that an element of the scheme covers performance on material with which participants are routinely familiar.

The subjectivity of the assessment is converted to numerical data. Four assessors mark independently with 5 being the maximum score from each. The marks are then totalled out of 20 with 12 being considered the minimum acceptable mark. The scoring criteria are adjusted in accordance with improvements in the field.

The questionnaire on methodology returned by participants yields valuable data that can be analysed against the scores. Because of the complexity of immunocytochemical techniques, monitoring of results against reagents can give only indications of how certain individual components and particular methods perform. Nevertheless, it is possible to highlight techniques and reagents that are less efficient, especially when employed by a large number of users.

AVIDIN–BIOTIN LABELLING

In the late 1970s (Heggeness & Ash 1977) and early 1980s (Hsu et al 1981) the use of avidin–biotin as a labelling system for immunocytochemistry was reported on. Avidin is a glycoprotein which contains hydrophobic pockets that can act as a binding site for biotin. The avidin–biotin complex technique consists of a complex (or conjugate) that is linked to the primary antibody via a biotinylated antibody (bridge) against immunoglobulin. A further modification replaces avidin with the bacterial version streptavidin. The neutral isoelectric point and lack of glycosylation was reported by Buckland (1986) to reduce non-specific binding on tissue sections.

With commercialization, this technology has not only become widely available, but is now the system of choice for most diagnostic immunocytochemistry laboratories. Bains et al (1988) compared peroxidase-labelled avidin–biotin techniques with the indirect peroxidase and peroxidase-antiperoxidase methods and reported that avidin–biotin was not only by far the most sensitive, but found it allowed good demonstration of light chain immunoglobulin, and especially mantle zone staining on formalin-fixed paraffin wax embedded sections. This is confirmed by UK NEQAS data (Fig. 6.1). Later Happerfield et al (1993) compared 11 avidin–biotin systems from six different sources and found that overall, whilst there were differences in sensitivity and cost, all the commercial systems were of high quality.

FIXATION AND IMMUNOCYTOCHEMISTRY

In the UK formol saline fixation, based on various formulae, is widely used and only replaced by fixatives such as Bouin's fluid or formol mercury for special needs. In the experience of the authors the latter two fixatives are not as effective for broad-spectrum immunocytochemistry. However, because of the toxicity of formalin and other traditional fixatives and with current health and safety legislation, it is conceivable that a robust non-toxic replacement for formalin may be required in future.

Formalin fixation and paraffin processing have contributed to a number of technical difficulties in identifying antigens. Even with the aid of trypsin (Huang et al 1976) and other proteolytic enzymes, primary antibodies useful to the diagnostic histopathologist have been limited. The main reagents

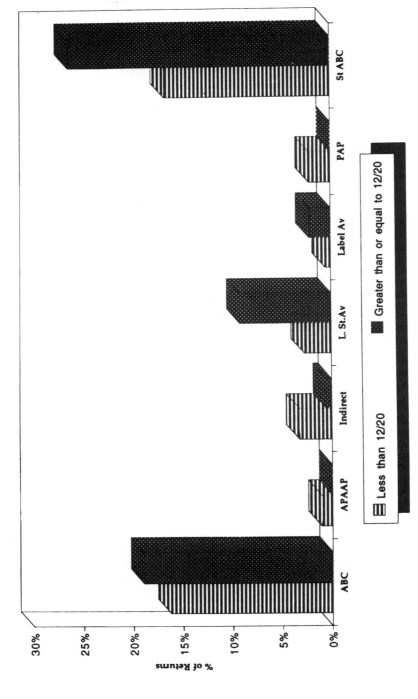

Fig. 6.1 UK NEQAS analysis of anti-kappa light chains on run 21. The histogram compares immunostaining technique (mostly peroxidase labelled) employed against the scores obtained by participants. 12/20 is the minimum acceptable mark. ABC = avidin–biotin complex; APAAP = alkaline phosphatase anti-alkaline phosphatase; L St Av = labelled St avidin; Label av = labelled avidin; PAP = peroxidase anti-peroxidase; St ABC = St avidin–biotin complex.

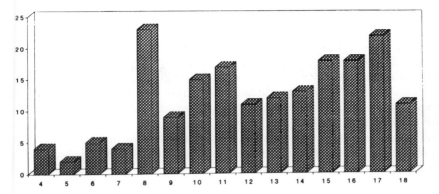

Fig. 6.2 UK NEQAS frequency histogram from run 21. This shows the distribution of scores achieved when demonstrating anti-kappa light chain immunoglobulin on formalin-fixed paraffin-embedded tonsil sections supplied by the scheme. Over 55% scored 12/20 or greater (passed).

include antibodies to cytokeratin, leukocyte-related antigens, protein S100 and desmin. However, with the advent of antigen recovery using microwave oven heating (see below) the number of useful antigens now detectable in paraffin sections is on the increase.

Over the past year the UK NEQAS for Immunocytochemistry has been assessing sections provided by the scheme and material supplied by the participating laboratories. Results indicate that the in-house material suffers from variable fixation and processing which in turn reflects on the quality of immunocytochemistry. Run 21, carried out in late 1992, showed that when staining for kappa light chain immunoglobulin using UK NEQAS sections participant performance improved (Fig. 6.2) compared with when participants' own material was used (Fig. 6.3). Not all antigens, such as immunoglobulin, are so susceptible to poor fixation. Nevertheless, there is no doubt that good-

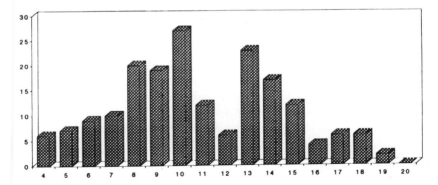

Fig. 6.3 UK NEQAS frequency histogram from run 21. This shows the distribution of scores achieved when demonstrating anti-kappa light chain immunoglobulins on formalin-fixed paraffin-embedded control lymphoid tissue (mostly tonsil), prepared by participating laboratories ('in-house sections'). Less than 40% scored 12/20 or greater (passed).

quality immunocytochemistry can only be achieved once fixation and process-ing procedures are optimized. Through the UK NEQAS for immunocy-tochemistry it has been shown that fresh lymphoid tissue sliced immediately prior to fixation in good-quality 10% formol saline is essential for producing subsequent high-quality immunocytochemistry. Standards for fixation and pro-cessing of specimens for histopathology need to be raised to enable any ensuing immunocytochemical investigation to contribute to the diagnosis. Problems that need attention include avoiding delay in fixing, slicing of large specimens to allow penetration of the fixative and monitoring fixative quality. Unbuffered formal saline becomes acidic over a peroid of weeks and is subsequently deleterious to antigen demonstration.

DEMONSTRATION OF LIGHT CHAIN IMMUNOGLOBULIN ON PARAFFIN SECTIONS

In practice, methodology for light chain immunoglobulin demonstration is optimized on formalin-fixed paraffin-embedded tonsil sections as this is a readily available source of lymphoid tissue in most hospitals. Fresh tonsils are sliced, fixed in 10% formol saline for a period of 12–48 hours, and routinely processed to paraffin wax; sections (3 μm) are cut onto clean glass slides and dried at 56°C. Proteolytic digestion using freshly prepared 0.1% trypsin in 0.1% calcium chloride at 37°C for 5–20 minutes on preheated slides enables good light chain immunoglobulin demonstration on tonsil sections when using an avidin–biotin system. Plasma cells, follicle centre cells and mantle zone cells are readily stained in correctly processed tonsil sections (Fig. 6.4a). Overdigestion (Fig. 6.4b) is seen by the excessive staining of reticulin and often some cells are removed from the slide. Underdigestion (Fig. 6.4c) is seen when only plasma cells are demonstrated. To achieve mantle zone staining it is important to use a relatively high concentration of primary antibody, which may result in some non-cellular elements being stained.

Some primary antibodies for immunoglobulin light chain demonstration on paraffin sections are less suitable than others. The UK NEQAS for Immuno-cytochemistry data, although not covering the whole range of antibodies available for light chain immunoglobulins, indicate that polyclonal reagents generally perform better than monoclonal antibodies (Fig. 6.5). This may be because polyclonal antisera are able to recognize more than one light chain epitope. Furthermore, UK NEQAS data indicate that proteolytic digestion using trypsin contaminated with quantities of chymotrypsin (Fig. 6.6) enables optimal demonstration of immunoglobulin light chain on formalin-fixed paraffin sections.

NEW LABELLING SYSTEMS

With the imposition of financial constraints on health care, commercial suppliers of immunocytochemical reagents have become increasingly aware that three-stage techniques are costly in terms of staff resources. The

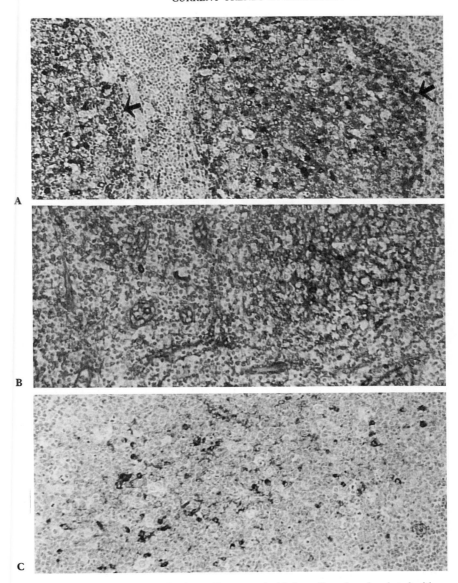

Fig. 6.4 UK NEQAS formalin-fixed paraffin-wax-embedded tonsil sections incubated with anti-kappa light chain immunoglobulin and labelled using an avidin–biotin peroxidase–DAB technique. **A** Plasma cells (dark cells), follicle centre B cells and mantle zone cells (arrowed) are clearly demonstrated. Score: 18/20. **B** This section demonstrates excessive proteolytic digestion as the connective tissue matrix is stained whilst much of the morphology is destroyed. Antigen staining is impaired. **C** This section shows essentially plasma cell staining only as too little proteolytic digestion is employed to unmask much of the immunoglobulin.

production of a novel direct method (Dako Ltd, UK) which overcomes the lack of sensitivity of the traditional direct techniques is an example of how

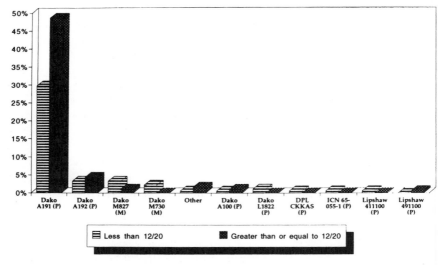

Fig. 6.5   UK NEQAS histogram of run 21 comparing scores of anti-kappa light chain immunoglobulin staining on formalin-fixed paraffin-embedded sections of tonsil with the source and code number of primary antibody employed. 12/20 is considered the minimal acceptable score. Monoclonal reagents appear to be less efficient. M = monoclonal antibody; P = polyclonal antisera. (See Appendix on p. 119 for suppliers' addresses.)

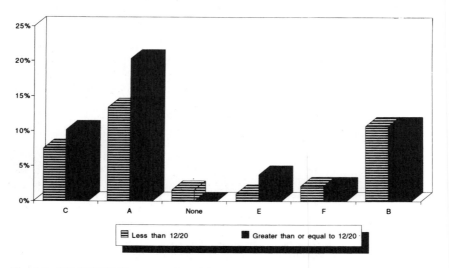

Fig. 6.6   UK NEQAS histogram of run 22 comparing results with antigen retrieval (proteolytic enzymes) employed and when no pretreatment (none) is used on formalin-fixed paraffin-embedded sections of tonsil. Antigen retrieval pretreatment appears to be essential. *NB* Only retrieval systems used by 3 or more participants are shown. C = Difco Trypsin: 0152; A = ICN Trypsin: 150213; E = Sigma Chymotrypsin: C4129; F = Sigma Trypsin: T0646; B = Sigma Trypsin: T8128.

immunocytochemistry is adapting to the financial pressures. The enhanced polymer one-step staining technique (EPOS) uses a polymer backbone to attach a larger number of peroxidase molecules to the primary antibody than was previously achieved with the traditional direct methodology.

Laboratories in which immunocytochemistry techniques are based on optimally diluting concentrated reagents in order to adapt to local fixation are able to obtain similar results using EPOS (Fig. 6.7). Prediluted reagents, however, do have the drawback of offering a fixed dilution and incubation time not attained on local material. By altering the incubation time this methodology can be turned to local conditions, and with two fewer steps and no dilutions much time is saved compared with most avidin–biotin techniques. This will enable laboratories to meet the increase in demand for immunocytochemistry without the need to recruit more immunocytochemists.

IMMUNOCYTOCHEMISTRY ON RESIN-EMBEDDED TISSUES

Clear morphology provided by semithin resin sections has not gained widespread use, especially for lymph node biopsies, because of the difficulty

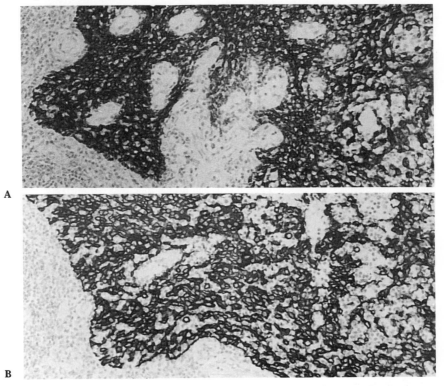

Fig. 6.7 Squamous epithelium demonstrated in formalin-fixed paraffin-embedded sections of tonsil stained with an anticytokeratin (MNF 116) using **A** the EPOS staining technique, and **B** an avidin–biotin labelling system.

of obtaining consistently good immunocytochemistry. Ferrell & Beckstead (1990) reported that the acrylic resin glycol methacrylate allowed a wide range of immunocytochemistry, but this has not been our experience. However, methyl methacrylate, an excellent embedding medium for bone, has been shown by Hand & Morrell (1990) to be a suitable plastic embedding medium for immunocytochemistry and this has been confirmed by Johns & Fish (1992). The gold standard of immunoglobulin light chain mantle zone staining is achievable, provided the sections are at least 2 µm thick (Fig. 6.8).

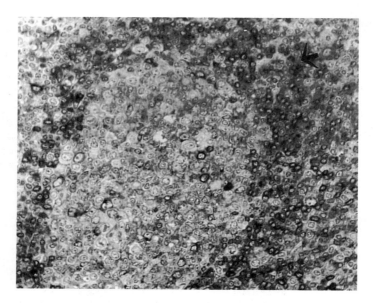

Fig. 6.8   Formalin-fixed and methyl methacrylate resin-embedded 2 µm thick tonsil section showing that plasma cells, follicle centre B cells and mantle zone cells (arrowed) are stained for kappa light chain immunoglobulin.

AUTOMATION OF IMMUNOCYTOCHEMISTRY

Instrumentation for immunocytochemistry is currently gathering momentum with the launch of several instruments offering various levels of automation. The instruments currently popular in the UK are the Sequenza (Fig. 6.9; Life Sciences International (Europe) Ltd, offering partial automation, and the HistoStainer (Fig. 6.10; Leica Ltd), providing a high degree of automation.

In addition, there are three other instruments either available or about to be launched in Europe at the time of writing: the Cadenza (Life Sciences International, UK), the Ventana (Ventana Medical Systems, Inc., USA) and one from BioGenex (USA).

Assessment of performance levels of automation is being monitored by UK NEQAS for Immunocytochemistry (Fig. 6.11).

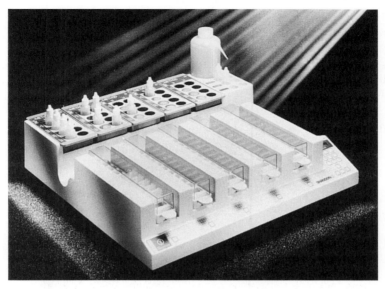

Fig. 6.9 The Sequenza, offering partial automation of the immunocytochemical technique (supplied by Life Sciences International (Europe) Ltd under the trade name of Shandon Scientific Ltd).

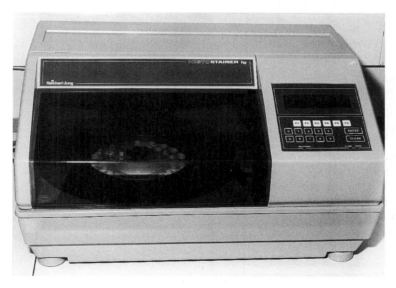

Fig. 6.10 The HistoStainer Ig, offering considerable automation of the immunocytochemical technique (supplied by Leica UK Ltd).

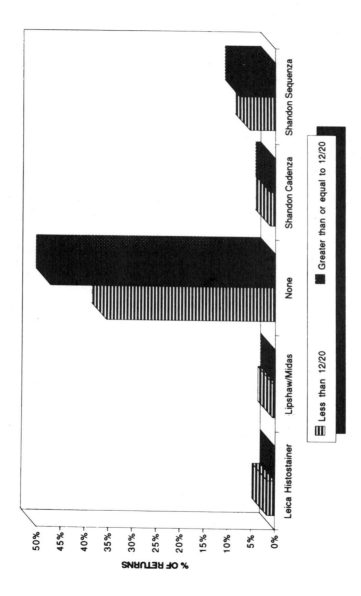

Fig. 6.11 UK NEQAS analysis of anti-kappa light chains on run 21. The histogram compares manual staining (none) and the instruments employed against the scores obtained by participants. 12/20 is considered the minimum acceptable mark.

MICROWAVE ANTIGEN RECOVERY

Shi et al (1991) described a microwave antigen recovery technique requiring the boiling of dewaxed sections in a heavy metal solution prior to immuno-staining. Acceptance of this technology was slow as it went against established theories that excessive heat destroyed antigenicity. Momose et al (1993) found there was no advantage in using heavy metal antigen recovery with microwave oven heating when compared to traditional techniques. Gerdes et al (1992) reported that the use of 0.01 M sodium citrate buffer without heavy metals gave excellent results for the demonstration of the Ki67 antigen on routinely processed paraffin-embedded sections. Subsequently, Singh et al (1993a) compared routine methodology, using proteolytic digestion when appropriate, with heating dewaxed sections in a glass coplin jar containing 0.01 M citrate buffer (pH 6.0) for 10–15 minutes in a microwave oven. For most of the antibodies tested (Table 6.1) the results (Table 6.2) showed that the microwave oven recovery was a considerable improvement on traditional immunocytochemical pretreatments. Since then, it has been discovered that CD21 (IF8) and placental alkaline phosphatase (8B6) are not easily stained after microwave oven heating.

A limitation of the glass coplin jar microwave method is that it allows only two slides to be heated at a time. Additional slides interfere with antigen exposure leading to non-uniform staining. This is overcome by microwave oven heating of ten slides using a plastic rack (Sigma A3807) in an Addis microwaveable container (Addis 9400; available from most department stores). The Addis container allows a considerable height of citrate buffer above the slides and less topping-up is needed. The heating time is increased to 40 minutes as a larger volume (500 ml) of citrate buffer is used.

Singh et al (1993b) reported that heating times in the microwave oven were uniform regardless of fixation time, even when tissues were left in fixative up

Table 6.1   Antibodies and dilutions used

Antibody	Type	Source	Dilution
Ki67	Polyclonal	Dako	1/50
MIB1	Monoclonal	Binding site	1/100
LCA/PD7 + 2B11	Monoclonal	Dako	1/20
CD20/L26	Monoclonal	Dako	1/100
CD3	Polyclonal	Dako	1/100
CD5	Monoclonal	Dr D. Mason (Oxford, UK)	1/10
CD8	Monoclonal	Dr D. Mason (Oxford, UK)	1/2
CD15/LeuM1	Monoclonal	Becton Dickinson	1/20
CD30/BerH2	Monoclonal	Dako	1/10
bc12–100	Monoclonal	Dako	1/20
IgM	Polyclonal	Dako	1/1000
IgD	Polyclonal	Dako	1/500
IgA	Polyclonal	Dako	1/1000
IgG	Polyclonal	Dako	1/4000
Oestrogen/ID5 receptor	Monoclonal	Dako	1/20

Table 6.2   Comparison of traditional immunocytochemistry (using proteolytic digestion where appropriate) with microwave antigen recovery

Antibody	Traditional immunocytochemistry	Antigen recovery with microwave
Ki67	–	+ + +
MIB1	–	+ + +
CD20	+ +	+ + +
CD3	+ +	+ +
	Inconsistent	Consistent
CD5	–	+ +
CD8	–	+ +
CD15	+ +	+ + +
CD30	+ +	+ + +
bcl2	+	+ + +
IgM	+ + +	+ + +
	Inconsistent	Consistent
IgD	+ –	+ + +
IgA	+ +	+ +
	Inconsistent	Consistent
IgG	+ +	+ +
	Inconsistent	Consistent
Oestrogen receptor	–	+ + +

to 2 months (Fig. 6.12). Proteolytic digestion, in contrast, has to be increased as fixation times increase with possible loss of morphological detail. Consequently, as rate of fixative penetration and size of specimen vary greatly, it is almost impossible to establish optimal digestion for most specimens at the first attempt. Microwaving not only overcomes this phenomenon, but exposes antigens previously thought lost to paraffin processing and enhances staining of many other antigens (e.g. CD20) that do not require pretreatment with proteolytic digestion (Fig. 6.13).

Microwave antigen recovery method

1. Paraffin sections are cut onto Vectabond coated slides (Vector Laboratories Ltd, UK) and dried at 56–60°C for a minimum of 1 hour.
2. After dewaxing the sections, endogenous peroxidase activity is inhibited with freshly prepared 0.5% hydrogen peroxide in methanol for 10 minutes.
3. Slides are washed thoroughly in tap water, then rinsed in distilled water and transferred to a coplin jar containing 0.01 M sodium citrate buffer (pH 6.0). The jar is covered with cling-film (ventilated) and heated in a 600 W microwave oven for 10 minutes at full power, pausing only to top-up the fluid lost through evaporation. At no time should the sections be allowed to dry when heated. Glass beads at the bottom of the jar reduce the loss of fluid.
4. After heating, the coplin jar is removed from the oven and the slides are placed in distilled water. Once cooled the sections are rinsed in tris buffered saline and immunostained.

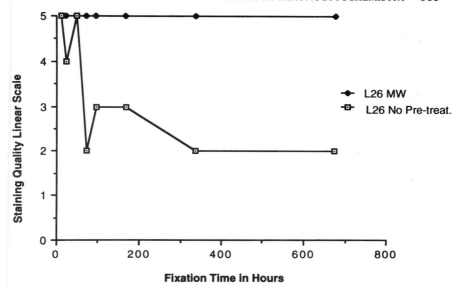

Fig. 6.12   CD20 (L26): microwave oven heating versus no pretreatment on paraffin-embedded sections of tonsil fixed in formol saline for various lengths of time (up to 672 hours). A standard pretreatment using microwave antigen recovery (see text) was carried out for 10 minutes in a coplin jar whilst a parallel set of sections received no pretreatment. Subsequently, all slides were immunostained identically using the monoclonal L26 antibody directed against the CD20 antigen. The staining quality was scored on a linear scale of 1–5. The graph shows that pretreatment for a standard time (10 minutes) with microwave oven heating enables excellent demonstration of the CD20 antigen regardless of fixation time. Sections of tonsil fixed for prolonged lengths of time and having no pretreatment show a decrease in staining quality.

(An alternative method allowing more slides to be processed is described previously.)

Recent work by Merz et al (1993) suggests that a combination of modified antigen retrieval, employing urea and trypsin, improves the reproducibility of light chain immunoglobulin staining on paraffin sections. In our hands, this technique has not proved better than the traditional method. However, Sandison & Smith (1993) have shown that a combination of citrate buffer microwaving followed by 30 seconds of trypsin digestion dramatically improves the detection rate of light chain restriction in bone marrow trephine biopsies (Fig. 6.14) involving myeloma. This plasma cell dyscrasia, in which the demonstration of light chain restriction is crucial, has proved difficult or sometimes impossible to stain for immunoglobulin using a trypsin method.

Jessup and Griffiths (1993) have shown that a similar combination of microwave followed by 30 seconds of trypsin digestion allows greater access to light chain immunoglobulins involved in renal amyloidosis of AL type in formalin-fixed paraffin-embedded sections (Fig. 6.15). Current studies on paraffin-embedded renal biopsies have shown that access to immunoglobulin and complement involved in glomerular disease is improved using the same

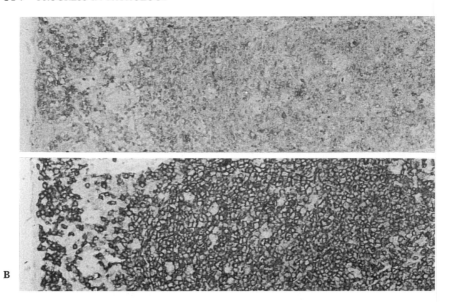

Fig. 6.13 Formalin-fixed (72 hours) paraffin-embedded tonsil sections stained with monoclonal antibody L26 directed against the CD20 antigen, using an avidin–biotin peroxidase DAB method. **A** No pretreatment to expose the antigen was employed. Staining is very weak. **B** Microwave oven pretreatment was employed for 10 minutes. Staining is intense.

combination of microwave and trypsin. Previously trypsin digestion alone has not always been successful as some biopsies suffered from prolonged fixation.

Lebrun et al (1992) suggested that if CD15 was labelled using an IgM bridge reagent in place of a multi-immunoglobulin bridge the number of positive Reed–Sternberg cells per section in Hodgkin's disease is increased. Charalambous et al (1993) not only confirmed the finding, but also went on to report that microwaving with citrate buffer also enhanced CD15 and CD30 staining.

Pressure cooker antigen recovery

Norton (1993) reported that a domestic stainless steel pressure cooker was more efficient than the microwave oven. At the time of writing the pressure cooker method achieved excellent staining for the markers described in Tables 6.1 and 6.2 and is similar to that described for the microwave oven coplin jar method except for step 3. After washing thoroughly in tap water, the slides are transferred to a slide rack. There must be a minimum space of 5 mm between the slides to allow for even heating. The racks are then immersed in boiling citrate buffer, the pressure cooker lid is restored and sealed. Once full pressure is achieved the cooking time is set for 1–2 minutes. The pressure is then released and the pressure cooker is cooled in cold

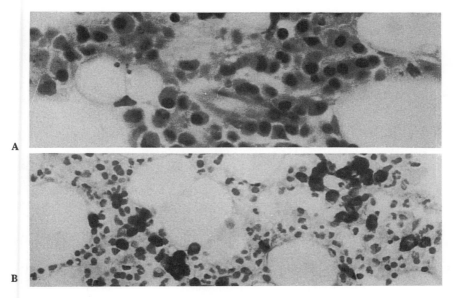

Fig. 6.14   Formalin-fixed, formic acid decalcified, paraffin wax processed bone marrow trephine biopsy sections. **A** Section stained with haematoxylin and eosin, showing many suspicious plasma cells present. **B** Shows clear lambda light chains using an avidin–biotin peroxidase–DAB method. Pretreatment for 10 minutes with microwave oven heating was followed by 30 seconds of trypsin. Kappa light chain immunoglobulin was absent.

running tap-water. The slides are washed in running tap water and subsequently immunostained.

CONCLUSION

Immunocytochemistry, having made a considerable impact as a diagnostic aid for the histopathologist in the 1980s, is continuing to improve in the 1990s. Major advances include microwave oven heating, which is expanding the range of useful antibodies on routinely processed paraffin sections, automation developments and improved methods such as EPOS. As a consequence, the use of antibodies to assist with identifying disease remains at the forefront as a diagnostic tool. As immunocytochemistry is relatively inexpensive in comparison to the expense of patient management, its use is very cost effective.

Difficulties still remain, and the National External Quality Assessment Scheme for Immunocytochemistry is stressing that fixation standards, choice of primary antibody and selection of technique need to be improved in order that a consistently high level of diagnostic information can be obtained. Overall, immunocytochemistry external quality assessment schemes with an educational element can assist all concerned with immunocytochemistry, especially medical laboratory scientists/technologists. By monitoring ad-

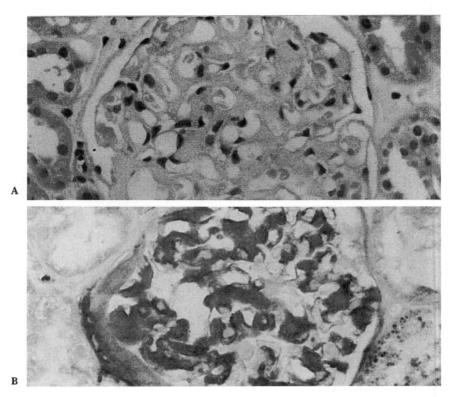

Fig. 6.15 Formalin-fixed paraffin wax processed sections of renal biopsy. **A** Haematoxylin and eosin stain. The renal biopsy has amyloid (AL type) deposition in the glomerulus. **B** Shows lambda light chain immunoglobulin present in AL amyloid deposited in the glomerulus using a peroxidase–antiperoxidase DAB method. Kappa light chain immunoglobulin was absent.

vances, monitoring the efficiency of individual immunocytochemical reagents, commenting on results and giving assistance with difficulties, standards can only improve.

NAMES AND ADDRESSES OF MANUFACTURERS AND SUPPLIERS

A list of manufacturers and suppliers can be found in the Appendix at the end of the chapter on p. 119.

REFERENCES

Bains RM, Miller KD 1988 Peroxidase labelling in immunocytochemistry: a critical comparison of five systems. Med Lab Sci 45: 240–244
Buckland RM 1986 Strong signals from streptavidin–biotin. Nature 557–558

Charalambous C, Singh N, Isaacson P 1993 Immunohistochemical analysis of Hodgkin's disease using microwaves. J Clin Pathol 46: 1085–1088

Coons AH, Creech HJ, Jones RN 1941 Immunological properties of an antibody containing a fluorescent group. Proc Soc Exp Biol Med 47: 200–202

Cordell JL, Falini B, Erber W et al 1984 Immunoenzymatic labelling of monoclonal antibodies using immune complexes of alkaline phosphatase and monoclonal anti-alkaline phosphatase (APAAP) complexes. J Histochem Cytochem 32: 219–229

Ferrell LD, Beckstead JH 1990 Plastic embedding: use of glycol methacrylate-embedded biopsy material at the light microscope level. Pathol Annu 25: 341–360

Gerdes J, Becker MHG, Key G 1992 Immunohistological detection of tumour growth fraction [Ki-67 antigen] in formalin-fixed and routinely processed tissues. J Pathol 168: 85–87

Graham RC, Karnovsky MJ 1966 The early stages of absorption of injected horseradish peroxidase in the proximal tubules of mouse kidney: ultrastructural cytochemistry by a new technique. J Histochem Cytochem 14: 291–302

Hand NM, Morrell KJ 1990 Immunocytochemistry on plastic sections for light microscopy: a new technique. Proc R Microsc Soc 25: 111

Happerfield LC, Bobrow LG, Bains RM et al 1993 Peroxidase labelling immunocytochemistry: a comparison of eleven commercially available avidin–biotin systems. Br J Biomed Sci 50: 21–26

Heggeness MH, Ash JF 1977 Use of the avidin–biotin complex for the localization of actin and myosin with fluorescence microscopy. J Cell Biol 73: 738–783

Hsu SM, Soban E 1982 Colour modification of diaminobenzidine (DAB) precipitation by metallic ions and its application to double immunocytochemistry. J Histochem Cytochem 30: 1079–1082

Hsu SM, Raine L, Fanger H 1981 Use of avidin–biotin–peroxidase complex (ABC) in immunoperoxidase techniques: a comparison between ABC and unlabeled antibody (PAP) procedures. J Histochem Cytochem 29: 577–580

Huang S, Minassian H, More JD 1976 Application of immunofluorescent staining improved by trypsin digestion. Lab Invest 35: 383–391

Jessup E, Griffiths M 1993 Personal communication

Johns L, Fish DKW 1992 Personal communication

Kohler G, Milstein C 1975 Continuous cultures of fused cells producing antibody of pre-defined specificity. Nature 256: 495–497

Lebrun DP, Kamel OW, Dorfman RF et al 1992 Enhanced staining for Leu M1 [CD15] in Hodgkin's disease using a secondary antibody specific for immunoglobulin M. Am J Clin Pathol 97: 135–139

Mason DY, Cordell J, Brown M et al 1989 Detection of cells in paraffin-wax embedded tissue using antibodies against a peptide sequence from the CD3 antigen. J Clin Pathol 42: 1194–1200

Merz H, Rickers O, Schrimel S et al 1993 Constant detection of surface and cytoplasmic immunoglobulin heavy and light chain expression in formalin-fixed and paraffin embedded material. J Pathol 170: 257–264

Momose H, Mehta P, Battifora H 1993 Antigen retrieval by microwave irradiation in lead thiocyanate: comparison with protease digestion retrieval. Appl Immunohistochem 1: 77–82

Nakane PK, Pierce GB 1966 Enzyme-labeled antibodies: preparation and application for the localisation of antigens. J Histochem Cytochem 14: 929–931

Norton A 1993 Personal communication

Sandison A, Smith MEF 1993 Personal communication

Shi R-R, Key ME, Kalra KL 1991 Antigen retrieval in formalin-fixed, paraffin embedded tissues; an enhancement method for immunohistochemical staining based on microwave oven heating of tissue sections. J Histochem Cytochem 39: 741–748

Singh N, Miller KD, Isaacson PG 1993a Microwave antigen retrieval: a new experience. J Pathol 169 (Suppl): Abstract 221

Singh N, Wotherspoon AC, Miller KD et al 1993b The effect of formalin fixation time on the immunocytochemical detection of antigen using the microwave. J Pathol 170 (Suppl): 382A

Sternberger LA, Hardy PH, Cuculis JJ et al 1970 The unlabeled antibody enzyme method of immunohistochemistry: preparation and properties of soluble antigen-antigen complex (horseradish peroxidase–anti-horseradish peroxidase) and its use in the identification of spirochaetes. J Histochem Cytochem 18: 315–333

Straus W 1982 Imidazole increases the sensitivity of the cytochemical reaction for peroxidase with diaminobenzidine at a neutral pH. J Histochem Cytochem 30: 491–493

APPENDIX

Names and addresses of manufacturers and suppliers

Dako Ltd, 16 Manor Courtyard, Hughenden Avenue, High Wycombe, Bucks HP13 5RE, UK

Difco Laboratories Ltd, PO Box 14B, Central Avenue, West Molesey, Surrey KT8 2SE, UK

Diagnostic Products Limited (DPL), 22 Blacklands Way, Abingdon Business Park, Abingdon, Oxon OX14 1DY, UK

ICN Biomedicals Ltd, Eagle House, Peregrine Business Park, Gomm Road, High Wycombe, Bucks HP13 7DL, UK

Leica UK Ltd, Davey Avenue Knowlhill, Milton Keynes MK5 8LB, UK

Life Sciences International (Europe) Ltd, Chadwick Road, Astmoor, Runcorn, Cheshire WA7, UK

Lipshaw Immunoproducts: see Life Science International (Europe) Ltd

Sigma Chemical Company Ltd, Fancy Road, Poole, Dorset BH17 7NH, UK

United Kingdom National External Quality Assessment Scheme for Immunocytochemistry, Histopatholog, University College London Medical School, London WCIE 6JJ, UK. Organizer: K. D. Miller

Vector Laboratories Ltd, Laboratories Ltd, 16 Wulfric Square, Bretton, Peterborough, Cambs PE3 8BR, UK

---

7. The molecular basis of development

C. L. Berry

'Given the molecular forces in a mutton chop, deduce Hamlet or Faust therefrom.' (see Huxley 1918)

In characteristic style, Huxley presented in this way a radical extension of the views of the physicist Tyndall. The latter, at the height of the Darwinian debate had given an address to the British Association for the Advancement of Science in 1896 suggesting that the mind/brain problem would soon be resolved, given the power of the new biological thought. Our new biology has given us additional insights and has altered our thinking about development, growth and differentiation more rapidly than changes have taken place in our understanding of the mind/brain relationship. Vertebrate development is now seen to be a process driven mainly by cellular interaction rather than direct genetic instruction. In particular, it has become clear that the processes involved in development have been conserved over an enormous timescale, are limited in their variety, are identical or closely related to those processes disturbed in neoplasia and are capable of disturbance by environmental factors. All of these characteristics make them of significance to pathologists. For those who have rashly allowed their embryology to slip an excellent general account is that of Gilbert (1992) and a number of the basic cellular processes to be discussed are described in the text of Alberts et al (1989).

EARLY DEVELOPMENT

This chapter will concentrate on the events in later development (embryogenesis) but earlier changes are of interest in terms of the involvement of growth factors. For many years, indeed since 1878, when Whitman suggested that each identified cell in the early embryo is developmentally distinct, embryology was taught as an essentially deterministic subject. Each identified blastomere and the clone of its descendent cells was thought to play a specific predestined role in later development as part of a rigorously programmed sequence of events. I have described in another text the evolution and characteristics of such rigorously defined systems where they exist (see Berry 1994), but it is worth noting that the identification of organizers (Spemann & Mangold 1924) and the phenomenon of induction (Nieuwkoop 1969) altered this view of developmental biology irretrievably. However, it is important to realize that it was not until 1970 that the concepts of a detailed plan for embryo building, of *local* organization as the basis for organogenesis and of signals passed from one part of the embryo to another were all identified.

The cellular events which control these early phenomena have become clear only in this decade. Members of the fibroblast growth factor (FGF), transforming growth factor-β (TGF-β) and *Wnt* gene families — acting as signalling factors over short distances — are effective in causing the undifferentiated ectoderm of the animal hemisphere to form mesoderm. Basic FGF (bFGF) like the rest of the family is a secreted protein that binds to the cell surface and extracellular glycosaminoglycans; this binding appears to restrict the distribution of the protein markedly, making this group excellent candidates as localizing signals. bFGF can induce most, if not all, mesodermal cell types and the presence of the gene and its transcripts can be demonstrated in the early embryo (Schmid et al 1991). Activin is the most potent inducing agent in the TGF-β family and may induce brain and eyes in explants, although it may be the mesoderm induced by the protein which actually has this effect on the ectoderm (Sokol et al 1990). In Kimelman's elegant model, a number of overlapping systems involving these three families may determine not only induction but also the precise pattern of distribution of mesoderm in the developing blastocyst. These data allow us to begin to answer questions about how genes actually work in development, but immediately the conservatism of the entire process is evident. From the data of Schmid et al (1991) it is clear that the TGF-β family of polypeptides is used not only in this phase but also later in development in the phase of branchial arch differentiation, formation of the lung and in the formation of the bones of the face, as examples. In general it is true to say that many growth-control and cell-signalling mechanisms are used repeatedly in development, often in different ways at different stages. An important characteristic of developmental mechanisms is that there often appears to be considerable redundancy in the operating systems — a point pathologists should recognize when they identify particular gene products as 'characteristic' of particular cell types. In a number of cases of apparent redundancy the additional mechanism may be effective in increasing the specificity of a process, acting as a form of 'fine tuning' of a regulatory process (Wolpert 1992); an analogy would be the differing processes which contribute to the effective monitoring of the fidelity of DNA reproduction. An example of this tuning is seen in the development of *Drosophila*, where genes determining anterior and posterior characteristics of an embryo interact with genes having localized non-polar expression, to produce graded concentrations of gene products which may have activating or repressive effects. As Wolpert has pointed out, some cases of redundancy may be evolutionary relics where genes have persisted for millions of years because they present no selection disadvantages.

AXIS FORMATION AND POLARITY

In discussing these and other events certain terms will be used which should be defined here. The *lineage* of a cell is a term used to denote its mitotic history and the *genealogy* of a cell is its position in the lineage. *Invariant lineages* are those which follow a prescribed pattern; *conditional lineages* may or may not, depending on other interactions. The process of *gastrulation* occurs at the end of the cleavage divisions (which occur in the blastular stage) and results in the conversion of a flat disc of cells into a three-dimensional structure in which morphogenetic movement occurs.

In a number of relatively simple animals such as the nematodes, deuterostomes and neogastropods, all initial cleavage is invariant and the lineages derived from specific blastomeres display predictable invariant fates. One embryonic axis is established by the time of fertilization (in general terms, by the site of penetration of the egg by the sperm) and the second within the first few cleavage cycles (Ransick & Davidson 1993). Some cell lineages are *autonomously* determined and will not vary whatever cell a blastomere finds itself next to, while others are *conditional*; the blastomere gives rise to different cells depending on local signalling. These embryos were classified as type I by Davidson (1991) in an important essay on early development; a major characteristic is a direct relationship between the polarity of the egg and an axial feature of the body plan. Importantly, cell-type specification precedes any large-scale embryonic cell migration.

Vertebrate and insect embryos differ from Davidson type I embryos. No vertebrate embryo has an invariate cell lineage and given structures are always composed of cells with differing lineages. Even after a significant number of cell divisions there remain cells which can give rise to a number of cell types (demonstrated for the zebrafish, chick and mouse). As an example, consider the neural crest where the fate of individual cells is largely determined by influences acting during their migration — the route the cell takes in leaving the crest, for example. In this type of embryo, cell-type specification generally occurs after gastrulation and cell-type specific molecular markers of differentiation can only be detected at gastrulation or later. There is a mechanism for regional identification, which is important since many of the cell types appear in all regions. This is mediated by diffusible intercellular morphogens such as FGF, TGF-β and retinoic acid. After the specification of regions such as the neural plate, head, and dorsal and ventral mesoderm the morphogenetic programmes begin to act. These embryos are in Davidson's type II which clearly includes man.

Because of certain differences in the use of conserved genes it is worth considering Davidson's type III embryos, in particular the insects. In insects initial development takes place in a syncytium. Cellular interaction cannot occur and after cellularization the subsequent cell lineage is invariant. The mechanisms described for type I and type II embryos are not available to insects but the end-point is identical; in Davidson's words, 'the generation of an assembly of spatially organised cells according to the body plan, that can now mount the intercellular functions required for cell type specification and morphogenesis'.

In type I embryos regional control functions will only be used in postembryonic development; lineage, cleavage pattern and gastrulation determine early form. In type II embryos long-range diffusible morphogens apparently determine the broad organization of body plan, and morphogens such as retinoic acid exert their effects by homeobox gene activation; TGF-β and bFGF are necessary for the initial axial specification of mesoderm with subsequent homeobox activity (for a more detailed account of the role of homeobox genes in development see Berry 1992). In type III embryos a different process is followed avoiding diffusible growth factors, short-range cell interactions or lineage determined events. Homeobox genes generate the body plan ab initio rather than being used to continue morphogenesis after the establishment of this plan by other means; these include the control of expression of ligands and receptors. This is a good example of how identical regulatory genes are used in a different mode in different species; homeobox genes exist in the most primitive metazoans (the cnidarians, e.g. jellyfish, anemones) and show a pattern of multiple functions in different vertebrates indicating a pattern of gene duplication, divergence and co-option for new functions. Other regulatory genes such as the steroid receptor gene family show analogous patterns of evolutionary change.

In general homeobox genes act by repressing the activity of other genes, removing some aspect of a primitive feature. In insects they prevent features of more anterior or posterior segments being expressed in the 'wrong' segment. Acting in this way the genes have acted on a multisegmented head region converting it into a single compound structure where modified appendages have acquired new functions. 'New' structures can develop in this way and malformation complexes such as the DiGeorge syndrome (absence of the thymus, parathyroids and heart, and great vessel anomalies) are readily explained if the mode of the development of the mesenchyme of the branchial arches is understood. Fig. 7.1 illustrates how homeoboxes act in the development of the hindbrain to produce a segment-restricted code of *Hox* expression in the neuroepithelium and the adjacent presumptive neural crest. This expression is maintained during the migration of the neural crest cells resulting in an identifiable pattern of expression in the cranial ganglia and branchial mesenchyme that indicates the rhombomere of origin. Finally, *Hox-2* expression occurs in the surface ectoderm in contact with the neural crest derived branchial mesoderm. Thymic, parathyroid, cardiac and great vessel abnormalities resembling those seen in the DiGeorge syndrome can be reproduced by targeted disruption of the *Hox 1.5* gene (Chisaka & Capecchi 1991). It is perhaps worth pointing out that the smooth muscle cells of the great arteries are neural crest derived.

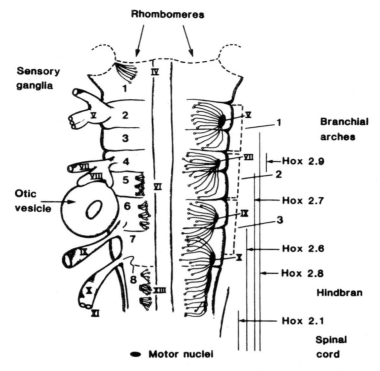

Fig. 7.1   The diagram shows the close association between the position of each branchial motor nucleus and the rhombomeric pattern (rhombomeres are the segmental equivalent of the somites in the head and neck region). The branchial arch lies ventral to the pair of rhombomeres in which the corresponding motor neuron cell bodies are located with a clear 2:1 relationship. The exit points of the cranial nerves occupy distinct positions in relation to individual rhombomeres. Further, each branchial motor nucleus occupies a distinct position with regard to rhombomere boundaries.

The segmental expression of *Hox* genes is shown on the right. As the *Hox* genes are expressed in mesoderm and ectoderm it is easy to see how complex malformations such as the DiGeorge syndrome and perhaps other anomalies of the face and neck may be affected by disturbance in their expression.

Based on Lumsden & Keynes (1989), Wilkinson et al (1989) and Stern & Keynes (1988).

DEVELOPMENTAL STRATEGIES

In the formation of the embryo, two broad strategies are available to the organism: to generate gross patterns of cells forming tissues or organs with cell diversity being generated later; or to generate cell diversity first, independently of any pattern, and allow patterns to form on the basis of interactions between specialist cells. In different tissues different strategies may be followed.

If diversity is to be generated, the cells must first be divided into domains by mechanisms that do not depend simply on divisions and a critical number in the anlage, since experiments have shown that there is clearly a capacity for modification of the effects of interference. It is probably worth repeating that the *lineage* of a cell denotes its mitotic history and the *genealogy* of a cell is its position in the lineage. As has been made clear, genealogy will not necessarily determine what a cell becomes; this may be modified by various cell–cell interactions. An example of this is the non-exclusiveness of restriction of tissue-type potential to the germ layers, long thought to be universal to all higher animals. In the tiny nematode worm *Caenorhabditis elegans* with its 959 characterized somatic cells, four muscle cells are produced by the ectoderm and four glial cells by the ectoderm. These exceptions occur at the site of penetration of another germ layer by the exceptional cells, but this type of interaction is not neccessary for this type of variation in vertebrates where similar non-exclusivity is also seen (Le Douarin 1980). There is another mechanism which will modify form: cells have the 'option' of dying rather than differentiating. In *C. elegans* 17% of embryonic cells die in this way and apoptotic cell death is a major feature of vertebrate organogenesis.

Even in an animal with fewer than 1000 cells the number of genes controlling cell identities in specific domains, lineages or cell types is surprisingly high (probably more than 40); many such genes exist in vertebrates.

EXTRINSIC CONTROLS AND THE DEVELOPMENTAL PROCESS

Many of the factors that are of critical importance in development of organs act by mechanisms that are not direct in terms of an effect on the lineage or genealogy of their anlage. These effects may be mediated via the extracellular matrix, the cytoskeleton or cell junctions.

The extracellular matrix

The extracellular matrix (ECM) may regulate development in three ways:

1.   The ECM may differ significantly in composition at different locations in ways that are permissive or restrictive to cell adhesion, division or mobility.

2.   Cell surface receptors for different components of the matrix may be the regulating factors in these functions and are clearly expressed differentially in different cell groups.

3.   Growth factors may bind to the matrix selectively, affecting local concentrations. This may affect the production of local matrix components or the controlled release of the factors by, say, variable rates of degradation (see Adams & Watt 1993).

A puzzling aspect of development may be explained by invoking the intervention of the ECM. It is evident that there are three well-defined axes for the vertebrate body: anteroposterior, dorsoventral and left–right. This later asymmetry is most evident in the development of the gut and the heart (asymmetry in man is first seen in the heart). Yost (1992) has suggested that changes in the ECM may be critical in determining left–right axes perhaps due to an inherent handedness of the fibrillary proteins that comprise much of it, presenting an asymmetric surface to the anlage. Elongation of the embryo anteroposteriorly may impose strains on the matrix and allow this handedness to develop. Recent descriptions of genes for situs inversus showing that laterality is disturbed by an active process suggest that this may be a reasonable hypothesis; an epigenetic mechanism normally acts on a neutral genetic state in which no particular 'handedness' is preferred (Hoyle et al 1992).

Cell junctions and associated proteins

The kidney provides a good model of how these factors operate. After the beginning of glomerulogenesis condensation occurs in the renal mesenchyme. As condensation occurs and the renal tubule develops a number of epithelial associated antigens such as laminin, type IV collagen and keratin are expressed. Garrod & Flemming (1990) have shown that apart from these expressions, regarded by the authors as epiphenomena in development, various desmosomal proteins can also be identified at early stages. They point out that this observation suggests an important early role for cell junctions in the condensation process, perhaps binding the tubular cells tightly together and facilitating the formation of tubules. This finding is in agreement with the general suggestion by Edelman (1988) of a precedence hypothesis in which morphogenesis is thought to be dependent on cell adhesion molecule (CAM) dependent cell association and later specialized cell junction formation.

There is clearly a great deal of cellular differentiation occurring while these morphogenetic events take place. At least 14 epithelial cell types develop from the metanephric mesenchyme, from multipotent stem cells that can generate three distinct cell types: glomerular, proximal and distal epithelia (Herzlinger et al 1992). These events are dependent on the changes in stromal associated molecules.

Changes in cytoskeletal and other proteins

Changes in individual proteins can cause significant changes in cellular architecture when raising their concentrations produces a change in the assembly of macromolecular networks. Examples are seen in the stable network formed by the cytoskeletal self-assembly of red blood cells, the production of microvilli, which is triggered by the appearance of the single protein villin, and the development of polarity in epithelial cells. This latter process is dependent on the calcium-sensitive protein E-cadherin (L-CAM, uvoromorulin) which produces a redistribution of the cytoskeleton and the membrane associated sodium pump when transfected into fibroblasts (McNeill et al 1990). The fundamental point in all of these rearrangements is that there is no change in the rate of production of the proteins, only a change in their configuration as macromolecular networks formed from pre-existing components. Such a change underlies the ability of synapsin to generate the complex structures and vesicles of synapses (Kelly 1991).

Here we have another example of using a conserved mechanism to different effect at different stages of development; some evidence suggests that this type of cytoskeletal phenomenon underlies the formation of the primary germ layers. The ventral furrow, posterior midgut invagination and other morphogenetic movements in *Drosophila* occur where the regular cobblestone-like appearance of the ectoderm is disturbed by rows of cells which undergo apical constriction forming a groove (Sweeton et al 1991). Nuclear positions in the cells in the groove change and eventually, as a result of the process of cell shortening which appears to occur in a stochastic manner, accumulated changes in cell form result in invagination. The groove is produced not by a grand genetic plan but by local changes in the cellular environment, which at a given stage in the genealogy affect the cytoskeleton.

Clausi & Brodland (1993) have carried out some very convincing computer simulations of the process of neurulation. The process of neural tube closure has been of major interest in embryology and dysmorphogenesis and is clearly dependent on changes of the kind described in the work of Sweeton et al (1991), but a great many variables have been shown to influence the process. Their method allows for the non-isometric properties of tissue and cells and for the large strain values exhibited by some biological materials in the construction of a 'virtual' embryo. They have shown that when uniform isotropic circumferential microfilament bundle (CMB) constriction and cephalocaudal elongation act together on a simulated circular neural plate it becomes keyhole shaped, resembling the neural plate, and that when these forces act on a spherical (amphibian) embryo dorsal surface flattening occurs. CMB constriction can produce sequential formation of neural ridges, narrowing and thickening of the neural plate and neural tube closure. This series of events is produced by mechanical changes alone; no cellular divisions or non-mechanical cell–cell interactions are necessary. Multiple 'redundant' mechanisms are necessary to produce an effective result; it is interesting to note the comments of Wolpert (above) in this context.

CELLULAR RECEPTORS AND POSITIONAL INFORMATION

I have already indicated that different organs and tissues may use different strategies of development. A combination of direct involvement of lineage and genealogically determined events and interactions with the ECM and with receptors will be involved in many tissues and the limbs provide a good example.

Experiments primarily concerned with the establishment of the morphological pattern of the limbs have shown that in early development the mesenchyme of the limb bud is apparently composed of a single cell type, but from later stages (stage 24 in the chick) mesenchymal cells differentiate into muscle, cartilage, bone and connective tissue cells. Kieny and her co-workers, in a long series of studies on the developing limb bud (see, for example, Chevallier et al 1977) have shown that the limb skeleton, tendons and dermis develop from the somatopleural mesoderm whereas muscle develops from the somite.

Each segment of the vertebrate limb is made from these same cell types but they are arranged in different spatial patterns. These differences depend on the fact that the cells, although similar, are in fact non-equivalent; they possess positional values that regulate the process of pattern formation in the limbs. This activity is determined by homeotic genes which occur in complexes. Each of these complexes consists of a string of related genes all coding for transcription factors containing a homeobox sequence. The genes in the box are brought into action obeying the rule that the further the gene lies from the beginning of the complex in the chromosome the more posterior its expression domain along the body axis. Mammals have at least four *HOM* gene complexes homologous to those of insects and two of these complexes, *Hox*-2 and *Hox*-5 are expressed in the central body axis of vertebrates in the same way as in insects, so that the chromosomal extent of *Hox* expression provides cells with an indication of their craniocaudal position (Graham et al 1989). In a massive study Dollé et al (1989) mapped the expression of five members of the *Hox*-5 gene complex by in situ hybridization at different stages of development. Each gene had a specific spatial domain and time of activation with these spatial domains of activation nested like a set of Babushka dolls in the order of the occurrence of the gene on the chromosome. Later, at the sites of potential joints the genes are down-regulated in a manner which suggests the activation of later-acting gene products.

Other data suggest that two different mechanisms define the anteroposterior and proximodistal positional values in the limb. The anteroposterior values are determined by a morphogen produced by the cells of the polarizing zone at the distal posterior margin of the limb bud (Brickell & Tickle 1989). Cells which lie close to this zone receive a high dose of morphogen (retinoic acid) and form structures which are posterior in type, such as little fingers. At the opposite end of the gradient they will form thumbs. Grafting experiments show that this pattern can be manipulated readily by the transposition of groups of cells from the polarizing zone or by implantation of beads loaded with retinoic acid; receptors for this morphogen are found in the limb bud at appropriate sites and stages. Proximodistal positional information depends on an effect of the apical ectodermal ridge at the distal end of the limb bud which maintains the mesoderm deep to it in a state where the cells display an autonomous tendency to become progressively more distal in their positional behaviour with time. As the limb grows, groups of cells become displaced from this specialized mesoderm and their positional value is thus fixed.

The way in which these systems interact is not yet clear. It seems probable that retinoic acid may regulate homeotic gene expression and that this compound may be able to reset positional values experimentally (Lewis & Martin 1989). Cells in the posterior part of the limb bud that will give rise to posterior structures such as little fingers are found to express all of the homeobox genes in the *Hox*-4 complex in the chick, while cells from which anterior structures develop only *Hox*-4.4.

GENETIC CHANGE AND DISEASE

It is clear that a number of malformation complexes are produced by inappropriate expression of homeobox and other regionally expressed genes. The example of the DiGeorge syndrome is discussed above and the work of Wolgemuth et al (1989) in inducing overexpression of the homeobox gene *Hox*-1.4 in the mouse has resulted in a phenocopy of Hirschsprung's disease with failure of the innervation of the large bowel manifest as hypoganglionosis and megacolon, apparently due to failure either of neural crest cell migration or more probably from failure of gut mesenchyme to provide appropriate signals for migration (the gene is also expressed in mesenchyme; see Berry 1993 for discussion). Do single genes of large effect produce malformations? Abnormal development will certainly follow mutations in type 1 collagen genes, as an example; osteogenesis imperfecta and Ehlers–Danlos disease type VII are examples caused by mutations in COL1A1 and COL1A2 respectively, but it is interesting to note that other tissues containing collagen (other than bone and skin) are apparently unaffected. It is clear that it is the precise biochemical change which has produced the particular phenotypic effect observed; in COL1A2 mutations the abnormal collagen can still be properly mineralized, so the bones are fine, but the failure of normal gap and overlap relationships in the altered collagen molecules produces the changes in mechanical properties which in turn produce the skin and joint changes of the syndrome (Kadler 1993).

It seems probable, for a number of reasons, that relatively few common malformation syndromes are produced by single genes of large effect. Those genes with products involved in pattern formation and positional information are more promising candidates and are being identified at a rapid rate, using the techniques of the new biology.

CONCLUSIONS

Development is a process in which highly conserved mechanisms are used in a number of ways to assemble groups of cells in appropriate numbers at well-defined sites. The cells must have defined mitotic histories and adequate positional information to allow a large number of epigenetic influences to operate on them in a flexible way to produce functional systems and assemblies. Much of this activity is subject to multiple and often apparently redundant control mechanisms and cell death is a major developmental mechanism in this control system. There is often some astonishment that such a complex system works so efficiently; there is, after all, a population explosion of apparently normal individuals. The answer is that it does not work; the outcome of the vast majority of zygotic fusions in vertebrates is death of the conceptus. This alone is a major clue to the redundancy seen and to the essential evolutionary conservativism — if it works it has a selection advantage. A limited number of growth factors, positional information genes and matrix proteins are found in the animal kingdom — even *Hydra* has a homeobox.

REFERENCES

Adams JC, Watt FM 1993 Regulation of development and differentiation by the extracellular matrix. Development 117: 1183–1198
Alberts B, Bray D, Lewis J et al 1989 Molecular biology of the cell. 2nd edn. Garland Publishing, New York
Berry CL 1992 What's in a homeobox? The development of pattern during embryonic growth. Virchows Arch A 420: 291–295
Berry CL 1993 Intestinal neuronal dysplasia: does it exist or has it been invented? Virchows Arch A 422: 183–184
Berry CL 1994 Building an embryo with limited resources. Recent Adv Pediatr (in press)
Brickell PM, Tickle C 1989 Morphogens in chick limb development. Bioessays 11: 145–149
Chevallier A, Kieny M, Mauger A 1977 Limb–somite relationship: origin of the limb musculature. J Embryol Exp Morphol 41: 245–258
Chisaka O, Capecchi MR 1991 Regionally restricted developmental defects resulting from targeted disruption of the mouse homeobox gene Hox 1.5. Nature 350: 473–479
Clausi DA, Brodland GW 1993 Mechanical evaluation of theories of neurulation using computer simulations. Development 118: 1013–1023
Davidson EH 1991 Spatial mechanisms of gene regulation in metazoan embryos. Development 113: 1–26
Dollé P, Izpisua-Belmonte J-C, Falkenstein H et al 1989 Coordinate expression of the murine Hox-5 complex homoeobox-containing genes during limb pattern formation. Nature 342: 767–772
Edelman GM 1988 Morphoregulatory molecules. Biochemistry 17: 3533–3543
Garrod DR, Flemming S 1990 Early expression of desmosomal components during kidney tubule morphogenesis in human and murine embryos. Development 108: 313–321
Gilbert SF 1992 Developmental biology. 3rd edn. Sinauer Associates, Sunderland, MA
Graham A, Papalopulu N, Krumlauf R 1989 The murine and *Drosophila* homeobox genes have common features of organisation and expression. Cell 57: 367–378
Herzlinger D, Koseki C, Mikawa T et al 1992 Metanephric mesenchyme contains metanephric stem cells whose fate is restricted after induction. Development 114: 565–572
Hoyle C, Brown N, Wolpert L 1992 Development of left/right handedness in the chick heart. Development 115: 1071–1078
Huxley L 1918 Life and letters of Sir Joseph Dalton Hooker. vol 2, p 119, Murray. Cited by Desmond A 1992 Darwin. Penguin, London
Kadler KE 1993 Learning how mutations in type I collagen genes cause connective tissue disease. Int J Exp Pathol 74: 319–323
Kelly RB 1991 A system for synapse control. Nature 349: 650–651
Le Douarin N 1980 Migration and differentiation of neural crest cells. In: Moscona AA, Monray A (eds) Current topics in developmental biology. Academic Press, New York, vol 16, pp 31–85
Lewis J, Martin P 1989 Vertebrate development. Limbs: a pattern emerges. Nature 342: 734–735
Lumsden A, Keynes R 1989 Segmental patterns of neuronal development in the chick hindbrain. Nature 337: 424–428

McNeill H, Ozawa M, Kemler R et al 1990 Novel function of the cell adhesion molecule uvomorulin as an inducer of cell surface polarity. Cell 62: 309–316

Nieuwkoop PD 1969 The formation of mesoderm in urodelean amphibians. I. The induction by the endoderm. Wilhelm Roux Arch Entwicklungsmech Org 162: 341–373

Ransick A, Davidson EH 1993 A complete second gut induced by transplantation micromeres in the sea urchin embryo. Science 259: 1134–1138

Schmid P, Cox D, Bilbe G et al 1991 Differential expression of TGF B1, B2 and B3 genes during mouse embryogenesis. Development 111: 117–130

Sokol S, Wong G, Melton DA 1990 A mouse macrophage factor induces head structure and organises body axis in *Xenopus*. Science 249: 561–564

Spemann H, Mangold H 1924 Uber Induction von Embryonanlagen durch Implantation artfremder Organis Atoren. Wilhelm Roux Arch Entwicklungsmech Org 175: 199–220

Stern CD, Keynes RJ 1988 Spatial patterns of homeobox gene expression in the developing mammalian. Trends Neurosci 11: 190–192

Sweeton D, Parks S, Costa M et al 1991 Gastrulation in *Drosophila*: the formation of the ventral furrow and posterior mid-gut invaginations. Development 112: 775–789

Whitman CO 1878 The embryology of Clepsin. Q J Microsc Sci 18: 215–315

Wilkinson DG, Bhatt S, Cook M et al 1989 Segmental expression of Hox-2 homeobox containing genes in the developing mouse hindbrain. Nature 341: 405–409

Wolgemuth DJ, Behringer RR, Mostoller MP et al 1989 Transgenic mice overexpressing the mouse homeobox-containing gene Hox-1.4 exhibit abnormal gut development. Nature 337: 464–467

Wolpert L 1992 Gastrulation and the evolution of development. Development (Gastrulation Suppl): 7–13

Yost HJ 1992 Regulation of vertebrate left–right symmetries by extracellular matrix. Nature 357: 158–161

8. The molecular basis of metastasis

R. G. Vile   I. R. Hart

A cancer eventually causes death because of a variety of damaging effects induced by the expanding number of neoplastic cells. The primary tumour cell population may pose relatively little direct threat to the patient, especially if the tumour mass is located where it can be resected surgically without the loss of crucial organ or tissue bulk. Potentially, therefore, the most dangerous genetic damage that can occur to tumour cells activates genes that promote, or inactivates genes which suppress, their spread from the site of origin to distant regions of the body.

The conversion of a single cell into a tumour frequently requires a timescale of years and the acquisition of multiple genetic and epigenetic changes. These include mutations which activate cellular proto-oncogenes and inactivate tumour suppressor genes (Fearon & Jones 1992, Vogelstein & Kinzler 1993). The progression from the partially transformed state (essentially a benign tumour mass) to the metastatic state also is considered to involve distinct, but interdependent, mutational events. It is possible that the genetic mutations for metastasis actually have accrued over the period of tumour development but can only manifest themselves after full growth transformation has taken place. Therefore, just as growth transformation is dependent upon many genetic changes, so metastasis can be viewed as a multifactorial process, which can be divided into several distinct stages. Tumour cells must accomplish each of these stages to spread and colonize distant sites separate from the location of the primary growth. The genetic mutations which contribute to the individual stages of the metastatic cascade (Hart & Saini 1992, Aznavoorian et al 1993, Yeatman & Nicolson 1993) are now increasingly tractable to study using modern molecular biology techniques. However, it should be remembered that metastasis is not only the result of multiple genetic changes but that it occurs within the context of the whole body. The power of molecular biology lies primarily in the reductionist approach. Care must be taken not to overinterpret findings based upon molecular manipulations within oversimplistic model systems which may not reflect adequately the complete spectrum of in vivo influences to which potentially metastatic cells are normally exposed. It is unlikely that metastasis is controlled by alterations in only a single molecule. Rather there are likely to be multiple genetic routes by which cells can arrive at a metastatic phenotype, thus implying a redundancy which means that the presence or absence of any particular genetic factor found to be important in one system may be insignificant in another. Indeed, the well-documented phenomenon of tumour heterogeneity (Nicolson 1987) means that even cells from within the same primary tumour may achieve the metastatic phenotype via a variety of different molecular changes. While these caveats apply, it is clear that recent developments in the understanding of the molecules involved in the metastatic cascade are providing new insights into the basis of tumour spread and providing new ideas for potential therapeutic strategies.

THE METASTATIC CASCADE

Tumour cell invasion and chemotaxis

The first step in metastatic spread involves the localized invasion of surrounding host tissue (Fig. 8.1, steps 1 and 2). Cells encroach into this local tissue by an active process involving lysis of host cells and degradation of the extracellular matrix (ECM) by proteolysis (Liotta et al 1991, Aznavoorian et al 1993). It has been proposed that a cascade of degradative enzymes clears a

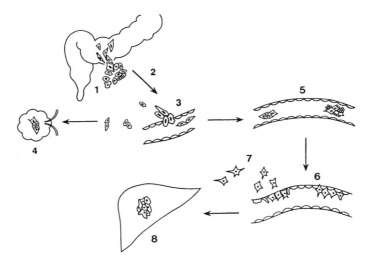

Fig. 8.1 The metastatic cascade. Growth transformed cells of the primary tumour separate from each other (1), invade the local tissue and move through the surrounding stroma using proteolysis and active cell motility (2). On reaching a vessel wall, they penetrate to the lumen (3) and are distributed via the lymphatic system (4) or in the blood (5), at which stage they are most vulnerable to immune attack. Surviving cells arrest at capillary beds, or in lymph nodes, using specific adhesion receptors or by simple entrapment of tumour cell aggregates (4,6). Following extravasation (7), cells move to sites where appropriate growth factors are present to support the growth of a secondary tumour (8).

path at the advancing edges of invasive tumours, into which the tumour cells move (Mignatti et al 1986). In this model, inactive proenzyme forms of the degradative enzymes are secreted locally, and become activated by the action of other regulatory enzymes which are produced either by the tumour cells themselves or the surrounding stromal cells (fibroblasts, mast cells, etc). Such enzymes include plasminogen activators, heparanases and matrix metallopro-teinases. The matrix metalloproteinases have been studied most extensively and consist of a multimembered family of enzymes which operate at neutral pH, and which differ according to their individual substrate specificities (Liotta et al 1991). The source of these metalloproteinases need not be the neoplastic cells themselves but may arise from stromal fibroblasts in response to tumour factors (Grey et al 1989). Stromelysin 3, for example, is overexpressed specifically in breast carcinomas (Basset et al 1990). Messenger RNA was expressed by stromal cells in all of the invasive breast carcinomas tested by this group but only in the direct vicinity of the neoplastic cells. Presumably the transformed cells secrete a factor that induces expression of stromelysin 3 from the stromal fibroblasts and allows progression of the expanding tumour cell mass through the ECM into surrounding tissue. Increasing evidence suggests that this mechanism of metalloproteinase activation is restricted neither to breast tumours nor to stromelysin 3 but may be applicable to many members of this enzyme family in a variety of tumour types (Poulsom et al 1992).

As well as the degradative enzymes produced by the neoplastic cells and/or the stromal fibroblasts, these same cell types elaborate tissue inhibitors of metalloproteinases which bind to, and inactivate, both the latent proenzyme and the active enzyme (Khokha & Denhardt 1989). Presumably the pro-teolytic activity of a tumour is a consequence of the balance between the production and secretion of enzymes and inhibitors in the local environment. Given that serum contains a relatively high concentration of protease inhibitors, how can this balance ever be tipped towards proteolytic activity? In part, this may be as a consequence of the enzymes functioning within protected microenvironments at the site of direct cell contact with the extracellular matrix proteins; the micropockets formed by these cell–substrate attachments may physically exclude the protease inhibitors. In this regard, it is interesting that expression of one of the integrin receptors (see below), the $\alpha v \beta 5$ vitronectin receptor, has been associated with localization of proteolytic activity and receptor-mediated endocytosis of vitronectin, resulting in extra-cellular matrix degradation (Panetti & McKeown-Longo 1993). Results such as this, and the demonstration of specific receptors for the urokinase-type plasminogen activator (Escheicher et al 1989, Koretz et al 1993), suggest that localization of proteolytic enzymes to the cell surface plays an important role in determining cancer-mediated proteolysis. For more detailed analysis of this important area, the interested reader should consult some of the excellent reviews on proteolysis that have appeared in recent years (e.g. Aznavoorian et al 1993, Liotta et al 1991, Matrisian 1990).

Aside from promoting the degradation of surrounding stroma, tumour cells must also be able to move into the regions cleared by the actions of these enzymes. Tissue-specific, chemotactic (soluble) and haptotactic (insoluble) factors have been identified which enhance tumour cell motility (see Fig. 8.1, step 2). The significance of tumour cell motility was noted over 40 years ago (Enterline & Coman 1950) and early studies showed that tumour cell lines known to be more highly invasive and metastatic were also more highly motile as assessed by criteria of pseudopod extension and vectorial translation (Mohler et al 1987). Several agents have been shown to stimulate motility in tumour cells in vitro, including tumour secreted factors (Liotta et al 1986, Ohnishi et al 1990, Stracke et al 1992), host derived scatter factor (Weidner et al 1990, Rosen et al 1991), growth factors (Kahan & Kramp 1987, Kohn et al 1993) and basement membrane components such as collagen, laminin and fibronectin (McCarthy & Furcht 1984, Wewer et al 1987). Conversely, other factors have been shown to suppress melanoma cell motility and, accordingly, their metastatic potential (Ikeyama et al 1993).

The molecular mechanisms underlying the action of motility factors are not fully understood. Tumour cells move in an amoeboid-like fashion by the extrusion of pseudopodia, similar to the movement of leukocytes (Hosaka et al 1979, Mohler et al 1987). This requires coordinated progression through repeated steps of formation of cell–matrix adhesions at the leading edge with the release of 'old' adhesions at the trailing edge. Therefore, the cellular network of polymerized actin filaments must be progressively disassembled (to allow protrusion) and then reassembled to stabilize the resulting extension. Very little is known of the biochemical regulation of these processes, except that some cytokines influence cell motility (Stoker & Gherardi 1991). Motility factors may affect the distribution of the receptors on the cell surface which mediate the cell–cell or cell–matrix interactions during pseudopodia movements and/or they may alter the ligand binding affinities of the receptors to allow the repeated cycles of adhesion and de-adhesion. The cellular receptor for the hepatocyte growth factor/scatter factor molecule, which is a defined motility factor for tumour cells, is a transmembrane tyrosine kinase the c-*met* proto-oncogene. Under certain conditions, c-*met* can be activated to become a dominantly acting transforming oncogene, suggesting that motility and growth control are closely linked (Rosen et al 1991). Despite the lack of understanding about the regulation of tumour cell motility, interference of this process might be employed as an antimetastatic therapy. Accordingly, Liotta and his colleagues have proposed that inhibitors of the motility-related signal transduction pathways may have therapeutic potential. They are currently testing the efficacy of a family of synthetic substituted imidazoles and triazoles which selectively block non-voltage and calcium influx and arachidonate release through the phospholipase A2 pathway. The active compounds inhibit the anchorage independent growth of a variety of tumour cell lines and oral administration to nude mice blocks the growth of established metastases and primary tumours from H-*ras* transfected fibroblasts and several human tumour lines (Kohn et al 1992).

Tumour cell separation

Clearly, separation of cells from the primary tumour mass must occur for long-range spread to be possible (see Fig. 8.1, step 1). Detachment of single cells or clumps of cells may be directly related to a decreased level of cell adhesiveness in tumour populations. One possibility is that this may be a cell-cycle regulated property. It has long been accepted from tissue culture studies that tumour cells have lost the property of contact inhibition which prevents normal cells from continuing to divide when they contact their nearest neighbours. Such a phenomenon in vivo could help cells to slough off from the body of the tumour mass during proliferation. Moreover, the release of lytic enzymes may contribute to collagenolytic degradation of the intercellular matrix that normally cements a tissue together. Disruption of a tumour mass during surgery could also provide a mechanical means by which cells break free prior to moving to distant sites.

At the molecular level, important molecules involved in controlling tumour cell–tumour cell adhesion are those of the cadherin family. These are calcium-dependent transmembrane adhesion molecules which bind to one another in homophilic interactions (Takeichi 1991). The three best characterized members of the family are: E-cadherin, found in adult epithelial cells; N-cadherin, found in adult neural and muscle tissue; and P-cadherin, found predominantly in placenta and epithelium. The cytoplasmic domain of cadherins interacts with the cytoskeleton via binding to cytoplasmic proteins known as catenins and the cadherin–catenin complexes localize to the zonula adherens of the cell to stabilize junction formation. As such, cadherins are important for maintaining multicellular structures throughout all stages of development.

Early evidence showed that disruption of intercellular adhesion between canine epithelial cells, by an antibody to E-cadherin, resulted in the acquisition of an invasive phenotype by these cells (Behrens et al 1989). A direct role for cadherins in regulating tumour invasion was provided by the demonstration that transfection of the cDNA for E-cadherin into cells of an invasive carcinoma cell line decreased their invasive capacity, an observation made by several groups (Vleminckx et al 1991, Chen & Obrink 1991, Navarro et al 1991). Analysis of a range of carcinoma cell lines revealed an association between the ability to invade collagen gels and the loss of E-cadherin expression (Vleminckx et al 1991). Immunohistochemical studies of human tumours have supported the notion that E-cadherin may function as an invasion suppressor, with loss of differentiation and E-cadherin expression correlating well with increased invasive behaviour (Shimoyama & Hirohashi 1991). These results indicate that loss of cadherin expression/function is correlated with increased invasiveness, at least in transformed epithelial cells (Birchmeier et al 1993).

Surface proteins other than cadherins are also likely to be involved in homotypic adhesion of tumour cells and modification of their expression may play a major part in determining tumour spread. For example, a gene which is deleted in many more advanced colorectal carcinomas (*DCC*) (Fearon et al 1990) encodes a molecule with homology to the adhesion protein N-CAM (an immunoglobulin superfamily member). Loss of this gene from tumour cells may, therefore, be associated with decreased cell–cell cohesion and an increased ability to move away from the primary tumour.

Simple loss, down-regulation or inactivation of the genes encoding for adhesion molecules expressed at the cell surface are not the only means whereby cell–cell adhesion may be abrogated. Thus, mutations for genes encoding for accessory adhesion molecules may be just as effective in altering the binding capacity of tumour cells. For example, function inactivating mutations in the catenins (Stappert & Kemler 1993) or the cell adhesion regulator (*CAR*) gene (Pullman & Bodmer 1992) could perturb cell–cell binding to an extent sufficient to permit lack of cohesion despite the presence of normal levels of associated cell surface adhesion proteins.

Movement of disseminating tumour cells clearly requires regulated inter-actions with the underlying substrata. Members of the integrin family of adhesion receptors (Hynes 1987, 1992, Ruoslahti 1991) involved in mediating these interactions have been examined closely. Integrins are heterodimeric glycoproteins consisting of a single α chain non-covalently associated with a single β chain. While, to date, 14 α and eight β subunits have been identified, only a few of the potential α/β combinations occur naturally. Integrins not only bind specifically to extracellular matrix proteins such as collagens, laminin, fibronectin, von Willebrand's factor, vitronectin and tenascin, but also mediate cell–cell interactions, often binding to counterreceptors of the immunoglobulin superfamily of adhesion receptors. The arginine–glycine–aspartic acid (RGD) sequence found in many adhesive glycoproteins (Ruo-slahti & Pierschbacher 1987) frequently serves as the minimal recognition site for a number of integrins. The potential importance of this motif is demonstrated by the ability of RGD-containing peptides to inhibit the lung-colonizing potential of tumour cells *in vivo* (Humphries *et al* 1986).

Promotion of metastasis via integrins could, paradoxically, be served either through loss or gain of function and expression. For example, decreased cellular adhesion to basement membrane or matrix proteins (by loss of particular integrins) could allow increased motility. Alternatively, enhance-ment of specific interactions with the matrix (by expression of certain integrins) might also allow increased cell spreading and motility over the matrix (Weitzman et al 1993). Thus, transformed fibroblasts show loss of expression of the fibronectin receptor ($\alpha5\beta1$) and invasive epithelial tumours sometimes demonstrate decreased $\alpha6\beta1$, $\alpha6\beta4$ receptor expression, while increased expression of the vitronectin receptor on melanoma cells can also be associated with increased invasiveness (Albelda 1993). These apparently contradictory results show the difficulty in making generalizations about even a single molecule in a process as complex as metastasis.

Blood vessel invasion

Intravasation into a blood or lymph vessel is required for the migrating cells to gain access to a distribution system which provides them with a conduit throughout the body (see Fig. 8.1, step 3). The action of the degradative enzymes that allow local invasion can also lead to destruction of the endothelial walls of small blood vessels. Equally, the expanding tumour mass may penetrate to the lumen by pressure alone, or single tumour cells that have broken free from the tumour mass may pass through the endothelial cell wall with little damage to the vessel.

Tumour cell distribution

Distribution of cells from the initial site of invasion of a vessel to distant organs may occur by one of two principal routes, i.e. the blood or the lymphatic system (see Fig. 8.1, steps 4 and 5). It has been noted that carcinomas tend to spread via the lymphatic system, while sarcomas tend to spread via the blood. However, these routes are not mutually exclusive and precise utilization may be governed by the proximity of a blood or lymph vessel to the site of the primary tumour growth.

Tumour cell arrest

The presence of circulating tumour cells need not necessarily be related to poor prognosis if they cannot adhere to, or at least lodge at, any site to which they are carried. The complement of cell surface adhesion molecules expressed by the tumour cells is particularly important at this stage, since specific interactions with receptors on the endothelial walls may enhance the ability of circulating cells to arrest at specific target organ sites (see Fig. 8.1, step 6).

The integrin family of surface adhesion receptors (see above) is particularly important for this stage of the metastatic process (Zetter 1993, Albelda 1993). As already indicated, the ability of RGD-containing peptides to inhibit the lung-colonizing potential of tumour cells in vivo (Humphries et al 1986) underscores the involvement of these molecules in some aspects of tumour spread. In addition, transfection of poorly metastatic rhabdomyosarcoma cells with cDNAs encoding the VLA-2 integrin led to the enhancement of their malignant capacity (Chan et al 1991). Other studies have shown that melanoma progression is associated with elevated levels of $\alpha 4\beta 1$ and $\alpha V\beta 3$ (Albelda et al 1990). The role that these changes in integrin expression play in affecting the various stages of metastasis is not clear but, in at least one case, increased integrin expression may be directly responsible for tumour cell arrest at distant capillary beds. Some tumour lines adhere preferentially to cytokine-stimulated endothelial cells (Rice et al 1988). A cytokine-inducible member of the immunoglobulin superfamily of molecules, VCAM-1, has been identified on vascular endothelial cells which is the ligand for the VLA-4 integrin (α4β1) (Elices et al 1990, Osborn et al 1989). Interestingly, more malignant melanoma cells express higher levels of this integrin than do their less metastatic counterparts (Albelda et al 1990, Hart 1989). Possibly VCAM-1 is used as a tumour cell adhesion receptor by VLA-4-expressing melanoma cells prior to their extravasation and establishment of secondary tumour growths. It may be significant that some melanomas have been shown to produce and secrete cytokines which can modulate the expression of VCAM-1 on endothelial cells (Burrows et al 1991).

VLA-4 is found primarily on leukocytes and is normally involved in the interaction of white blood cells with the endothelium. Since many immune cells must also travel, via the circulation, to distant sites in the body (Springer 1990), it has been suggested that the normal mechanisms of trafficking of immune cells to sites of inflammation may be mimicked by metastasizing tumour cells (Ratner 1992). There is growing evidence that tumour cells express some of the same cell surface receptors that are used by these immune cells and that this may contribute to their metastatic spread. One such example is the lymphocyte homing molecule, CD44. CD44 is a widely distributed integral membrane protein which exists in a variety of forms ranging from 85 kDa to 160 kDa (Picker et al 1989). The 90 kDa form is the principal form of leukocytes and is believed to be important in lymphocyte homing, whereas the larger 160 kDa isoform is found on epithelial cells (Aruffo et al 1990). Several lines of evidence implicate CD44 as a metastasis-promoting molecule. An antibody specific for a rat pancreatic carcinoma cell line which had acquired an increased metastatic potential in vivo was used to identify a c-DNA that encoded a close homologue of CD44 (Gunthert et al 1991). The identified clone (pMeta-1) contained an additional extracellular domain encoding 162 amino acids, produced by alternative splicing, and this was sufficient to confer full metastatic behaviour to non-metastasizing cells (Gunthert et al 1991). This variant has been detected on aggressive human lymphomas (Koopman et al 1993) and highly metastatic non-Hodgkin's lymphomas (Horst et al 1990), while the epithelial form of CD44 was overexpressed in carcinomas relative to normal epithelia (Stamenkovic et al 1989). Recently the existence of the alternatively spliced metastatic form has been demonstrated in a range of human tumours of malignant characteristics (Matsumura & Tarin 1992), while the epithelial form has been reported as occurring more frequently in colon carcinomas and their metastases than in normal mucosa (Tanabe et al 1993).

Although these results would tend to suggest an association between the metastatic propensity and the presence of the larger-sized forms of CD44, this situation is neither clear-cut (Heider et al 1993) nor does it give any indication as to the underlying mechanism. The existence of variant CD44 on recently activated T cells is consistent with the possibility that tumour cells expressing this isoform can mimic the normal movement of lymphocytes into the lymph node (Arch et al 1992).

Expression of several other cell surface proteins has been associated with increased malignancy but roles for these molecules are even less well defined than for CD44. For example, overexpression of ICAM-1 is associated with progression of melanoma metastases (Johnson et al 1989), while expression of a 67 kDa laminin-binding protein appears to be enhanced in some human carcinomas (Liotta 1991). Cell surface carbohydrates also play a role in metastasis via mediation of cell–cell adhesion. Proteins that bind carbohydrates (lectins) have been used to select tumour cells with varying metastatic capacities while malignant transformation can be accompanied by changes in the carbohydrate profiles of tumour cells (Lotan & Raz 1988). Recently, a family of membrane proteins with lectin activity, called selectins, has been identified which is normally involved in leukocyte–endothelial cell interactions. The three known selectins, L-, E- and P-selectin, are calcium-dependent carbohydrate-binding proteins which contain an N-terminal lectin-like domain, followed by an epidermal growth factor-like domain with varying numbers of short consensus repeats (Bevilacqua 1993, Cummings & Smith 1992). L-selectin is expressed constitutively on lymphocytes, P-selectin on endothelial cells and activated platelets and E-selectin is expressed on activated endothelial cells. The carbohydrate moieties recognized by the selectins also differ: L-selectin on leukocyte surfaces interacts principally with sialylated fucosylated and sulphated carbohydrates found in activated endothelium and high endothelial venules, whereas P- and E-selectins recognize carbohydrates derived from sialyl Le^x antigen on neutrophils and monocytes (Bevilacqua 1993). Different groups have demonstrated a role for these molecules in tumour cell adhesion; experimental metastases have been reduced with an antibody against a galactoside-specific lectin of murine melanomas and fibrosarcomas, and the adhesive and metastatic properties of murine melanoma cells can be altered using drugs known to alter the glycosylation profile of cell surface glycoproteins (reviewed in Yeatman & Nicolson 1993). A soluble form of P-selectin binds tumour cells from a variety of tumour types (breast, lung, colon), suggesting it may be important in tumour cell arrest in the capillary beds (Aruffo et al 1992). Others have proposed that adhesion of colon carcinoma cells to endothelial cells is mediated by E-selectin (Dejana et al 1992, Lauri et al 1991).

While these receptor-mediated mechanisms by which circulating tumour cells become arrested at capillary beds currently attract much research, it should not be forgotten that mechanical processes may also influence the seeding of metastases. Indeed, simple entrapment of tumour cell aggregates may account for the majority of arrest of disseminating cells from solid tumours.

Tumour cell extravasation

Arrest of tumour cells must be followed by invasion of the wall of the vessel in a process which is presumably the reverse of that described earlier. Exit of tumour cells from the distributing vessel is called extravasation (see Fig. 8.1, step 7). The majority of tumour cells are killed rapidly following their arrest at a secondary site, as demonstrated by [125]IUdR labelling of circulating tumour cells (Shekhar et al 1993). Those cells which do survive may proliferate in the vessel and penetrate its wall as a consequence of pressure build-up. Alternatively, cells may pass between the endothelial cells of the vessel, possibly secreting lytic enzymes to disrupt endothelial intercellular adhesion, using active locomotory mechanisms. Finally, it has been suggested that tumour cells may actually pass through the endothelial cells in a manner reminiscent of the exit of haematopoietic cells from the bone marrow into the circulation or of immune cells exiting at sites of inflammation (Ratner 1992).

Arrest/seeding of tumour cells at the secondary site

Some tumour types metastasize to preferred organs suggesting that different tumour cells can only seed specific sites (Zetter 1990, Yeatman & Nicolson 1993, Nicolson 1991, 1993). Growth factor requirements probably ensure that not every tumour cell deposited in an organ will proliferate. Ability to respond to the local paracrine growth factors/inhibitors which are produced by the 'target' organ or tissue will determine secondary tumour formation (Nicolson 1991). Once established, the tumour cells themselves often release autocrine growth factors to enhance their local colonization (reviewed in Nicolson 1993) (see Fig. 8.1, step 8).

Paget (1889) proposed that site-specific metastasis is the result of the provision of a fertile environment (the soil) by the target tissue, in which compatible tumour cells (the seed) could proliferate. Alternatively, the anatomical location of the primary tumour could decide the haemodynamic consequences of tumour cell release and the mechanical entrapment of tumour cells in the nearest capillary beds (Ewing 1928). These theories are not mutually exclusive and experimental data support both possibilities. Additionally, organ preference is also partially mediated by selective attachment of tumour cells to organ-specific microvascular endothelium (Pauli & Lee 1988). Again, this may be an instance of tumour cells mimicking the homing mechanisms of lymphocytes to specific vascular addressins (Butcher 1991, Berlin et al 1993). An addressin possibly involved in tumour cell 'homing' has recently been identified as a 90 kDa protein expressed selectively on distinctive branches of lung vessels and on endothelial cells cultured on lung-derived extracellular matrix (Zhu et al 1991). Significantly, antibodies directed against this protein were able to inhibit the lung-colonizing potential of B16 melanoma cells (Zhu et al 1991).

No doubt, different tumour types will rely on these various mechanisms to different extents, making generalizations difficult.

Angiogenesis

Neovascularization is critical for tumour growth and tumours secrete factors that induce these processes both in the developing primary tumour as well as in metastatic deposits (Folkman & Shing 1992, Folkman et al 1989). These factors include fibroblast growth factors, transforming growth factors (Mahadevan & Hart 1990) and vascular endothelial cell growth factor (Leung et al 1989). The importance of the developing blood supply in metastatic progression is illustrated by the positive correlation of the number of microvessels detectable at the advancing front of the primary tumour and the incidence of metastatic disease (Weidner et al 1991, 1993). Apart from providing the necessary nutrient supply to the expanding cell mass, new capillaries dispersed through the tumour increase the chances of invasive cells reaching the circulation more quickly (Liotta et al 1974).

Inhibitors of angiogenesis, therefore, provide hope for a therapeutic approach that is not tumour type-specific (Folkman et al 1983, Ingber et al 1990).

Genetic controls of metastasis

Metastasis is a complex, multistep process involving many tumour cell–tumour cell, tumour cell–host cell and tumour cell–matrix interactions. However, metastatic cells show few characteristics that are unique to tumour cell behaviour other than the ability to proliferate at distant sites. Migration, proteolysis, adhesion and stimulation of angiogenesis are all characteristics exhibited by normal cells at different developmental stages. The pathology of tumour cell metastasis must, therefore, derive from imbalances of regulation of these normal processes, that is as a consequence of aberrant homeostasis (Fidler 1992). Identification of the genetic controlling principles behind each of the steps involved — adhesion, proteolysis, invasion, angiogenesis, immune evasion — could permit a targeted approach to new therapeutic interventions.

As well as being central to growth transformation of normal cells, mutations in some cellular proto-oncogenes appear to be able to control the metastatic phenotype. Expression of an activated *ras* oncogene in non-metastatic NIH 3T3 cells originally was shown to confer metastatic potential to the cells in vivo (Thorgeirsson et al 1985), while other *ras* oncogenes have produced similar effects in other cell types. Mutated forms of the *mos*, *raf*, *fms*, *src* and *fes* proto-oncogenes, as well as the p53 tumour suppressor gene, all have similar metastasis-enhancing properties when expressed in a range of transformed cell lines (reviewed in Aznavoorian et al 1993). Effector genes activated or suppressed by the action of *ras* include proteinases and motility-associated cytokines (Aznavoorian et al 1993) indicating that subtle differences in the pathways downstream of oncogene activation may account for variation between evoked changes in growth transformation and changes in disseminative capacity.

One gene which appears to be associated specifically with tumour spread is the metastasis suppressor gene *nm23*. Originally identified because its expression was down-regulated in highly metastatic sublines of a murine melanoma (Steeg et al 1988), *nm23* expression has been found to be reduced in association with lymph node metastasis of breast carcinoma (Bevilacqua et al 1989). Transfection of the gene into metastatic cell lines significantly reduced their metastatic potential (Leone et al 1991). The *nm23* gene product is highly homologous to nucleoside diphosphate kinases (Biggs et al 1990) which may be involved in the assembly/disassembly of microtubules and cell signalling through G proteins. This suggests that *nm23* may be associated with regulation of cell motility and, possibly, adhesion functions. Intriguingly, a nuclear transcription factor which binds to control regions upstream of the c-*myc* proto-oncogene, PuF, has been shown to be identical to the *nm23* metastasis suppressor gene (Postel et al 1993). These surprising data may help to explain the link between proto-oncogenes and the metastatic cascade, since a known negative regulator of metastasis can regulate the levels of expression of a proto-oncogene proved to have a central role in the genesis of several tumour types. Just how the nucleoside diphosphate kinase activity of *nm23* fits with its role as a transcription factor in the control of c-*myc* expression remains to be clarified. It should also be noted that the true significance of these *in vitro* studies and their relevance to cellular behaviour is not known at this time.

The cancer cell and the immune system

Tumour cells are usually accessible to cells of the immune system at most stages of the metastatic cascade. They are particularly exposed in the circulation and there is evidence that fewer than 1% of tumour cells that enter the circulation ever survive to form metastases (Fidler 1990) (see Fig. 8.1, steps 4 and 5). The proportion of tumour cell death attributable to immune clearance is not known, but it is assumed that it constitutes a significant part of this phenomenon.

Certainly cancer cells express determinants that can form the basis of an antitumour immune reaction (Boon et al 1992). The idea that tumour incidence is limited by the immunological defence mechanisms of the host is not new (Burnet 1970). Clinical evidence for specific antitumour immune activity is inferred from the very rare occasions when spontaneous disappearance of a cancer in a patient occurs and cannot be attributed to the treatment (Oliver & Nouri 1992). Such cases are cited as evidence that the immune system has mounted a successful attack against the cancer cells, and won (Rosenberg 1992). The nature of tumour antigens varies between tumours and may represent viral or cellular proteins expressed (1) at normal levels in altered forms (e.g. mutated oncoproteins such as activated RAS); (2) in normal forms at elevated levels (e.g. overexpressed proteins such as c-MYC); or (3) in normal forms but in a temporally or spatially inappropriate manner (e.g. the human melanoma tumour antigen MAGE). There is evidence that tumour cells can present these tumour antigens to the immune system (Jung & Schluesener 1991, Marchand et al 1993, Van der Bruggen & Van den Eynde 1992, Knuth et al 1992) so that efforts aimed at enhancing the immune system's recognition and destruction of emerging solid tumours now provide a focus for therapeutic intervention (Pardoll 1993) particularly using gene therapy for cancer (Russell 1993).

The tumour cell may evade the immune system by mechanisms which include loss of class I histocompatibility antigens, essential for cytotoxic T cell recognition of target cells (Browning & Bodmer 1992, Restifo et al 1993) and/or by production of immunosuppressive factors. What role these various checks and balances have in affecting tumour growth is unclear but it seems probable that metastasis, the process where cells are most susceptible to attack, is the aspect of tumour development most likely to be influenced by the immune system.

SUMMARY AND CONCLUSIONS

The metastatic process can now be summarized. Initially, normal cell–cell and cell–substratum adhesion must be disrupted to allow the release of tumour cells from the primary tumour mass. Loss of expression of cadherins and, perhaps, integrins are important at this stage, at least in epithelial tumours. Tumour cells must then be able to migrate through the extracellular matrix, which has been cleared partially by proteolysis, towards the vasculature. This step requires secretion of motility and degradative factors by both tumour and host cells and efficient cell–substratum interactions which are transient both spatially and temporally. Once in the lymphatics or vasculature, tumour cells must survive immune surveillance, which will detect any cells with grossly immunogenic determinants which can be recognized as non-self, as well as non-specific turbulence. Thereafter, strong and specific cell–cell contacts could enhance the arrest of tumour cells or clumps and these interactions are regulated by many adhesion molecules including the integrins, VCAM, CD44, carbohydrates, selectins, laminin-binding proteins and specific vascular addressins. Following cell arrest, cell–cell adhesion must be weakened to allow tumour cells to separate and move through the endothelium into the tissue parenchyma. Additional cell–substratum adhesions must promote the cell motility and invasion required to move the cells towards areas where growth factors and other molecules are available to promote the growth of the tumour cells in the new 'soil' which is the host tissue for the development of the secondary tumour deposit. Finally, release of angiogenesis factors and subsequent development of neovascularization is required in order that any tumour mass can grow beyond about 2 mm in any dimension.

Using molecular techniques to identify individual molecules which regulate separate steps would seem to offer therapeutic potential. However, such approaches also have inherent problems. Apparently conflicting data demonstrate that both enhanced or reduced tumour cell adhesion can promote metastasis but this is because of the experimental systems used and the individual stages examined. Hence, studies in which tumour cells are injected intravenously often show that greater adhesion leads to greater metastatic capabilities, because they select for tumour cells which form aggregates with cells in circulation and adhere to vascular walls. These studies completely bypass the early stages of the cascade. Alternatively, results obtained from implanted tumours which grow and metastasize spontaneously usually demonstrate that lower adhesive capacities lead to greater metastatic potential, reflecting the importance of release of tumour cells from the primary tumour. The important point is that sweeping generalizations should not be made from reductionist studies. Because the process of metastasis is complex and multifaceted, it will require the tumour cells to exhibit different properties at different stages. Molecular biology has great power to study the actions of single genes within simplified model systems. Metastasis is, however, undoubtedly a disease of the whole organism. The challenge for future research is to confirm that findings from the laboratory are relevant to human tumours and, if so, to use them to devise new therapeutic strategies.

REFERENCES

Albelda SM 1993 Role of integrins and other cell adhesion molecules in tumour progression and metastasis. Lab Invest 68: 4–17

Albelda SM, Mette SA, Elder DE et al 1990 Integrin distribution in malignant melanoma: association of the β3 subunit with tumour progression. Cancer Res 50: 6757–6764

Arch R, Wirth K, Hofmann M et al 1992 Participation in normal immune responses of a metastasis-inducing splice variant of CD44. Science 257: 682–685

Aruffo A, Stamenkovic E, Melnick M et al 1990 CD44 is the principal cell surface receptor for hyaluronate. Cell 61: 1303–1313

Aruffo A, Dietsch MT, Wan H et al 1992 Granule membrane protein 140 (GMP140) binds to carcinomas and carcinoma-derived cell lines. Proc Natl Acad Sci USA 89: 2292–2296

Aznavoorian S, Murphy A, Stetler-Stevenson WG et al 1993 Molecular aspects of tumour cell invasion and metastasis. Cancer 71: 1368–1383

Basset P, Bellocq JP, Wolf C et al 1990 A novel metalloproteinase gene specifically expressed in stromal cells of breast carcinoma. Nature 348: 699–704

Behrens J, Mareel MM, Van Roy FM et al 1989 Dissecting tumour cell invasion: epithelial cells acquire invasive properties after the loss of uvomorulin-mediated cell–cell adhesion. J Cell Biol 108: 2435–2447

Berlin C, Berg EL, Briskin MJ et al 1993 α4β7 integrin mediates lymphocyte binding to the mucosal vascular addressin MAdCAM-1. Cell 74: 1–20

Bevilacqua MP 1993 Endothelial–leukocyte adhesion molecules. Annu Rev Immunol 11: 767–804

Bevilacqua G, Sobel ME, Liotta LA et al 1989 Association of low nm23 RNA levels in human primary infiltrating ductal breast carcinomas with lymph node involvement and other histopathological indicators of high metastatic potential. Cancer Res 49: 5185–5190

Biggs J, Hersperger E, Steeg PS et al 1990 A Drosophila gene that is homologous to a mammalian gene associated with tumour metastasis codes for a nucleoside diphosphate kinase. Cell 63: 933–940

Birchmeier W, Weidner KM, Hulsken J et al 1993 Molecular mechanism leading to cell junction (cadherin) deficiency in invasive carcinomas. Semin Cancer Biol 4: 231–239

Boon T, De Plaen E, Lurquin C et al 1992 Identification of tumour rejection antigens recognised by T lymphocytes. Cancer Surv 13: 23–37

Browning MJ, Bodmer WF 1992 MHC antigens and cancer: implications for T-cell surveillance. Curr Opin Immunol 4: 613–618

Burnet FM 1990 The concept of immunological surveillance. Progr Exp Tumour Res 13: 1–27

Burrows FJ, Haskard DO, Hart IR et al 1991 Influence of tumour-derived interleukin-1 on melanoma–endothelial cell interactions in vitro. Cancer Res 51: 4768–4775

Butcher EC 1991 Leucocyte–endothelial cell recognition: three or more steps to specificity and diversity. Cell 67: 1033–1036

Chan BMC, Matsuura N, Takada Y et al 1991 In vitro and in vivo consequences of VLA-2 expression on rhabdomyosarcoma cells. Science 251: 1600–1602

Chen W, Obrink B 1991 Cell–cell contacts mediated by E-cadherin restrict invasive behaviour of L-cells. J Cell Biol 114: 319–327

Cummings RD, Smith DF 1992 The selectin family of carbohydrate-binding proteins: structure and importance of carbohydrate ligands for cell adhesion. BioEssays 14: 849–856

Dejana E, Martin-Padura I, Lauri D et al 1992 ELAM-1 dependent adhesion of colon carcinoma cells to vascular endothelium is inhibited by an antibody to Lewis fucosylated type 1 carbohydrate chain. Lab Invest 66: 324–330

Elices MJ, Osborn L, Takada Y et al 1990 VCAM-1 on activated endothelium interacts with the leukocyte integrin VLA-4 at a site distinct from the VLA-4/fibronectin binding site. Cell 60: 577–584

Enterline HT, Coman DR 1950 The amoeboid motility of human and animal neoplastic cells. Cancer 3: 1033–1038

Escheicher A, Wohlwend A, Belin D et al 1989 Characterisation of the cellular binding site for the urokinase type plasminogen activator. J Biol Chem 264: 1180–1189

Ewing J 1928 Neoplastic diseases. Saunders, Philadelphia

Fearon ER, Jones PA 1992 Progressing toward a molecular description of colorectal cancer development. FASEB J 6: 2783–2790

Fearon ER, Cho KR, Nigro JM et al 1990 Identification of a chromosome 18q gene that is altered in colorectal cancer. Science 247: 49–56

Fidler IJ 1990 Critical factors in the biology of human cancer metastasis. Cancer Res 50: 6130–6138

Fidler IJ 1992 Metastasis as a consequence of aberrant homeostasis. Clin Exp Metastasis 10: S5–S8

Folkman J, Shing Y 1992 Angiogenesis. J Biol Chem 267: 10931–10934

Folkman J, Langer R, Linhardt RJ et al 1983 Angiogenesis inhibition and tumour regression caused by heparin or a heparin fragment in the presence of cortisone. Science 221: 719–725

Folkman J, Watson K, Ingber D et al 1989 Induction of angiogenesis during the transition from hyperplasia to neoplasia. Nature 339: 58–61

Grey AM, Schor AM, Rushton G et al 1989 Purification of the migrating stimulating factor produced by foetal and breast cancer patient fibroblasts. Proc Natl Acad Sci USA 86: 2238–2242

Gunthert U, Hormann M, Rudy W et al 1991 A new variant of glycoprotein CD44 confers metastatic potential to rat carcinoma cells. Cell 65: 13–24

Hart IR 1989 Immune profile in metastasis. Curr Opin Immunol 1: 900–903

Hart IR, Saini A 1992 Biology of tumour metastasis. Lancet 339: 1453–1457

Heider KH, Hofmann M, Hors E et al 1993 A human homolog of the rat metastasis-associated variant of CD44 is expressed in colorectal carcinomas and adenomatous polyps. J Cell Biol 120: 227–233

Horst E, Meijer CJ, Radaszkiewicz T et al 1990 Adhesion molecules in the prognosis of diffuse large cell lymphoma: expression of a lymphocyte homing receptor (CD44), LFA-1, (CD11a/18), and ICAM-1 (C54). Leukaemia 4: 595–599

Hosaka S, Suzuki M, Sato H 1979 Leucocyte-like motility of cancer cells, with reference to mechanisms of extravasation in metastasis. GANN 70: 559–561

Humphries MJ, Olden K, Yamada KM 1986 A synthetic peptide from fibronectin inhibits experimental metastasis of murine melanoma cells. Science 233: 467–470

Hynes RO 1987 Integrins: a family of cell surface receptors. Cell 48: 549–554

Hynes RO 1992 Integrins: versatility, modulation, and signalling in cell adhesion. Cell 69: 11–25

Ikeyama S, Koyama M, Yamaoko M et al 1993 Suppression of cell motility and metastasis by transfection with human motility-related protein (MRP-1/CD9) DNA. J Exp Med 177: 1231–1237

Ingber D, Fujita T, Kishimoto S et al 1990 Synthetic analogues of fumagillin that inhibit angiogenesis and suppress tumour growth. Nature 348: 555–557

Johnson JP, Stade BG, Holzmann B et al 1989 De novo expression of intercellular adhesion molecule in melanoma correlates with increased risk of metastasis. Proc Natl Acad Sci USA 86: 641–644

Jung S, Schluesener HJ 1991 Human T lymphocytes recognise a peptide of a single point mutated, oncogenic ras protein. J Exp Med 173: 273–276

Kahan BW, Kramp DC 1987 Nerve growth factor stimulation of mouse embryonal cell migration. Cancer Res 47: 6324–6328

Khokha R, Denhardt DT 1989 Matrix metalloproteinases and tissue inhibitor of metalloproteinases: review of their role in tumorigenesis and tissue invasion. Invasion Metastasis 9: 391–405

Knuth A, Wolfel T, Meyer zum Buschenfelde K-H 1992 T cell responses to human malignant tumours. Cancer Surv 13: 39–52

Kohn EC, Holmes K, Liotta LA 1992 Signal transduction therapy of metastasis. Clin Exp Metastasis 10: 66–67

Kohn EC, Hollister GH, DiPersio JD et al 1993 Granulocyte macrophage colony stimulating factor induces human melanoma cell migration. Int J Cancer 53: 968–972

Koopman G, Heider KH, Horst E et al 1993 Activated human lymphocytes and aggressive non-Hodgkin's lymphomas express a homologue of the rat metastasis-associated variant of CD44. J Exp Med 177: 897–904

Koretz K, Moller P, Schwartz-Albiez R 1993 Plasminogen activators and plasminogen activator inhibitors in human colorectal carcinoma tissues are not expressed by tumour cells. Eur J Cancer 29A: 1184–1189

Lauri D, Needham L, Martin-Padura I et al 1991 Tumour cell adhesion to endothelial cells: ELAM-1 as an inducible adhesive receptor specific for colon carcinoma cells. J Natl Cancer Inst 83: 1321–1324

Leone A, Flatow U, King CR et al 1991 Reduced tumour incidence, metastatic potential, and cytokine responsiveness of nm23-transfected melanoma cells. Cell 65: 25–35

Leung DW, Cachianes G, Kuang WJ et al 1989 Vascular endothelial growth factor is a secreted angiogenic mitogen. Science 246: 1306–1309

Liotta LA 1991 Tumour invasion and metastases: role of the extracellular matrix. Cancer Res 46: 1–7

Liotta L, Kleinerman J, Saidel G 1974 Quantitative relationships of intravascular tumor cells, tumor vessels, and pulmonary metastases following tumor implantation. Cancer Res 34: 997–1004

Liotta LA, Mandler R, Murano G et al 1986 Tumor cell autocrine motility factor. Proc Natl Acad Sci USA 83: 3302–3306

Liotta LA, Steeg PS, Stetler-Stevenson WG 1991 Cancer metastasis and angiogenesis: an imbalance of positive and negative regulation. Cell 64: 327–336

Lotan R, Raz A 1988 Endogenous lectins as mediators of tumour cell adhesion. J Cell Biochem 37: 107–117

McCarthy JB, Furcht LT 1984 Laminin and fibronectin promote the haptotactic migration of B16 melanoma cells in vitro. J Cell Biol 98: 1474–1480

Mahadevan V, Hart IR 1990 Metastasis and angiogenesis. Acta Oncol 29: 97–103

Marchand M, Brasseur F, Van der Bruggen P et al 1993 Perspectives for immunisation of HLA-A1 patients carrying a malignant melanoma expressing gene MAGE-1. Dermatology 186: 278–280

Matrisian LM 1990 Metalloproteinases and their inhibitors in matrix remodeling. Trends Genet 6: 121–125

Matsumura Y, Tarin D 1992 Significance of CD44 gene products for cancer diagnosis and disease evaluation. Lancet 340: 1053–1058

Mignatti P, Robbins E, Rifkin DB 1986 Tumour invasion through the human amniotic membrane: requirements for a proteinase cascade. Cell 47: 487–498

Mohler JL, Partin AW, Coffey DS 1984 Prediction of metastatic potential by a new grading system of cell motility: validation in the Dunning R-3327 prostatic adenocarcinoma model. J Urol 138: 168–170

Navarro P, Gomez M, Pizarro A et al 1991 A role for the E-cadherin cell–cell adhesion molecule during tumour progression of mouse epidermal carcinogenesis. J Cell Biol 115: 517–533

Nicolson GL 1987 Tumor cell instability, diversification, and progression to the metastatic phenotype: from oncogene to oncofetal expression. Cancer Res 47: 1473–1487

Nicolson GL 1991 Tumour and host molecules important in the organ preference of metastasis. Semin Cancer Biol 2: 143–154

Nicolson GL 1993 Cancer progression and growth: relationship of paracrine and autocrine growth mechanisms to organ preference of metastasis. Exp Cell Res 204: 171–180

Ohnishi T, Arita N, Hayakawa T et al 1990 Motility factor produced by malignant glioma cells: role in tumor invasion. J Neurosurg 73: 881–888

Oliver RTD, Nouri AME 1992 T Cell immune response to cancer in humans and its relevance for immunodiagnosis and therapy. Cancer Surv 13: 173–204

Osborn L, Hession C, Tizard R et al 1989 Direct expression cloning of vascular cell adhesion molecule 1, a cytokine-induced endothelial protein that binds to lymphocytes. Cell 59: 1203–1211

Paget S 1889 The distribution of secondary growths in cancer of the breast Lancet 1: 571–573

Panetti TS, McKeown-Longo PJ 1993 The $\alpha v \beta 5$ integrin receptor regulates receptor-mediated endocytosis of vitronectin. J Biol Chem 268: 11492–11495

Pardoll DM 1993 Cancer vaccines. Immunol Today 14: 310–316

Pauli BU, Lee CL 1988 Organ preference of metastasis: the role of organ specifically modulated endothelial cells. Lab Invest 58: 379–387

Picker LJ, Nakache M, Butcher EC 1989 Monoclonal antibodies to human lymphocyte homing receptors define a novel class of adhesion molecules on diverse cell types. J Cell Biol 109: 927–937

Postel EH, Berberich SJ, Flint SJ et al 1993 Human c-*myc* transcription factor PuF identified as nm23-H2 nucleoside diphosphate kinase, a candidate suppressor of tumour metastasis. Science 261: 478–480

Poulsom R, Pignatelli M, Stetler-Stevenson WG et al 1992 Stromal expression of a 72 kDa type IV collagenase (MMP-2) and TIMP-2 mRNAs in colorectal neoplasia. Am J Pathol 141: 389–396

Pullman WE, Bodmer WF 1992 Cloning and characterisation of a gene that regulates cell adhesion. Nature 356: 529–532

Ratner S 1992 Exploring the boundaries between lymphocyte traffic and tumor metastasis. Invasion Metastasis 12: 61–65

Restifo NP, Esquivel F, Kawakami Y et al 1993 Identification of human cancers deficient in antigen processing. J Exp Med 177: 265–272

Rice GE, Gimbrone MA, Bevilacqua MP 1988 Tumor cell endothelial interactions. Am J Pathol 133: 204–210

Rosen EM, Knesel J, Goldberg ID 1991 Scatter factor and its relationship to hepatocyte growth factor and met. Cell Growth Differ 2: 603–607

Rosenberg SA 1992 The immunotherapy and gene therapy of cancer. J Clin Oncol 10: 180–199

Ruoslahti E 1991 Integrins. J Clin Invest 87: 1–5

Ruoslahti E, Pierschbacher MD 1987 New perspectives in cell adhesion: RGD and integrins. Science 238: 491–497

Russell SJ 1993 Gene therapy for cancer. Cancer J 6: 21–25

Shekhar PVM, Aslakson CJ, Miller FR 1993 Molecular events in metastatic progression Semin Cancer Biol 4: 193–204

Shimoyama Y, Hirohashi S 1991 Cadherin intercellular adhesion molecule in hepatocellular carcinomas: loss of E-cadherin expression in an undifferentiated carcinoma. Cancer Lett 57: 131–135

Springer TA 1990 Adhesion receptors of the immune system. Nature 346: 425–434

Stamenkovic I, Amit M, Pesando JM et al 1989 A lymphocyte molecule implicated in lymph node homing is a member of the cartilage like protein family. Cell 56: 1057–1062

Stappert J, Kemler R 1993 Intracellular associations of adhesion molecules. Curr Opin Neurobiol 3: 60–66

Steeg PS, Bevilacqua G, Kopper L et al 1988 Evidence for a novel gene associated with low tumour metastatic potential. J Natl Cancer Inst 80: 200–204

Stoker M, Gherardi E 1991 Regulation of cell movement: the motogenic cytokines. Biochim Biophys Acta 1072: 88–102

Stracke ML, Krutzsch HC, Unsworth EJ et al 1992 Identification, purification, and partial sequence analysis of autotaxin, a novel motility-stimulating protein. J Biol Chem 267: 2524–2529

Takeichi M 1991 Cadherin cell adhesion receptors as a morphogenetic regulator. Science 251: 1451–1455

Tanabe KK, Ellis LM, Saya H 1993 Expression of CD44R1 adhesion molecule in colon carcinomas and metastases. Lancet 341: 725–726

Thorgeirsson UP, Turpeenniemi-Hujanen T, Williams JE et al 1985 NIH3T3 cells transfected with human tumour DNA containing activated *ras* oncogenes express the metastatic phenotype in nude mice. Mol Cell Biol 5: 259–262

Van der Bruggen P, Van den Eynde B 1992 Molecular definition of tumor antigens recognised by T-lymphocytes. Curr Opin Immunol 4: 608–612

Vleminckx K, Vakaet L, Mareel M et al 1991 Genetic manipulation of E-cadherin expression by epithelial tumour cells reveals an invasion suppressor role. Cell 66: 107–119

Vogelstein B, Kinzler KW 1993 The multistep nature of cancer. Trends Genet 9: 138–141

Weidner KM, Behrens J, Vandekerckhove J et al 1990 Scatter factor: molecular characteristics and effect on invasiveness of epithelial cells. J Cell Biol 111: 2097–2108

Weidner N, Semple JP, Welch WR et al 1991 Tumour angiogenesis and metastasis — correlation in invasive breast carcinoma. N Engl J Med 324: 1–8

Weidner N, Carroll PR, Flax J et al 1993 Tumor angiogenesis correlates with metastasis in invasive prostate carcinoma. Am J Pathol 143: 401–409

Weitzman JB, Pasqualin R, Takada Y et al 1993 The function and distinctive regulation of the integrin VLA-3 in cell adhesion, spreading and homotypic cell aggregation. J Biol Chem 268: 8651–8657

Wewer UM, Taraboletti G, Sobel ME 1987 Role of laminin in tumour cell migration. Cancer Res 47: 5691–5698

Yeatman TJ, Nicolson GL 1993 Molecular basis of tumour progression: mechanisms of organ-specific tumour metastasis. Semin Surg Oncol 9: 256–263

Zetter BR 1990 The cellular basis of site specific tumour metastasis. N Engl J Med 322: 605–612

Zetter B 1993 Adhesion molecules in tumor metastasis. Semin Cancer Biol 4: 219–229

Zhu D, Cheng CF, Pauli BU 1991 Mediation of lung metastasis of murine melanomas by a lung-specific endothelial cell adhesion molecule. Proc Natl Acad Sci USA 88: 9568–9572

9 Cerebrovascular and neurodegenerative diseases — an approach for general histopathologists

J. Lowe

Establishing the precise diagnosis in cases of vascular and degenerative diseases of the nervous system has never been more important. At a time of unprecedented and increasing clinical and research interest, generalists in histopathology still have to perform the bulk of autopsies on affected patients. Unfortunately, these autopsies are commonly poorly focused as few general pathologists have had much exposure to clinical neuroscience and lack awareness of the main clinical issues involved.

Several pressures now exist to improve the quality of the autopsy service for the main diseases of the nervous system.

1. Primary and secondary stroke prevention strategies rely on detailed knowledge of the cause of cerebrovascular disease which is often not provided by an autopsy.

2. The clinical diagnosis of neurodegenerative processes is inaccurate; about 25% of clinical diagnoses are not confirmed pathologically and accurate diagnostic feedback is being sought for purposes of audit (Homer et al 1988, Marks et al 1988, Boller et al 1989). For example, in modern practice, most clinically diagnosed cases of 'multi-infarct dementia' turn out to be something else. Equally, cases diagnosed as depression, alcoholic dementia and Parkinson's disease may turn out on pathological examination to be Alzheimer's disease (Mendez et al 1991).

3. Many more diseases are recognized as having a genetic component and families are beginning to ask for counselling based on the nature of the degenerative process. It is common to go back to autopsy records and find that a brain was weighed, described as being small, sliced and returned to the body without histology. This is no longer acceptable.

4. The recent publicity surrounding Creutzfeldt–Jakob disease and its possible relation to bovine spongiform encephalopathy has highlighted public concerns over the cause of dementia as well as health and safety concerns over the transmissibility of these diseases at autopsy.

5. New approaches to therapy are being tried as the fundamental biological processes underlying neurodegenerative and vascular diseases are uncovered. Clinicians need to know if the right drug was given for the right disease.

Faced with these pressures an immediate question for the general pathologist is whether all cases should be seen by a neuropathologist. This is not possible in the immediate future as there is a limited capacity in established neuropathology departments even for examination of referred brain material.

If all cases are not referred for neuropathological examination should general pathologists be expected to develop an expertise in these areas of neuropathology? The problem is evident in the USA where general pathologists have been provided with guidelines for making the diagnosis of Alzheimer's disease (Mirra et al 1993). The problem is emerging in the UK with clinicians and pathologists already identifying a lack of provision of autopsy diagnosis in neuropsychiatric disorders.

These problems are unresolved yet the pressures to improve the diagnostic autopsy service are increasing. Whatever the outcome, it is evident that all general pathologists need to have greater awareness of neurological diseases and be prepared to provide part of a diagnostic autopsy service.

The purpose of this overview is to provide: a framework for performing autopsy examinations in cases of cerebrovascular disease which will improve the service provision to clinicians; a knowledge of neurodegenerative diseases which will provide background awareness for the pathologist to preserve appropriate tissues for neuropathological examination; a review of pathological features in the common neurodegenerative diseases which may whet the appetite of some pathologists to develop their own diagnostic service; and a knowledge of Creutzfeldt–Jakob disease which will allow appropriate health and safety measures to be implemented.

At the outset, it is important to state that brain examination by slicing in the fresh state can only at best give a crude indication of cerebral pathology. The vast majority of brain changes which directly cause death can be ascertained by external examination.

Those conditions that cannot be ascertained by external examination are likely to be subtle and will not be seen by slicing when fresh. It is always necessary to preserve the brain and examine it when fixed to ascertain the cause of neurological disease. Most cases, for example cerebrovascular disease, do not need referral for specialist neuropathological examination.

CEREBROVASCULAR DISEASE

Refinements in the diagnosis and classification of stroke have come about because of the development of clinical programs of secondary stroke prevention and rehabilitation.

The clinical diagnosis of stroke is based on criteria of sudden onset of non-traumatic focal neurological deficit which causes death or lasts for over 24 h. The terms minor stroke and reversible ischaemic neurological deficit are used when recovery of clinical features occurs after a period of time, usually defined as 7 days. Transient ischaemic attacks are defined as episodes of non-traumatic focal loss of cerebral or visual function lasting less than 24 hours.

STROKE IN THE GENERAL POPULATION

Stroke is mainly seen in the elderly population and is divided into two main groups: haemorrhagic and ischaemic causes. Meningeal-related haemorrhages (extradural, subdural and subarachnoid bleeding) will not be discussed in detail here but are potential causes of the clinical picture of stroke.

Haemorrhage

Parenchymal cerebral haemorrhages causing stroke are of two main types:

1. Central haemorrhages (main sites basal ganglia, thalamus pons and cerebellum) mainly associated with the presence of cerebral arteriosclerosis with the main associated risk factor of hypertension. Less common predisposing factors include bleeding diatheses, bleeding into tumour, vascular malformations, and bleeding from aneurysm.

2. Peripheral or lobar haemorrhages (seen in the periphery of cerebral hemispheres) are more commonly associated with the presence of cerebral artery amyloid composed of βA4 protein (as seen in Alzheimer's disease). This type, if associated with a better clinical outcome than central bleeds and in elderly populations, accounts for about 10% of cases of intracerebral bleeding (Itoh et al 1993, Wijdicks & Jack 1993, Yamada et al 1993). Peripheral haemorrhages are also caused by infective arteritis.

Ischaemia

Ischaemic cerebrovascular disease causing stroke is of four main types:

1. Large vessel disease causes regional infarction, the main mechanisms being embolism and thrombosis. Infarcts correspond to territories of supply of named cerebral arteries and their main branches.

2. Small vessel disease causes micro-infarcts (lacunar infarction) or ischaemic white matter degeneration (Binswanger's disease). Small vessel disease is especially seen in hypertensives and diabetics and is the result of arteriolosclerosis mostly affecting small perforating branches. The key sites for this pattern of infarction are the pons and the basal ganglia/internal capsule region (Fig. 9.1).

3. Global ischaemia, caused by reduction in cerebral blood flow such as seen in cardiorespiratory arrest, causes widespread neuronal necrosis and leads to laminar cortical necrosis. When global ischaemia is incomplete, infarction at arterial boundary zones occurs.

4. Venous infarction is uncommon, results in haemorrhagic infarction, and is usually related to thrombosis in a main cerebral venous sinus associated with an abnormal predisposititon to thrombosis.

The macroscopic and histological appearances of different patterns of infarction are well covered in standard textbooks.

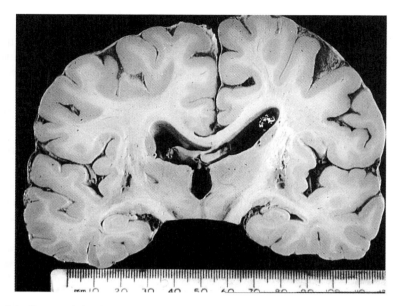

Fig. 9.1   Lacunar infarction. In this coronal slice of brain small cystic infarcts about 2–4 mm in size are seen in the basal ganglia and thalamus bilaterally. Similar areas will also be seen in the white matter if histology is performed. This type of infarction is particularly associated with the development of vascular dementia.

STROKE IN YOUNGER PATIENTS

The list of causes of strokes in younger patients is different to that seen in the elderly (Bevan et al 1990, Lisovoski & Rousseaux 1991, Stern et al 1991, Bogousslavsky & Pierre 1992, Toffol & Swiontoniowski 1992, Carolei et al 1993). Determining the cause of a stroke in a young patient is important as some diseases are heritable and amenable to therapy in affected relatives. About 40% of young strokes are the result of non-traumatic intracerebral haemorrhage; the main causes are hypertension, berry aneurysms, arterio-venous malformations, and bleeding into tumours. Cocaine abuse also predisposes to haemorrhage (Klonoff et al 1989). Some 20% of cases have subarachnoid haemorrhage, the majority being due to ruptured berry aneurysms or vascular malformations; 40% of cases have cerebral infarction with many associated causes or predisposing factors. Importantly, no cause is ascertained in about one-third of young-onset cerebral infarcts.

AUTOPSY IN CASES OF STROKE

In the general autopsy for cerebrovascular disease the following should be a routine minimal standard, including documentation of relevant negative findings.

- Careful examination for potential sources of emboli from the heart and great vessels.
- Opening the carotid vessels from their origin to the base of the skull will reveal the main sites of occlusion associated with atheroma, particularly stenosis at the region of the bifurcation.
- Opening the vertebral arteries throughout their length will reveal the cause of infarcts in the posterior territory (brain stem, cerebellum and occipital lobes). This is a simple procedure which adds 10–12 min to the standard autopsy. A simple technique using side-cutters has been published (Bromilow & Burns 1985). Failure to do this in an autopsy for cerebrovascular disease should be regarded in the same light as failing to examine the right coronary artery in cases of ischaemic heart disease.
- The anatomy of the circle of Willis should be defined and the state of vessels documented while the brain is in the fresh state, including tracing the middle cerebral arteries along to their main division in the depth of the sylvian fissure. Variation in the circle of Willis may account for unusual patterns of infarction. Blood clot should be removed from around the base of the brain and the leptomeninges in the fresh state as later examination of vessels after fixation is otherwise very difficult.
- Examination of the venous sinuses, particularly in cases of haemorrhagic cerebral infarction.
- The brain should be preserved in formalin and sliced after 3–4 weeks in the fixed state. This allows delineation of small lacunar infarcts as well as white matter degeneration. Histological sampling should be performed in all cases and will reveal abnormalities of vessels such as arteriosclerosis, amyloid angiopathy and, in unusual cases, vasculitis.

In providing a pathological evaluation of ischaemic cerebrovascular disease the following aspects require documentation:

- Pattern of disease. Although a large number of clinical syndromes related to brain stem infarction and occlusion of individual arteries are described, a more important practical distinction is to divide infarcts into those affecting the carotid territory (frontal, temporal, parietal lobes or basal ganglia/internal capsule) and those affecting the vertebrobasilar territory (occipital lobe, cerebellum or brain stem). The pattern of disease, whether due to large vessel occlusion or small vessel disease, should be determined.
- Mechanism of infarction: atheroma/thrombosis, cardioembolic, lacunar infarction, or haemodynamic cause.
- Pathology related to therapeutic intervention, particularly carotid endarterectomy and anticoagulant administration.
- Consideration of unusual cause for infarction, particularly in younger patients (see Table 9.1).
- Relation of infarction to cause of death. This may be direct (e.g. if swelling causes cerebral herniation and brain stem compression), or may be indirect such as predisposing to development of pneumonia.

Table 9.1   Causes of cerebral infarction in the young age group (<45 years)

Cause	Notes	References
Cardiogenic emboli	Important causes due to structural cardiac defects, particularly abnormalities of valves and patent foramen ovale	Ranoux et al 1993
Oral contraceptives and pregnancy	A main associated factor in vascular thrombosis in young women	Brick & Riggs 1989. Bevan et al 1990, Matias et al 1990, Lisovoski & Rousseaux 1991, Carolei et al 1993, Kokkinos & Levine 1993
Migraine-associated	Infarcts are well documented in patients with severe migraine, although there is suggestion that ischaemia may, on occasion, cause the migraine	Bevan et al 1990, Matias et al 1990, Schroth Tenner 1991, Bogousslavsky & Pierre 1992, Carolei et al 1993, Olesen et al 1993
Premature atherosclerosis	Predispose to infarction and may be associated with a defined atheroma risk factor	
Arterial dissection	May affect either carotid or vertebral territories	Lisovoski & Rousseaux 1991, Bogousslavsky & Pierre 1992, Carolei et al 1993
Recreational drugs	Increasingly associated with cerebral infarction and haemorrhage, especially cocaine	Klonoff et al 1989, Kaku & Lowenstein 1990, Sauer 1991, Kokkinos & Levine 1993
Vasculitis	May be localized to the nervous system or part of systemic disease and may also be associated with varicella zoster infection	Aghaji & Nzewi 1989
Fibromuscular dysplasia	Can present as cerebral infarction, especially in women	Mettinger 1982
Alcohol and smoking	Ethanol and cigarette smoking are important risk factors for young-onset stroke	Bevan et al 1990, Love et al 1990, Monforte et al 1990, Carolei et al 1993, Kokkinos & Levine 1993
Antiphospholipid antibodies	This syndrome is increasingly recognized as predisposing to thrombosis and cerebral infarction. Antibodies may be detected in postmortem blood samples	Montalban, et al 1991, Kittner & Gorelick 1992
Inflammatory bowel disease	This may predispose to vascular thrombosis and result in stroke	Johns 1991
Heritable conditions	Although uncommon causes of stroke, important to detect Hereditary vascular degenerations	Tournier et al 1991, Baudrimont et al 1993, Tournier et al 1993
	Fabry's disease Homocystinuria	Grewal & Barton 1992
	Mitochondrial cytopathy syndromes which may be detected by examination of skeletal muscle	Symposium 1992
	Congenital lack of inhibitors of coagulation protein C, protein S and antithrombin III (assays cannot readily be performed on postmortem blood)	Kohler et al 1990, Camerlingo et al 1991, Lagosky & Witten 1993, Martinez et al 1993

In providing a pathological evaluation in a case of non-traumatic intra-cerebral haemorrhage the following aspects require documentation:

- Pattern: divided into central or peripheral type.
- Vascular pathology: arteriosclerosis, amyloid, vasculitis, infective.
- Ascertain predisposing factors, particularly hypertension, bleeding diathesis.
- Consideration of unusual cause: for example, bleed from vascular malformation, aneurysm or tumour.
- Relation of haemorrhage to cause of death as for infarction above.

OVERVIEW OF MAIN NEURODEGENERATIVE PROCESSES

The main primary neurodegenerative diseases are those causing dementia syndromes, those causing movement disorders, and those causing motor weakness. Less common are specific heredofamilial diseases. This overview will not cover neurometabolic diseases which mainly present in childhood.

DEMENTIA SYNDROMES

Dementia is frequently defined as a global deterioration in intellectual function, yet it is really only true for end-stage disease. In the early stages of dementing illnesses, different diseases affect different cortical areas and result in distinct patterns of cortical abnormality, an understanding of which greatly facilitates intelligent reading of case notes. Disease of the frontal lobes produces abnormalities in regulation and is a major part of a the group of frontal lobe dementias. Disease of the parietal lobe gives rise disorders of manual dexterity or praxis, for example becoming unfamiliar with the use of an everyday object. Disease of adjacent regions of the parietal lobe leads to disorders of perception causing agnosias and spatial disorientation. Disease of the medial side of the temporal lobe leads to disorders of memory.

Dementia syndromes may also affect subcortical structures and lead to other neurological signs, the most common of which is development of parkinsonism.

This overview will cover the common causes of 'degenerative' dementia in the elderly population.

Alzheimer's disease

Alzheimer's disease is the most common cause of dementia which increases in incidence with age. It is possible to divide cases into four main groups, each beginning to be associated with distinct molecular genetic abnormalities: sporadic late onset (commonest); familial late onset (uncommon); familial early onset (rare); associated with Down's syndrome (Evenhuis 1990).

Macroscopic features

The brain in Alzheimer's disease is smaller than normal; brain weight is reduced and is evident as shrinkage of gyri and widening of sulci of the

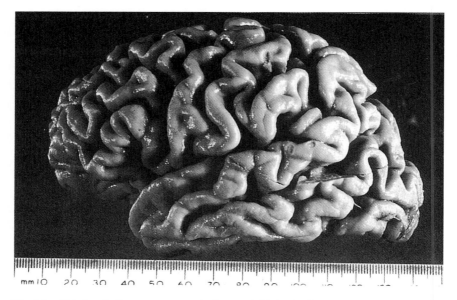

Fig. 9.2 Alzheimer's disease, macroscopic features. This brain shows cortical atrophy with wide sulci and thin gyri. This change affects frontal tempora! and parietal regions but spares the occipital lobe. Although the most common reason for this is Alzheimer's disease, identical changes are seen with other causes of dementia.

cerebral hemispheres (Fig. 9.2). Atrophy is most evident in the medial temporal regions, particularly the parahippocampal gyrus, but also affects frontal and parietal regions. The occipital lobe and the motor cortex are generally spared. This pattern of atrophy may be present in dementing diseases of diverse aetiology and is not specific for Alzheimer's disease. It is not unusual to find evidence of old or recent cerebral infarction in the brains of patients with Alzheimer's disease, and this does not by itself mean that a patient has multi-infarct dementia. The brain should be fixed for detailed assessment.

When the fixed brain is cut, reduction in the thickness of the cortical mantle is seen. There is also loss of the amount of white matter which is otherwise normal in appearance. With cerebral atrophy there is dilatation of the ventricular system which must not be confused with obstructive hydrocephalus. In the midbrain the substantia nigra shows normal pigmentation and this is an important distinction from cases of Lewy body dementia discussed below.

Histological features

Alzheimer's disease is characterized by the presence of several main abnormalities, none of which is pathognomonic:

- Intraneuronal inclusions termed neurofibrillary tangles composed of material which is generically termed paired helical filament protein (Fig. 9.3).
- Deposition of a specific amyloid in brain as senile plaques (Fig. 9.4).
- Distortion of neuronal processes to form structures termed dystrophic neurites and neuropil threads (Fig. 9.3).

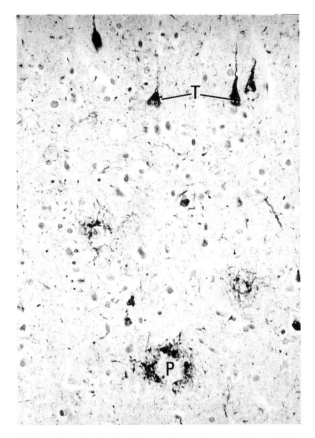

Fig. 9.3 Neurofibrillary tangles, dystrophic neurites and neuropil threads (tau immunostaining). Immunohistochemistry to detect tau protein is increasingly used as a standard technique (see Appendix). Neurofibrillary tangles are intraneuronal filamentous inclusions. They are composed of a microtubule-binding protein, tau protein, modified by phosphorylation. The classical tangle T is a flame-shaped skein of matted fine fibrils which occupies most of the cell body of the affected neurone. In H&E preparations tangles appear as a faint basophilic fibrillar structures. Tangles can also be detected with several silver staining methods (see Appendix). Tangles are not specific to Alzheimer's disease but can be seen in a number of other conditions as well as being normally present in the brains of elderly non-demented persons, particularly in the hippocampus and adjacent temporal cortex. Tau protein is also present in dystrophic neurites around senile plaques P as well as in the neuropil threads, seen as a background of fine twisted and distorted nerve cell processes in cerebral cortex, not associated with senile plaques. Abnormality of nerve cell processes in the cortex interferes with neuronal communication and contributes to the cortical deficits of the disease.

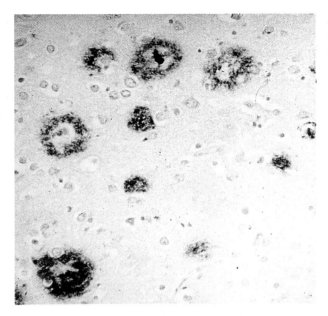

Fig. 9.4 Senile plaques (immunostaining for βA4 protein).   Senile plaques are aggregates of a specific amyloid protein (βA4 protein), typically 50–200 μm in diameter, within the neuropil. The nerve cell processes surrounding the amyloid become distorted and are termed dystrophic neurites, not seen with this stain. In addition to immunostaining, there are many other histological staining methods, the most reliable in use is the modified methenamine silver (see Appendix). Amyloid plaques are present in high number in Alzheimer's disease and Lewy body dementia. They are also common in the cortex in normal aging and may be present in high density in cognitively normal elderly patients.

- Amyloid is often deposited in cerebral arteries causing an angiopathy (congophilic angiopathy).

All of these changes can be found in the brains of normal elderly individuals in low density or restricted distribution. The diagnosis of Alzheimer's disease is based on the collective presence of lesions in high density in a patient with clinical dementia.

There is a marked loss of neurones (approx. 50%) from the cortex in Alzheimer's disease which particularly affects large pyramidal cells. This cell loss is most significant in patients younger than 80 years.

In some instances amyloid angiopathy may be responsible for cerebral haemorrhage, particularly in a peripheral (lobar) pattern and be a secondary cause of stroke in patients with an Alzheimer dementia (Itoh et al 1993).

Molecular pathology

Molecular pathology of Alzheimer's disease has recently been reviewed (Rossor 1993). Purification of tangles reveals at least two major protein constituents; tau protein and ubiquitin. Tau protein is a normal cell protein with roles in stabilizing the microtubular cytoskeleton in neurones. In Alzheimer's disease it is abnormally phophorylated. Ubiquitin is a normal cell protein with roles in targeting cell proteins for degradation. It is associated with a minority of all tangles.

Molecular analysis of the amyloid of Alzheimer's disease has lead to great insights into the disease. The precursor protein, termed Alzheimer amyloid precursor protein or APP, is a normal cell membrane protein of unknown function coded on chromosome 21. The protein found in the amyloid is a 40 amino acid fragment of APP referred to as amyloid β protein or A4 protein derived by proteolytic cleavage from APP.

Mutation in the APP gene has been found in early-onset familial Alzheimer's disease but this accounts for an extremely small number of cases. Linkage of some cases of Alzheimer's disease to chromosome 14 and chromosome 19 has been found.

The presence of apolipoprotein ApoE4, a normal form of apolipoprotein, predisposes to the development of late-onset Alzheimer's disease. This is found in both familial late-onset cases and probably accounts for linkage of Alzheimer's disease to chromosome 19 (Corder el at 1993). The presence of ApoE4 is also linked to sporadic late-onset cases. Penetrance in the 3% of the population who are homozygous for this apolipoprotein variant is believed to be 90%, while the 25% of the population who are heterozygous are at higher risk (Scott 1993). The finding that ApoE4 is linked with development of Alzheimer's disease will promote intense research into drugs which modify its activities in the brain.

In terms of treatment, neurochemical analysis has shown widespread transmitter defects in the brains of patients with Alzheimer's disease. particularly of acetylcholine. Treatment protocols which supplement cholinergic transmission are under trial to see if this alleviates disease.

Pathological diagnosis

There are problems in making a pathological diagnosis of Alzheimer's disease because the histological changes overlap with those seen in the normal elderly population and are not pathognomonic. Plaques are seen in the cortex with increased frequency in aging and tangles are seen in the hippocampus (Delaere et al 1993). Plaques may be seen with silver stains, the best being variants of methenamine silver, or immunohistochemistry for A4 protein (See Appendix, page 176). Tangles may be seen by several silver stains, the AgNOR method being perhaps most familiar to general laboratories, and also by immunohistochemistry for tau protein (See Appendix, page 176).

There is a growing trend to restrict the diagnosis of Alzheimer's disease to cases with both plaques and tangles in the hippocampus and neocortex in the presence of a history of dementia. Patients who have plaques and tangles in a restricted distribution or who are not clinically demented (Crystal et al 1988) are best classified as having Alzheimer changes as this does not prejudge the nature of their disease.

Guidelines for the histological diagnosis of Alzheimer's disease, adapted from those used by neuropathologists participating in the Consortium to Establish a Registry for Alzheimer's Disease, have been published and are easily used in a general pathology laboratory, including descriptions of reliable special staining techniques (Mirra et al 1993). Assessment of histological changes is by comparison with standard reference pictures included in the paper, making this particularly useful for non-specialists.

Lewy body dementia

Lewy body dementia has emerged as a common pathology, particularly in patients who have been clinically diagnosed either as Alzheimer's disease or as multi-infarct dementia. It has some of the pathology of Alzheimer's disease with some of the pathology of idiopathic Parkinson's disease.

The condition can be diagnosed in life and clinical diagnostic criteria have been proposed, particularly dementia associated with Parkinsonism, hallucinations and fluctuation in intellectual performance (Byrne et al 1989, 1991).

Macroscopic and histological features

The macroscopic appearances are similar to those seen in Alzheimer's disease. The key pathology is the presence of changes similar to idiopathic Parkinson's disease in the substantia nigra which is macroscopically pale. Classical Lewy bodies are seen in the substantia nigra and other pigmented neurones of the brain stem (Fig. 9.5). Inclusions termed cortical Lewy bodies can be seen in cortical neurones (Fig. 9.6) on haematoxylin–eosin staining. They are best seen with immunochemical staining for ubiquitin (Lennox et al 1989). Most patients also have histological features of plaques and tangles in the cortex warranting inclusion into the Alzheimer's disease group.

It is as yet uncertain if Lewy body dementia is aetiologically different from other forms of dementia having plaques and tangles and included as Alzheimer's disease. Whether it is a completely separate entity from sporadic late-onset Alzheimer's disease with association with ApoE4 remains to be evaluated.

Frontal lobe dementias

Patients who present with abnormality of frontal lobe function can be grouped together as having a frontal lobe dementia (Brun 1987, Neary et al 1988, Gustafson et al 1990, Knopman et al 1990). They differ from patients with Alzheimer's disease in that they have preserved parietal lobe function until very late in the disease process. From clinicopathological studies this group

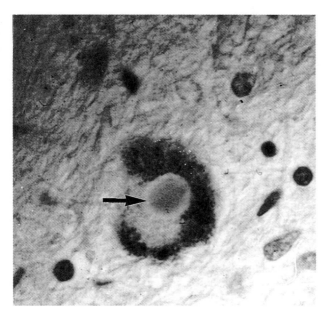

Fig. 9.5   Brain stem Lewy body. A Lewy body (arrow) is seen as an eosinophilic spherical inclusion in this neuromelanin-containing nigral neurone. These inclusions are based on aggregates of neurofilament proteins and ubiquitin. They are seen in idiopathic Parkinson's disease and Lewy body dementia.

accounts for up to 1 in 5 dementia cases. Importantly, many cases of frontal dementia are associated with an autosomal dominant pattern of inheritance.

Macroscopic and histological features

Macroscopically, most cases show severe frontotemporal atrophy, although some cases show minimal macroscopic atrophy.

Common to all forms is neuronal loss from the frontal cortex as well as the temporal lobes. On haematoxylin–eosin stains, spongy vacuolation and gliosis is seen in the outer cortical layers. becoming severe with increasing neuronal loss (Fig. 9.7). Three main subtypes are encountered (Mann, South et al. 1993).

1. Classical Pick's disease with rounded Pick bodies and swollen Pick cells in the cortex. These may be detected with silver stains and antibodies to tau protein.
2. Frontal lobe gliosis with swollen cells but no inclusions in cells.
3. Motor neurone disease dementia: a disease which pathologically resembles motor neurone disease affecting the non-motor cortex. Inclusions can only be detected by anti-ubiquitin. This group frequently develops late bulbar palsy and patients die of aspiration pneumonia.

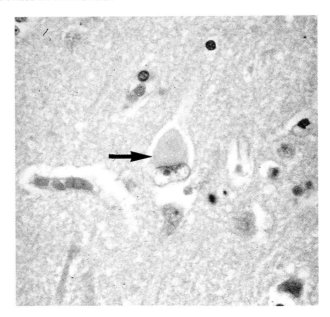

Fig. 9.6   Cortical Lewy body. The cortical Lewy bodies seen in Lewy body dementia appear as ill-defined eosinophilic inclusions (arrow) which push the neuronal nucleus to one side. They are mainly seen in the small neurones in layers 5 and 6 and are best seen in the cingulate gyrus, insular cortex and parahippocampal gyrus.

Vascular dementia

Vascular dementia, also termed multi-infarct dementia, describes global cognitive decline caused by cumulative effects of multiple episodes of cerebral ischaemia. This excludes cases of diffuse cerebral cortical damage caused by a single episode of severe hypoxia or global cerebral hypoperfusion.

Clinically, vascular dementia presents with early gait difficulties, strokes, urinary incontinence, parkinsonian features, pseudobulbar signs and cognitive impairment. Clinicians diagnose multi-infarct dementia on the basis of focal neurology consistent with the presence of strokes, a stepwise deterioration in condition suggestive of discrete insults to the brain, and day-to-day fluctuation in cognitive performance. These are embodied in a clinical rating scale called the Hachinski score which is frequently employed to assess whether a patient has multi-infarct dementia.

In clinicopathological studies it has been found that the Hachinski score is not a very specific tool, and that the clinical diagnosis of multi-infarct dementia is not substantiated by autopsy in about one-fifth of cases (Fischer et al, 1991). Very often patients have a changes of Alzheimer's disease plus strokes (mixed dementia); in other cases Lewy body dementia or Alzheimer's disease mimics the clinical features.

Imaging studies are also used to support a diagnosis of vascular dementia, particularly finding the abnormality of white matter termed leukoaraiosis.

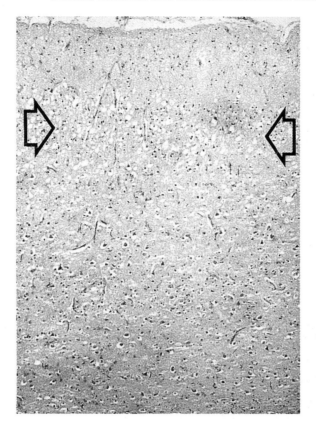

Fig. 9.7   Frontal dementia, spongy change. At low magnification (between arrows), vacuolation is seen in layer 2 of the frontal cortex, termed spongy change. This is a key feature of frontal dementias.

Pathological studies have shown that this is non-specific: it can be seen in normal elderly persons as well as associated with vascular risk factors and dementia (Ferrer et al 1990, Smith & Hendrie 1992).

For these reasons it is not safe to assume a clinical diagnosis of multi-infarct dementia, even if cerebral infarction is seen macroscopically, and histological validation is always required.

Neuropathological features

The pathology associated with vascular dementia is diverse. It is probable that large regional infarcts do not contribute to cognitive decline in the majority of patients. Cortical micro-infarcts, lacunar infarcts in basal ganglia (Fig. 9.1) and white matter and diffuse ischaemic white matter degeneration are all probably more related to intellectual decline (Munoz 1991). Dementia occurring in patients with small vessel disease is mainly due to ischaemic damage to white matter. The term 'lacunar dementia' has been proposed, instead of the less well-known terms 'Binswanger disease' and 'subcortical arteriosclerotic encephalopathy' (Roman 1985). Changes of Alzheimer's disease are not infrequent in clinically diagnosed cases, warranting a diagnosis of mixed dementia.

Unusual dementia syndromes

For the non-specialist, excluding a diagnosis of one of the common causes of dementia may leave the situation where there has been clinically diagnosed dementia but no firm pathological diagnosis. This may be accounted for three main reasons:

1. The most likely reason is that the clinical diagnosis of dementia is uncertain. Diagnosis by non-specialist clinicians may label confusional states as dementia. Depression in the elderly may have many of the clinical features of specific dementia syndrome. In these instances the situation is resolved by careful reading of the case notes to ascertain how the diagnosis of dementia was made and with what certainty.

2. In addition to the main conditions of Alzheimer's disease, Lewy body disease, frontal dementias, and vascular dementia, there are many uncommon forms of dementia. These are usually given descriptive terms related to neuropathological features seen on special staining (e.g. argyrophilic grain dementia). Descriptions of neuropathology in these rare forms is to be found in journal articles rather than in textbooks and so is outside the scope of this general review. Dementia syndromes are also seen in association with alcoholism.

Cognitive abnormalities are uncommonly associated with infective diseases, particularly HIV (human immunodeficiency virus). While this is at present an uncommon cause of dementia in the elderly, it is only a matter of time until this manifestation of HIV infection becomes more significant.

In the diagnosis of unusual cases of dementia referral to a specialist centre is advisable.

3. Rarely, a confident clinical diagnosis of dementia is not accompanied by morphological changes in the brain.

Autopsy in dementia syndromes

In cases clinically diagnosed as dementia the following is a minimal standard for autopsy assessment, including documentation of negative findings.

- Before starting, make sure that there are no features to warrant a clinical suspicion of a transmissible dementia such as Creutzfeldt–Jakob disease (see below).

- Detailed dissection of the extracranial arteries supplying the brain (carotid and vertebral vessels). Careful documentation of the state of the heart and great vessels should include assessment of potential sites for embolization.
- Macroscopic assessment of the brain including weight and pattern of atrophy.
- Fixation of brain for later histological assessment. If dysphagia or motor weakness has been present in the latter stages of disease the spinal cord should also be preserved. The brain is cut after fixation for a period of 4–6 weeks and blocks are taken for histological assessment. Alternatively the brain may be referred for examination to a specialist centre.
- The presence of disease of cerebral vessels (particularly arteriosclerosis and amyloid angiopathy), lacunar infarction and ischaemic white matter degeneration should be sought histologically.
- Histological examination is made of substantia nigra, temporal lobe, including hippocampus, frontal lobe and any areas of focal pathology seen externally or on cut surface. Large blocks are preferable to maintain anatomical relationships; however, diagnoses can be made on cassette-sized blocks.
- Haematoxylin–eosin staining will show neuronal loss, gliosis and Lewy bodies. Myelin stains show white matter degeneration. Staining for plaques and tangles is performed on cerebral cortex and will show changes of Alzheimer's disease and Lewy body dementia (See Appendix, p. 174). If a frontal dementia is suspected on histological examination then immunostaining to detect neuronal inclusions (anti-ubiquitin and anti-tau) is performed on frontal and hippocampal blocks.

TRANSMISSIBLE NEURODEGENERATIVE DISEASES

Creutzfeldt–Jakob disease

Creutzfeldt–Jakob disease is one of the rare transmissible neurodegenerative disorders along with scrapie in sheep and bovine spongiform encephalopathy in cattle. A familial human form of the disease if Gerstmann–Straussler–Scheinker syndrome which presents as a familial form of cerebellar ataxia. Clinical, pathological and molecular findings have been recently reviewed (Harrison & Roberts 1991). The agent causing Creutzfeldt–Jakob disease is believed to be a conformationally deviant form of a normal cell membrane protein termed prion protein. The precise mechanisms involved in disease pathogenesis are uncertain. The main risk to pathologists is from inoculation of material derived from the central nervous system, even from formalin-fixed material, as the agent is resistant to processes which normally inactivate conventional microbiological agents.

   In considering autopsies on patients with dementia, a diagnosis of Creutzfeldt–Jakob disease will usually have been suggested by clinicians on the basis of well-recognized features. It is uncommon to have cases of classical

Creutzfeldt–Jakob disease which are undiagnosed in life. The main features which clinically suggest a possible diagnosis of Creutzfeldt–Jakob disease are rapid progress of dementia leading to death in under a year, dementia with myoclonus, and the finding of characteristic EEG changes.

These features should be ascertained from case notes prior to undertaking an autopsy on a dementia case so that appropriate health and safety precautions can be taken if there is clinical suspicion of transmissible disease. Cases of other forms of transmissible neurodegenerative disease, such as Gerstmann–Straussler–Scheinker syndrome, are very uncommon and are unlikely to crop up as undiagnosed disease in non-specialist centres. Rarely, cases of atypical transmissible neurodegenerative disease are uncovered only at autopsy, having been diagnosed as something else (e.g. Alzheimer's disease).

It is common for a clinical diagnosis of transmissible dementia to be wrong because of confusion with other forms of neurodegenerative disease. Many patients with other forms of dementia develop myoclonus in the late stages of their illness but the disease will have been present for many years. Some cases of Lewy body dementia have a rapid progression and myoclonus. The possibility that many cases of undiagnosed dementia or dementia with atypical features might be caused by the same transmissible agent as Creutzfeldt–Jakob disease seems unlikely in the face of detailed studies on large numbers of cases (Brown et al 1993).

Neuropathology

The characteristic feature of Creutzfeldt–Jakob disease is a fine vacuolation in the neuropil associated with development of neuronal loss and gliosis (Fig. 9.8). The spongy change affects all layers of the cortex and may be either focal or diffusely present in the cortex. It may also affect the cerebellum and deep grey matter structures. In some forms of disease spongiform change is not seen; in others, plaques of amyloid composed of prion protein can be seen in cerebellar or cerebral cortex. Immunochemical detection of the abnormal prion protein is being used as a research tool but is not yet available for routine use.

Spongy change is not always diagnostic of transmissible prion dementia; it may be seen in restricted distribution in several neurodegenerative diseases, including Alzheimer's disease, Lewy body dementia and frontal dementias.

Autopsy

Autopsy validation of the diagnosis of Creutzfeldt–Jakob disease is important and may be safely carried out in a standard mortuary. A detailed protocol suitable for use in routine autopsy practice has been produced and is essential reading for all pathologists performing autopsies as it incorporates appropriate health and safety guidelines (Bell & Ironside 1993). During examination

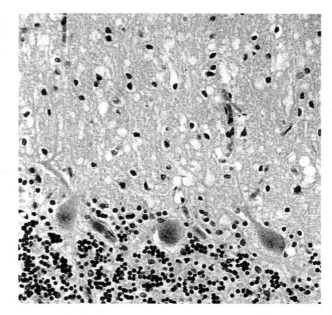

Fig. 9.8 Creutzfeldt–Jakob disease, spongiform change. In this section of cerebellum, fine vacuolation is seen in the neuropil characteristic of the spongiform change of Creutzfeldt–Jakob disease. It is likened to the development of fine champagne bubbles and contrasts with the coarse vacuolation seen in non-specific areas of vacuolation in other neurodegenerative diseases.

precautions are taken to avoid contamination of surfaces, and the brain is removed by sawing through the skull with the head and saw enclosed in a large polythene bag.

Autopsies on recipients of human-derived tissues or tissue extracts should also be considered as being in a high-risk category of carrying a transmissible agent, although not necessarily manifesting disease. The most important are patients who have received pituitary-derived hormones, and dura mater used in neurosurgical repairs. These features should be looked for in case notes prior to performing and autopsy in clinically relevant cases. Recipients of Kveim antigen are, at present, not recognized in this high-risk group.

The transmissble agent has been recently classified as a category III pathogen and must be handled according to appropriate health and safety requirements. Importantly, it is now possible to render tissues non-infectious by immersion in formic acid (Brown et al 1990). In the mortuary work surfaces and instruments may be sterilized with 2 N sodium hydroxide for 1 h. Glassware can be cleaned in sodium hypochlorite (20 000 p.p.m.).

In the UK, cases suspected of having Creutzfeldt–Jakob disease and those falling into high-risk categories are encouraged to be referred to the National

Creutzfeldt–Jakob disease Surveillance Team based in Edinburgh (Bell & Ironside 1991).

PARKINSONISM AND RELATED MOVEMENT DISORDERS

Parkinsonism is characterized by the clinical features of slow movement (bradykinesia), rigidity and tremor. Treatment with a variety of agents, notably L-DOPA, improves motor performance in some cases, and in others has no effect. This is because the parkinsonian syndrome may be caused by many disease processes, only one of which is regarded as classical Parkinson's disease. It is necessary to make a distinction between parkinsonism and Parkinson's disease. For practical purposes a clinical diagnosis of Parkinson's disease should be regarded as parkinsonism until histology of the brain has been performed. Even in the best centres, diagnosis on clinical features is unreliable at predicting pathology.

Neuropathology

There are several distinct neurodegenerative diseases which result in parkinsonism. *Classical Parkinson's disease* is characterized by cell loss from the substantia nigra with the formation of spherical intracellular inclusions composed of modified intermediate filaments and ubiquitin termed Lewy bodies.

Multiple system atrophy causes an akinetic/rigid syndrome but is due to an abnormality in glial cells in the absence of Lewy bodies (Papp et al 1989). Cell loss and gliosis are seen in the substantia nigra, basal ganglia, pons, cerebellum and spinal cord. When parkinsonism is predominant, cases are termed striatonigral degeneration. Additional neurological features to those of parkinsonism are often present, particularly postural hypotension, leading to a clinical diagnosis of Shy–Drager syndrome. In cases with postural hypotension it is essential to preserve the spinal cord as this is the seat of pathology as a result of loss of sympathetic neurons in the cord.

Corticobasal degeneration is a disease causing an akinetic rigid syndrome frequently misdiagnosed as Parkinson's disease in non-specialist centres. The pathology includes cell loss from the substantia nigra as well as the presence of large swollen cells in the cerebral cortex. Inclusions similar to neurofibrillary tangles are seen in some neurones (Gibb et al 1990).

Progressive supranuclear palsy is clinically characterized by parkinsonism and impairment of eye movements, particularly vertical upgaze. Histologically there is cell loss and neurofibrillary tangles in the substantia nigra as well as in neurones in nuclei controlling eye movements (Kristensen 1985). Post-encephalitic parkinsonism is characterized by tangles and loss of nigral neurons (Geddes et al 1993). This is thought to be the result of a past episode of infective encephalitis.

Small vessel disease may cause lacunar infarction in basal ganglia leading to vascular pseudoparkinsonism. Some cases of clinically diagnosed Parkinson's disease have neuropathological features of Alzheimer's disease. Drug-induced parkinsonism may be clinically misinterpreted as Parkinson's disease. Parkinsonism may be seen in neurodegeneration associated with repeated head trauma as in boxers (Roberts et al 1990). Wilson's disease associated with disordered copper metabolism may cause a parkinsonian syndrome, usually in young individuals. Several rare neurodegenerative diseases have prominent parkinsonism as a component.

Because of this pathological heterogeneity, histological validation of the cause of Parkinsonism if always desirable.

Autopsy

The brain should be preserved as a minimum autopsy procedure. If hypotension has been associated with parkinsonism it is also necessary to save the spinal cord to look at sympathetic neurones in the intermediolateral columns. Histology of the substantia nigra should be performed to look for Lewy bodies and if these are present it is usually safe to make a diagnosis of idiopathic Parkinson's disease. Histology of the basal ganglia, brain stem nuclei and other regions may reveal unusual causes of parkinsonism associated with other neurodegenerative processes.

MOTOR NEURONE DISEASE

Motor neurone disease is being seen more frequently as a result of the competitive nature of human mortality — as we don't die of other diseases. Disease is characterized by loss of motor neurones from brain, brain stem and spinal cord. Depending on the pattern of cell loss, different clinical subtypes are seen.

Most cases are clinically diagnosed in life, the most common manifestation is as amyotrophic lateral sclerosis or progressive bulbar palsy. Variants such as primary lateral sclerosis (due to restricted loss of neurones from the cerebral motor cortex) and pure progressive muscular atrophy (due to restricted loss of neurones from the spinal cord) are uncommon. Patients who are diagnosed will usually have developed weakness leading to paralysis and have died of respiratory problems (respiratory failure or aspiration pneumonia) within 4 years of onset. Affected patients are occasionally only discovered at autopsy, often those who have developed rapid bulbar involvement, clinically interpreted as cerebrovascular disease.

Motor neurone disease probably has a much wider clinical phenotype than previously realized. It has recently been discovered that some cases of frontal lobe dementia syndrome have the pathology of motor neurone disease, with characteristic inclusion bodies in non-motor cortex as well as in brain stem motor neurones. In a similar way, some patients with motor neurone disease develop a frontal lobe dementia syndrome (Neary et al 1990, Gunnarsson et al 1991, Mann et al 1993). Importantly, many cases of motor neurone disease are familial.

Neuropathology

The brain is usually macroscopically unremarkable. The spinal cord may show atrophy of anterior nerve roots. Histology shows cell loss from the motor cortex, brain stem motor nuclei or spinal anterior horns, depending on clinical type of disease (Hirano 1991). There is loss of myelin and degeneration of motor tract, best seen in the lateral corticospinal tracts of the spinal cord, although in cases with death due to severe early bulbar involvement this may be subtle or absent. Inclusion bodies specific for motor neurone disease can be seen in spinal anterior horn cells if anti-ubiquitin immunostaining is used (Fig. 9.9), but are not otherwise easily visible (Lowe et al 1988, 1989, Leigh & Swash 1991, Schiffer et al 1991).

Autopsy

It is essential to preserve the brain and spinal cord in all cases of motor weakness clinically suspected of being motor neurone disease. Because of clinical diagnostic uncertainty in cases of motor weakness, it is also essential

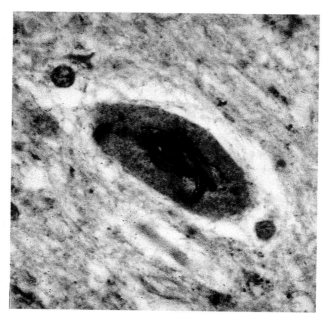

Fig. 9.9 Motor neurone disease inclusion (ubiquitin immunostaining). This is one of the skein-like filamentous inclusions seen in motor neurones in motor neurone disease. They can only be readily seen with anti-ubiquitin staining.

to save samples of skeletal muscle (deltoid and quadriceps) as well as peripheral nerve (sural, lumbar plexus and brachial plexus are readily accessible). In an ideal world, nerve and muscle should be sampled and preserved as for biopsy specimens, with snap-freezing of muscle for frozen section assessment and fixation of nerve in glutaraldehyde for assessment in resin sections.

The brain and spinal cord should be examined after fixation for several weeks. As a minimal assessment, histological examination of spinal cord, medulla and motor cortex should be performed. Myelin stains will identify gross tract degeneration secondary to motor neurone loss. Immunostaining with anti-ubiquitin is now used routinely to detect the pathognomonic inclusion bodies in remaining neurones. In cases where motor neurones and motor tracts are not affected, additional pathology accounting for motor weakness can be sought in muscle or nerves.

HEREDOFAMILIAL NEURODEGENERATIVE DISEASES

Many neurodegenerative diseases have long been recognized as being familial and it is vital to obtain pathological confirmation of the nature of the disease for the purpose of refining genetic counselling to surviving family members. In some of these conditions, for example Huntington's disease, it is possible to test directly for an abnormal gene or enzyme activity.

At autopsy, the extent of investigation is, in part, determined by the degree of confidence in the clinical diagnosis. Tissue should be kept frozen to facilitate search for genetic abnormalities, or to characterize abnormally stored material in all cases that have not been genetically worked up, to allow future genetic counselling if required. The main conditions coming to autopsy are listed in Table 9.2.

Table 9.2 Main heredofamilial neurodegenerative diseases coming to autopsy and minimum samples to save for examination

Huntington's disease	Brain
Multiple-system atrophies (olivopontocerebellar atrophy, Shy–Drager syndrome, striatonigral degeneration)	Brain, spinal cord and peripheral nerves
Familial dementia syndrome	Brain, spinal cord and peripheral nerves
Spinocerebellar degenerations	Brain, spinal cord and peripheral nerves
Leukodystrophies	Brain, spinal cord, and peripheral nerves and adrenal glands
Storage disorders	Brain, spinal cord peripheral nerves
Unexplained severe mental retardation	Brain and spinal cord

REFERENCES

Aghaji MA, Nzewi C 1989 Stroke syndrome in the young due to obliterative arteritis of extracranial carotid arteries. Clinical pathological profiles. J Neurosurg Sci 33: 333–337

Baudrimont M, Dubas F et al 1993 Autosomal dominant leukoencephalopathy and subcortical ischemic stroke. A clinicopathological study. Stroke 24: 122–125

Bell J, Ironside J 1991 Department of Health National Surveillance of Creutzfeldt–Jakob disease. Bull R Coll Pathol 74: 9–10

Bell J, Ironside J 1993 How to tackle a possible Creutzfeldt–Jakob disease necropsy. J Clin Pathol 46: 193–197

Bevan H, Sharma K et al 1990 Stroke in young adults. Stroke 21: 382–386

Bogousslavsky J, Pierre P 1992, Ischemic stroke in patients under age 45. Neurol Clin 10: 113–124

Boller F, Lopez O L et al 1989 Diagnosis of dementia: clinicopathologic correlations. Neurology 39: 76–79

Brick J F Riggs J E 1989 Ischemic cerebrovascular disease in the young adult. Emergence of oral contraceptive use and pregnancy as the major risk factors in the 1980s. W V Med J 85 (1): 7–8

Bromilow A, Burns J 1985 Technique for removal of the vertebral arteries. J Clin Pathol 38: 1400–1402

Brown P, Wolff A et al 1990 A simple and effective method for inactivating virus infectivity in formalin-fixed tissue samples from patients with Creutzfeldt–Jakob disease. Neurology 40: 887–890

Brown P, Kaur P et al 1993 Real and imagined clinicopathological limits of 'prion dementia', Lancet 341: 127–129

Brun, A 1987 Frontal lobe degeneration of non-Alzheimer type. I. Neuropathology. Arch Gerontol Geriatr 6: 193–208

Byrne E J, Lennox G et al 1989 Diffuse Lewy body disease: clinical features in 15 cases. J Neurol Neurosurg Psychiatry 52: 709–717

Byrne E, Lennox G et al 1991 Dementia associated with cortical Lewy bodies: proposed clinical diagnostic criteria. Dementia 2: 283–284

Camerlingo M, Finazzi G et al 1991 Inherited protein C deficiency and nonhemorrhagic arterial stroke in young adults. Neurology 41: 1371–1373

Carolei A, Marini C et al 1993 A prospective study of cerebral ischemia in the young. Analysis of pathogenic determinants. The National Research Council Study Group. Stroke 24: 362–364

Corder E, Saunders A et al 1993 Gene dose of apolipoprotein E type 4 allele and the risk of Alzheimer's disease in late onset families. Science 261: 921–923

Crystal H, Dickson D et al 1988 Clinico-pathologic studies in dementia: nondemented subjects with pathologically confirmed Alzheimer's disease. Neurology 38: 1682–1687

Delaere P, He Y et al 1993 Beta A4 deposits are constant in the brain of the oldest old: an immunocytochemical study of 20 French centenarians. Neurobiol Aging 14: 191–194

Evenhuis H M 1990 The natural history of dementia in Down's syndrome. Arch Neurol 47: 263–267

Ferrer I, Bella R et al 1990 Arteriolosclerotic leucoencephalopathy in the elderly and its relation to white matter lesions in Binswanger's disease, multi-infarct encephalopathy and Alzheimer's disease. J Neurol Sci 98: 37–50

Fischer P, Jellinger K et al 1991 Prospective neuropathological validation of Hachinski's Ischaemic Score in dementias. J Neurol Neurosurg Psychiatry 54: 580–583

Geddes JF, Hughes AJ et al 1993 Pathological overlap in cases of parkinsonism associated with neurofibrillary tangles. A study of recent cases of postencephalitic parkinsonism and comparison with progressive supranuclear palsy and Guamanian parkinsonism–dementia complex. Brain 116: 281–302

Gibb WR, Luthert PJ et al 1990 Clinical and pathological features of corticobasal degeneration. Adv Neurol 53: 51–54

Grewal RP, Barton NW 1992 Fabry's disease presenting with stroke. Clin Neurol Neurosurg 94: 177–179

Gunnarsson LG, Dahlbom K et al 1991 Motor neuron disease and dementia reported among 13 members of a single family. Acta Neurol Scand 84: 429–433

Gustafson L, Brun A et al 1990 Frontal lobe dementia of non-Alzeimer type. Adv Neurol 51: 65–71

Harrison PJ, Roberts GW 1991 'Life, Jim, but not as we know it'? Transmissible dementias and the prion protein. Br J Psychiatry 158: 457–570

Hirano A 1991 Cytopathology of amyotrophic lateral sclerosis. Adv Neurol 56: 91–101

Homer AC, Honavar M et al 1988 Diagnosing dementia: do we get it right? Br Med J 297: 894–896

Itoh Y, Yamada M et al 1993 Cerebral amyloid angiopathy: a significant cause of cerebellar as well as lobar cerebral hemorrhage in the elderly. J Neurol Sci 116: 135–141

Johns Dr 1991 Cerebrovascular complications of inflammatory bowel disease. Am J Gastroenterol 86: 367–370

Kaku DA, Lowenstein DH 1990 Emergence of recreational drug abuse as a major risk for stroke in young adults. Ann Intern Med 113: 821–827

Kittner SJ, Gorelick PB 1992 Antiphospholipid antibodies and stroke: an epidemiological perspective. Stroke 62(6): 529–536

Klonoff DC, Andrews BT et al 1989 Stroke associated with cocaine use. Arch Neurol 46: 98–993

Knopman DS, Mastri AR et al 1990 Dementia lacking distinctive histologic features: a common non-Alzheimer degenerative dementia Neurology 40: 251–256

Kohler J, Kasper J et al 1990 Ischemic stroke due to protein C deficiency. Stroke 21: 1077–1080

Kokkinos J, Levine SR 1993 Stroke Neurol Clin 11: 577–590

Kristensen MO 1985 Progressive supranuclear palsy—20 years later. Acta Neurol Scand 71: 177–189

Lagosky S, Witten CM 1993 A case of cerebral infarction in association with free protein S deficiency and oral contraceptive use. Arch Phys Med Rehabil 74: 98–100

Leigh PN, Swash M 1991 Cytoskeletal pathology in motor neuron diseases. Adv Neurol 56: 115–124

Lennox G, Lowe J et al 1989 Anti-ubiquitin immunocytochemistry is more sensitive than conventional techniques in the detection of diffuse Lewy body disease. J Neurol Neurosurg Psychiatry 52: 67–71

Lisovoski F, Rousseaux P 1991 Cerebral infarction in young people. A study of 148 patients with early cerebral angiography. J Neurol Neurosurg Psychiatry 54: 576–579

Love BB, Biller J et al 1990 Cigarette smoking. A risk factor for cerebral infarction in young adults. Arch Neurol 47: 693–698

Lowe J, Lennox G et al 1988 A filamentous inclusion body within anterior horn neurones in motor neurone disease defined by immunocytochemical localisation of ubiquitin Neurosci Lett 94: 203–210

Lowe J, Aldridge A et al 1989 Inclusion bodies in motor cortex and brainstem of patients with motor neurone disease are detected by immunocytochemical localisation of ubiquitin. Neurosci Lett 105: 7–13

Mann DM, South PW et al 1993 Dementia of frontal lobe type: neuropathology and immunohistochemistry. J Neurol Neurosurg Psychiatry 56: 605–614

Marks WA, Shuman RM et al 1988 Cerebral degenerations producing dementia: importance of neuropathologic confirmation of clinical diagnoses. J Geriatr Psychiatry Neurol 1: 187–198

Martinez HR, Rangel GR et al 1993 Ischemic stroke due to deficiency of coagulation inhibitors. Report of 10 young adults. Stroke 24: 19–25

Matias GJ, Alvarez J et al 1990 Ischemic stroke in young adults. II. Analysis of risk factors in the etiological subgroups. Acta Neurol Scand 81: 314–317

Mendez MF, Mastri AR et al 1991 Neuropathologically confirmed Alzheimer's disease: clinical diagnoses in 394 cases. J Geriatr Psychiatry Neurol 4: 26–29

Mettinger K 1982 Fibromuscular dysplasia and the brain II: current concepts of disease. Stroke 13: 53–59

Mirra SS, Hart MN et al 1993 Making the diagnosis of Alzheimer's disease. A primer for practicing pathologists Arch Pathol Lab Med 117: 132–144

Monforte R, Estruch R et al 1990 High ethanol consumption as risk factor for intracerebral hemorrhage in young and middle-aged people. Stroke 21: 1529–1532

Montalban J, Codina A et al 1991 Antiphospholipid antibodies in cerebral ischemia. Stroke 22: 750–753

Munoz DG 1991 The pathological basis of multi-infarct dementia. Alzheimer Dis Assoc Disord 5: 77–90

Neary D, Snowden JS et al 1988 Dementia of frontal lobe type. J Neurol Neurosurg

Psychiatry 51: 353–361

Neary D, Snowden JS et al 1990 Frontal lobe dementia and motor neuron disease. J Neurol Neurosurg Psychiatry 53: 23–32

Olesen J, Friberg L et al 1993 Ischaemia-induced (symptomatic) migraine attacks may be more frequent than migraine-induced ischaemic insults. Brain 116: 187–202

Papp M, Khan J et al 1989 Glial cytolasmic inclusions in the CNS of patients with multiple system atrophy (striatonigral degeneration, olivopontocerebellar atrophy, and Shy-Drager syndrome). J. Neurol Sci 94: 79–100

Ranoux D, Cohen A et al 1993 Patent foramen ovale: is stroke due to paradoxical embolism? Stroke 24: 31–34

Roberts GW, Allsop D et al 1990 The occult aftermath of boxing. J Neurol Neurosurg Psychiatry 53: 373–378

Roman GC 1985 The identity of lacunar dementia and Binswanger disease. Med Hypotheses 16: 389–391

Rossor M 1993 Molecular pathology of Alzheimer's disease. J Neurol Neurosurg Psychiatry 56: 583–586

Sauer CM 1991 Recurrent embolic stroke and cocaine-related cardiomyopathy. Stroke 22: 1203–1205

Schiffer D, Autilio GL et al 1991 Ubiquitin in motor neuron disease: study at the light and electron microscope. J Neuropathol Exp Neurol 50: 463–473

Schroth S, Tenner S 1991 When migraine is more than a headache. Stroke in a young patient. Postgrad Med 89: 87–89

Scott J 1993 Apolipoprotein E and Alzheimer's disease. Lancet 342: 696

Smith RR, Hendrie HC 1992 Leuko-araiosis: description and clinical correlates. Compr Ther 18: 7–16

Stern BJ, Kittner S et al 1991 Stroke in the young. Part II Md Med J 40: 565–571

Symposium 1992 Mitochondrial encephalomyopathies. Brain Pathol 2: 111–162

Toffol GJ, Swiontoniowski M 1992 Stroke in young adults. A continuing diagnostic challenge. Postgrad Med 91: 123–128

Tournier LE, Iba ZM et al 1991 Autosomal dominant syndrome with strokelike episodes and leukoencephalopathy. Stroke 22: 1297–1302

Tournier LE, Joutel A et al 1993 Cerebral autosomal dominant arteriopathy with subcortical infarcts and leukoencephalopathy maps to chromosome 19q12. Nature Genet 3: 256–259

Wijdicks EF, Jack CJ 1993 Intracerebral hemorrhage after fibrinolytic therapy for acute myocardial infarction. Stroke 24: 554–557

Yamada M, Itoh Y et al 1993 Subarachnoid haemorrhage in the elderly: a necropsy study of the association with cerebral amyloid angiopathy. J Neurol Neurosurg Psychiatry 56: 543–547

APPENDIX

Staining techniques useful in the assessment of dementia:

- Standard H&E staining is still the most useful way of assessing the brain but requires practice to detect subtle changes. Special stains make changes obvious to the infrequent neuropathologist.
- The easiest myelin stain to establish in a laboratory is the solochrome cyanin technique. This can be used to assess tract and white matter degeneration.
- The HAGA methenamine silver technique is very sensitive for detection of plaques but only detects a few tangles (Neuropathol Appl Neurobiol 1989, 15: 531–542).
- The AgNOR technique, as used in proliferation studies, fortuitously detects both plaques and tangles in sections but picks up neuronal nuclei and some normal cell processes (Pathol Res Pract 1991; 187: 1045–1049).

- Recent modifications of Bielshowski or Bodian stains will detect both plaques and tangles but are less sensitive for detection of subtypes of plaques composed of fine amyloid fibrils (Neuropathol Appl Neurobiol 1989, 15: 563–578).
- The Gallyas technique is a superb method for detecting tangles, neuropil threads and dystrophic neurites but is technically demanding (Brain Pathol 1991; 1: 213–216).
- Simple staining with Congo red or Sirius red is used to detect amyloid angiopathy.
- Immunostaining can be performed to detect βA4 (DAKO) in the amyloid of plaques as well as in walls of cerebral blood vessels. This must be preceded by formic acid treatment of sections to reveal antigen in the amyloid (DAKO).
- Immunostaining for ubiquitin (DAKO) is useful to detect cortical Lewy bodies as well as the inclusions in motor neurone disease. This will only detect a proportion of tangles.
- Immunostaining for tau protein (Sigma) is a reliable way to detect tangles and dystrophic neurites in Alzheimer's disease.
- Immunostaining for glial fibrillary acidic protein is useful to detect astrocytic gliosis.

10A. The atypical naevus: a clinician's viewpoint

J. A. Newton Bishop

Clinically atypical naevi characterize individuals with an increased susceptibility to cutaneous melanoma whether within melanoma families or in the general population.

An association between unusual melanocytic naevi and an increased risk of melanoma within families was first recognized by Norris in 1820. The condition was first explored in detail, however, by Clark et al (1978). They described two families with an increased risk of melanoma, in whom susceptibility to melanoma was associated with the presence of many atypical naevi, as the 'BK mole syndrome' (named after the two families).

Clark was impressed by the histological appearances seen in biopsied naevi from these families and described the so-called 'dysplastic naevus', as a result, as a distinct clinicopathological entity. This naevus was described as a naevus larger than 5 mm in diameter with an irregular border and variable colour (Fig. 10.1). There was usually both a macular and a raised component. Histologically there was said to be architectural atypia, with atypical proliferation of the melanocytes at the dermoepidermal junction. There was

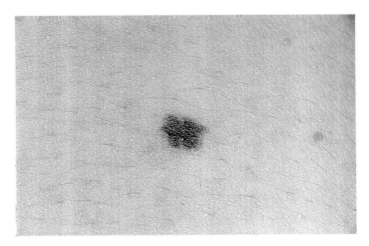

Fig. 10.1 A dyplastic naevus. Such naevi are defined by us as naevi greater in diameter than 5 mm, with an irregular or blurred edge, and irregular colour.

179

cytological atypia and, finally, a stromal reaction with a lymphocytic reaction, vascular changes and condensation of collagen in the dermis (Fig. 10.2).

Within the BK mole families large numbers of such naevi occurred in family members who developed melanoma, and the histological atypia of their naevi lead Clark to suggest that these naevi were not only markers of risk for melanoma, but that they were precursors of melanoma. Clark and others thought that the naevi were clinically and pathologically distinct and were diagnostic of familial susceptibility to melanoma. He renamed the syndrome the 'dysplastic naevus syndrome'. Subsequently, the Leiden group (Bergman et al 1986) have used the term 'FAMMM syndrome' (familial atypical mole and malignant melanoma syndrome); we prefer the term the 'atypical mole syndrome' (AMS) as was suggested by the Consensus Conference in 1991 (NIH Consensus Development Conference Statement 1992).

In subsequent genetic linkage studies to find the underlying tumour suppressor gene for melanoma, the definition used for the syndrome phenotype was the presence of two histologically proven dysplastic naevi. In recent years, much controversy has followed the use of this definition. The type of discussion and the degree of hysteria that has surrounded it has proved detrimental to our understanding of the very real familial melanoma syndrome and to our management of patients with these naevi. In fact, we now know a good deal about the epidemiology of these atypical naevi which enables us to understand the origin of this controversy.

The first problem with the 'two histologically proven dysplastic naevi' definition of the AMS phenotype was that, contrary to initial expectations, these naevi showed poor clinicopathological correlation (Clark & Ackerman 1989, Black & Hunt 1990, Piepkorn et al 1989). Clinically very atypical naevi

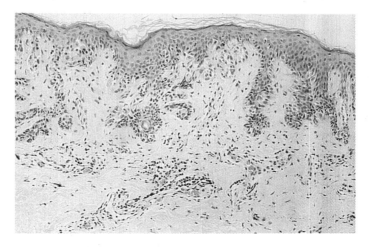

Fig. 10.2 The histological appearance of a dysplastic naevus with atypical melanocytic hyperplasia, cytological atypia and a stromal reaction.

were shown to be banal histologically and some authors reported the changes said to be characteristic of dysplastic or atypical naevi in randomly biopsied banal naevi in normal individuals (Klien & Barr 1990).

The second problem was that clinically atypical naevi proved to be much more common in the normal population than had previously been supposed. In studies from the UK, New Zealand (Cooke et al 1989) and France, an estimated 8% of the normal population were said to have small numbers of these atypical naevi. In Sweden the estimate was higher at around 19% (Stierner et al 1990). In our UK study it was around 2% (Newton et al 1993). Therefore, practising clinicians and pathologists commonly come across such naevi, especially in pigmented lesion clinics. Few of them occur in individuals with a family history of melanoma and therefore this proved to be another cause of confusion. What did it all mean?

Even within families the 'two dysplastic naevi' definition has proved inadequate. Not all melanoma patients within these families have atypical naevi. In the Leiden study only 54% of the melanoma patients had the so-called FAMMM phenotype, and in our UK studies a very similar percentage (56%) of melanoma patients were found to have abnormal naevi. There is, in addition, variation in the types of naevi seen between families and within families. Some individuals, for example, have very large numbers of naevi but they are otherwise banal (Fig. 10.3). Others have small numbers of naevi but they are individually clinically atypical and occur in unusual sites such as on the scalp (Fig. 10.4).

We have seen that atypical features of melanocytic naevi are not specific to familial melanoma, and that they do not occur in all familial melanoma patients. Furthermore, as a definition of phenotype the presence of atypical naevi alone is rather subjective even if we try to define them carefully. We have attempted to develop a more objective definition of the phenotype based on experience in the Royal London Hospital familial melanoma clinic. We have evaluated this system in a population-based case-control study of melanoma cases and in family studies to determine if we can better understand the significance of atypical naevi.

Definition of the AMS phenotype: the London Hospital AMS scoring system

In the familial melanoma clinic we observed that patients from melanoma prone families had naevi that were numerous, individually atypical and/or occurred in unusual sites such as on the scalp, buttocks (Crutcher 1988), dorsa of the feet and even in the iris (Newton 1993, Roderiguez-Sains 1986) (Fig. 10.5). We have developed a clinical scoring system to describe these clinical characteristics, known as the AMS scoring system (Table 10.1). Each observation merits 1 point up to a maximum of 5, a score of 3 being necessary for the individual to be said to have the AMS phenotype. This scoring system was designed to be as specific to the AMS patient as possible but yet to

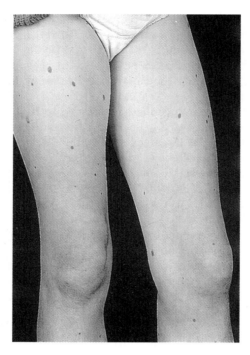

Fig. 10.3 A child from a family prone to melanoma who had numerous naevi but none was classically dysplastic. © The Royal London Trust.

describe as many patients with the very variable AMS phenotype as possible. It was also hoped that the scoring system would be very much more robust than others previously used, that observers would achieve a greater level of agreement in AMS score than they would, for example, in counting atypical naevi. This has been shown to be the case (Bataille et al 1994).

The scoring system has been used within the families we are studying in genetic linkage studies, and in a case-control study of cutaneous melanoma in the UK. In the case-control study which began in 1989, 266 melanoma patients and 305 controls were examined. Their naevi were carefully documented and described, and the AMS scoring system was retrospectively

Table 10.1 The AMS phenotype scoring system

100 or more naevi larger in diameter than 2 mm, or 50 or more if >50 years	1
2 or more clinically atypical naevi	1
1 or more naevi on the buttocks, or 2 or more on the dorsa of the feet	1
Naevi in the anterior scalp	1
Pigmented lesions of the iris	1

The patient is said to have the phenotype if they score 3 out of a maximum of 5.

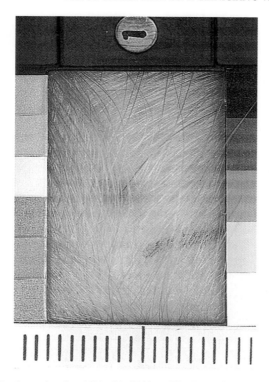

Fig. 10.4 Naevi in the scalp of a child with AMS. © The Royal London Trust.

used to determine the relative percentages of those with the AMS phenotype in the two groups. If individual components of the AMS scoring system are considered (Table 10.2), it can be seen that the presence of clinically dysplastic naevi, numerous naevi and an abnormal distribution of naevi were all significantly more common in cases than controls and were therefore risk

Table 10.2 Individual components of the AMS score in a case-control study of 266 melanoma patients in the NE Thames region of the UK

Observation	% cases	% controls
> 100 naevi bigger than 2 mm	24	10
≥ 2 atypical naevi	14	2
Naevi on buttocks or dorsa feet	46	25
Naevi in anterior scalp	7	7
A pigmented lesion of the iris	20	12

Clinically atypical naevi, numerous naevi and naevi on the buttocks are significantly more common in melanoma patients and are all risk factors for melanoma as clinical signs of the AMS syndrome.

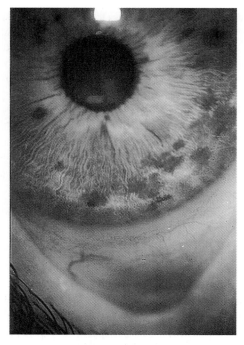

Fig. 10.5 Pigmented lesions of the iris in a patient who developed her first melanoma in 1954.

factors for cutaneous melanoma (as has been shown in other case-control studies). The presence of increasing numbers of individual variables (an increasing AMS score) was associated with an increased risk of melanoma, here expressed as the odds ratio (Table 10.3). The presence of a score of 3 or more (the AMS phenotype) is a powerful risk factor for melanoma.

The study's principal conclusions were therefore:

1. Only 2% of the general population have the AMS phenotype as defined by us. The definition is therefore relatively specific to melanoma patients.

Table 10.3 The AMS score in cases and controls in the NE Thames case-control study. An increasing AMS score carries an increasing risk of melanoma

AMS score	% cases	% controls	Odds ratio (adjusted)
0	38	58	1.00*
1	31	29	1.60
2	16	8	2.54
3	11	2	8.48
4	4	0	19.30

The odds ratios are given relative to an AMS score of 0.

2. The presence of unusual characteristics of naevi, whether it be clinically atypical naevi, numerous naevi or unusually distributed naevi, are risk factors for melanoma even in the unselected, i.e. non-familial, population.

3. Compared with other risk factors for melanoma — perhaps better known risk factors, such as hair colour — the risk factors for atypical moles are an order of magnitude greater. In case-control studies from around the world the relative risk for melanoma for fair hair, for example, is usually around 2, and for the presence of freckles, around 3.

The odds ratio for melanoma of the AMS phenotype (score 3 or 4) was 11 in this study. In the UK, with an incidence of melanoma at about 10 per 100 000 per annum, individuals have an approximate lifetime risk of 1 in 200 of a melanoma. With the AMS phenotype the lifetime risk is significantly increased to 1 in 20. Thus, the presence of the phenotype in apparently non-familial circumstances should not be dismissed as irrelevant. The phenotype implies an increased risk of melanoma. Detection of the phenotype in the pigmented lesion clinic identifies patients at risk of melanoma. It is likely that they would benefit from counselling about sun avoidance and self-examination of naevi with the aim of early detection of melanoma.

Whether within a family or not, then, the presence of atypical naevi implies an increased risk of melanoma. The detection clinically of such features is therefore important in terms of health education and the prevention of disease.

The AMS scoring system in AMS families

We have undertaken detailed studies of melanocytic naevi in families prone to melanoma. Over 100 families were recruited to the study from England and Wales, 13 of the most informative families being selected for linkage studies. There were 61 melanomas in 37 patients, 9 patients having multiple tumours. The pattern of melanomas within the families was consistent with an autosomal dominant gene. Efforts were made to see all relatives without selection; all were examined and the AMS score was determined (Newton et al 1994). The correlation between the AMS phenotype, as defined by us, and susceptibility to melanoma was not absolute. In two families with 4 and 2 melanoma cases, respectively, there were insufficient features to make the diagnosis of AMS. In the 11 other families, 4 melanoma patients had normal moles, although other individuals from those same families had recognizable AMS phenotype. Fig. 10.6 and 10.7 show the clinical appearances of patients from a familial melanoma pedigree (Fig. 10.8).

In summary, the AMS scoring system identified individuals with abnormal moles in a pattern consistent with an autosomal dominant gene. Expression of the AMS gene appeared to be very variable, however, even within families.

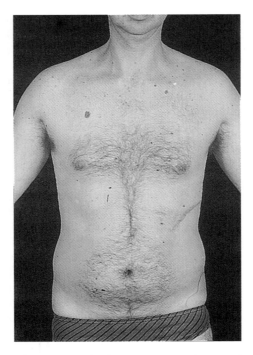

Fig. 10.6 This patient from pedigree BAC 526 has had 3 primary melanomas and his mother had 6. Both had the AMS phenotype. This picture shows an increased number of naevi, and clinically dysplastic naevi. © Tower Hamlets Health Authority.

The AMS scoring system appeared to work as well as any other, perhaps better, in categorizing gene carriers in families (Fig. 10.8), but because of incomplete penetrance of the phenotype, use of the scoring system imperfectly identifies gene carriers. Laboratory tests will, in the end, probably be preferable as an absolute indication of who is at risk of melanoma. In the meantime in family studies using formal assessment of naevi, and comparing the findings with population norms as in our AMS system, it is possible to give a reasonable, if imperfect, estimate of who is a gene carrier and who is not.

Summary

We have attempted to define the AMS phenotype by developing a simple system which can be used readily in the clinic. The scoring system had to:

— be as specific as possible to melanoma patients,
— define as many melanoma patients from AMS
    families as possible, i.e. it had to include, for example, patients with
    huge numbers of moles yet who did not have clinically dysplastic naevi,
— be as objective as possible.

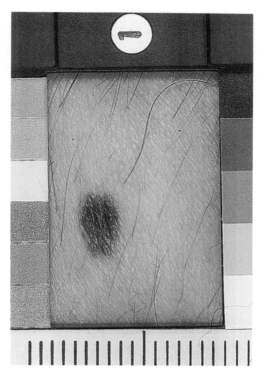

Fig. 10.7   This is a melanoma arising in a dysplastic naevus removed from the same patient as in Fig. 10.6. © Tower Hamlets Health Authority.

The scoring system appeared to function in these respects reasonably well, and its use identified a population of patients at high risk of melanoma. In patients without a family history of melanoma the lifetime risk of that tumour in the UK is 1 in 20. In the presence of a family history, the lifetime risks are considerably higher.

Although there remains confusion about the relationship between clinically atypical naevi and melanoma, it is clear that recognition of these naevi is important in identifying a reasonably large cohort of patients at increasd risk of melanoma. Melanoma is becoming increasingly common in Northern Europe and it is desirable to limit this increase. The recognition of patients with the AMS phenotype enables us to identify a group of patients who would benefit from targeted education and some degree of surveillance.

The role of the pathologist

It is my view that there is no value in biopsying naevi to 'confirm' the clinical diagnosis of a dysplastic naevus because it has been shown that the presence

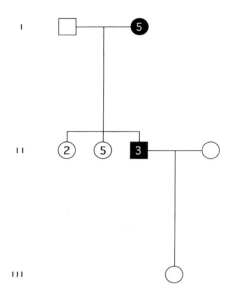

Fig. 10.8   The BAC pedigree, showing good agreement between the AMS score and risk of melanoma; both the AMS phenotype and melanoma appear to be inherited in an autosomal dominant pattern.

of clinically atypical naevi is the most potent risk factor for melanoma. There is no evidence that histologically dysplastic naevi carry any greater risk.

How should we view, as clinicians, a pathology report which describes a dysplastic naevus? I would interpret this in the same way as I would the clinical observation of atypia. The clinician should examine the patient and if there are other features of the AMS then the paitent should be counselled about sun avoidance and self-examination of naevi. Most importantly, too, a careful family history should be taken of other cancers as well as melanoma because there is some evidence that patients with other family cancer syndromes, such as the Li–Fraumeni syndrome, may present in this way (Newton 1993). Patients with a positive family history would benefit from referral to specialist clinics with genetic input.

ACKNOWLEDGEMENT

This research was funded by the Imperial Cancer Research Fund (ICRF). Veronique Bataille, an ICRF research fellow, worked on case control and family studies with Elizabeth Pinney. Jane Squire and Kairen Griffiths also contributed. The analyses were carried out by Peter Sasieni, D Timothy Bishop and Jack Cuzick.

REFERENCES

Bataille V, Newton Bishop J A, Sasieni P, Cuzick J 1994 (in preparation)
Bergman W, Palan A, Went L N 1986 Clinical and genetic studies in six Dutch kindreds with the dysplastic nevus syndrome. Ann Hum Genet 50: 249–258
Black WC, Hunt WC 1990 Histologic correlations with the clinical diagnosis of dysplastic nevus. Am J Surg Pathol 14: 44–52
Clark WH, Ackerman AB 1989 An exchange of views regarding the dysplastic nevus controversy. Semin Dermatol 18: 229–250
Clark WM, Reimer RR, Greene M et al 1978 Origin of familial malignant melanomas from hereditable melanocytic lesions: 'the B.K. mole syndrome'. Arch Dermatol 114: 732–738
Cooke KR, Spears GFS, Elder DE et al 1989 Dysplastic naevi in a population-based survey. Cancer 63: 1240–1244
Crutcher WA 1988 The dysplastic nevus and its clinical management. Adv Dermatol 3: 187–204
Klien LJ, Barr RJ 1990 Histologic atypia in clinically benign nevi. A prospective study. J Am Acad Dermatol 22: 275–282
Newton JA 1993 Familial melanoma. Clin Exp Dermatol 18: 5–11
Newton JA, Bataille V, Griffiths et al 1993 How common is the atypical mole syndrome phenotype in apparently sporadic melanoma? J Am Acad Dermatol 29: 989–996
Newton JA, Bataille V, Pinney E et al 1994 Familial Melanoma. Melanoma Res (in press)
NIH Consensus Development Conference Statement 1992. Volume 4 (9) National Institutes of Health, Bethesda
Norris W 1820 A case of fungoid disease. Edinb Med Surg J 16: 562–565
Piepkorn M, Meyer LJ, Golgar D et al 1989 The dysplastic melanocytic nevus: a prevalent lesion that correlates poorly with clinical phenotype. J Am Acad Dermatol 20: 407–415
Roderiguez-Sains RS 1986 Ocular findings in patients with dysplastic nevus syndrome. Ophthalmology 93: 1994 661–665
Stierner U, Augustsson A, Rosdahl I et al 1990 Regional distribution of common and dysplastic naevi in relation to melanoma site and sun exposure. A case control study. Melanoma Res 1: 367–375

10B. The atypical naevus: a histopathologist's viewpoint

N. Kirkham

HOW DO YOU MAKE THE HISTOPATHOLOGICAL DIAGNOSIS OF A DYSPLASTIC NAEVUS?

The time has now passed when the histopathologist should be asked to diagnose a dysplastic naevus in isolation. In the early days of the dysplastic naevus syndrome it was recommended that two representative lesions be removed from a patient to confirm a clinical diagnosis of the dysplastic naevus syndrome. The first part of this chapter has shown how this is no longer considered necessary by dermatologists. The diagnosis of the dysplastic or atypical mole syndrome is made on clinical grounds using clinically defined criteria.

Dermatologists are now more likely to excise a pigmented lesion to exclude the possibility of melanoma. The task of the histopathologist is therefore to make an accurate subclassification of the lesion into one of six possible categories. These are:

1. Dysplastic naevus;
2. A junctional or compound naevus without diagnostic features of a dysplastic naevus;
3. A naevus of special type, such as a pigmented spindle cell naevus;
4. Malignant melanoma in radial growth phase (including melanoma in situ);
5. Malignant melanoma in vertical growth phase;
6. Something completely different.

HISTOPATHOLOGY

The basis of any histopathological diagnosis is the careful examination of the gross specimen, the appropriate 'cut up' or 'trimming' of the specimen and the subsequent preparation of well-cut and well-stained sections. This may seem self evident but is worth emphasizing. Many of the difficulties that histopathologists experience can be resolved by having better quality sections.

GROSS EXAMINATION

Clinically dysplastic naevi have been described as being greater than 4 mm in diameter, with a macular component, and with or without a papular component (Elder et al 1980, Elder 1985, Elder et al 1993). This minimum diameter criterion is an important one, allowing smaller lesions to be excluded. The dysplastic naevi show border irregularity and lack the well-defined border usually seen in radial growth phase melanoma, but instead often have a fuzzy or hazy border. Within the lesion there is colour variegation ranging in shades from tan to dark brown. Pink areas may also be present. The black or blue/black commonly seen in melanoma is usually absent. Skin markings are accentuated over the surface of the lesion. The specimen will usually be an excision biopsy consisting of a skin ellipse containing a pigmented lesion.

The length, width and thickness of the specimen should be measured in millimetres. The lesion should also be described, including the maximum diameter and a description of the colour and degree of variation present. The whole of the lesion must be examined microscopically. The best way of achieving this is to use a fresh, sharp blade to cut the specimen transversely into a series of parallel slices, each less than 2 mm thick. These can usually be processed in one cassette to make one block. It is important to use a sharp blade. If the knife blade is blunt then the delicate melanocytes in the junctional component of the lesion may become disrupted when the specimen is sliced, literally increasing at a stroke the problems of diagnosis.

The alternative method of cutting one transverse slice through the centre of the biopsy and two 'cruciate' slices from the ends of the biopsy should be abandoned. Too often this leads to a clear view of the margins of excision at the price of severe disruption of the lesion itself. The report can say whether or not the lesion is completely excised, but may not be able to say what the lesion was. The margins of excision are far less important than the nature of the lesion. Most dermatologists are capable of performing an adequate excision biopsy most of the time. If the diagnosis of melanoma is made then a further excision of the biopsy site is likely to be performed anyway.

It is important to cut multiple sections from the block. One way of doing this is to cut the block at three levels. This decreases the chances of missing a significant abnormality in the biopsy.

MICROSCOPICAL EXAMINATION

'Dysplastic naevus'

The alleged problems with the term 'dysplastic naevus' have been over emphasized. The detractors have pointed out that the words 'dysplasia' or 'dysplastic' have different meanings in different contexts (Ackerman & Milde 1992). This criticism applies to many words in the English language. Indeed practically all words have more than one meaning: it is the context that defines the meaning in the particular circumstance. For instance the same voices that have objected to the use of 'dysplastic' have not raised any objection to the use of 'mole' to describe a particular group of skin lesions, even though the same word describes a small hairy mammal that spends most of its time underground, but may emerge to disrupt your carefully tended garden. The word 'dysplastic' is used in histopathology to indicate a combination of cytological atypia, architectural irregularity and a likelihood of premalignant potential. In the context of dysplastic naevus this is exactly what is required in the chosen descriptive term.

Criteria for diagnosis

The accurate subclassification of pigmented lesions depends upon the careful application of simple diagnostic criteria. When strict criteria are used for both clinical and pathological diagnoses then a more reproducible classification can be achieved (Barnhill & Roush 1991, Clemente et al 1991, Cochran 1994, Duncan et al 1993, Duray et al 1992, Maiweg et al 1992).

The problem for the histopathologist is to identify these lesions reliably and at the same time not confuse them with truly benign simulants or true melanomas. The only practical approach is to adhere to strict diagnostic criteria. The history of histopathology is not overburdened with diagnostic criteria that can be used in an infallible way by all and sundry. Nevertheless there are some criteria that should be useful in this context.

In all forms of tumour pathology diagnosis it is important to identify characteristics and classify changes in tissue architecture and also changes in cellular detail. The dysplastic naevus is no different. A melanocytic lesion of the skin can only be classified as a dysplastic or atypical naevus if it shows the requisite architectural and cytological features. Variability is the key in both clinical and pathological classification of these lesions. The naevi are variable in size, in shape, and in colour, both between lesions and within each lesion. There is both architectural and cellular variability. The combination of variability of all of these features points towards the correct diagnosis. The use of just a few criteria can never distinguish accurately between the common naevus and the dysplastic naevus (Hastrup & Hou-Jensen 1993). It is the combination of many factors that leads to the appropriate classification. This is perhaps why the diagnosis has posed so many problems. The criteria are:

1. Diameter;
2. Host lymphocytic response;
3. Lentiginous and nesting melanocytic proliferation;
4. Random cytological atypia;
5. Delicate elongation of rete ridges and fusion of adjacent rete;
6. Narrow elongated spindle-shaped melanocytes orientated horizontally;
7. Lamellar fibroplasia around rete ridges;

1. Diameter. The architectural features include, firstly, the diameter of the lesion. This feature has been largely overlooked in previous debates about the definition and diagnosis of dysplastic naevi (Hastrup et al 1994). Opinions vary a little but it is generally agreed that the lesion should have a diameter of at least 4 mm, with the majority now suggesting 5 mm as the cut off. The diameter should be taken into account by the dermatologist before taking the biopsy. Nevertheless it is a feature that can be easily measured microscopically, preferably by using the Vernier stage micrometer of the microscope to make a measurement accurate to a tenth of a millimetre (Kirkham & Cotton 1984, Cotton & Kirkham 1991).

The diameter of the lesion is an important measurement to make. Lesions less than 4 or 5 mm in diameter may have some of the other defining features of dysplastic naevi, but fail at the first hurdle. Smaller lesions are more likely to be classified as junctional or compound naevi. Alternatively it is possible for a nodular melanoma with a Breslow depth of 2 mm to be only 2 mm in diameter. When lesions are larger than 8 mm in diameter then they are more likely to have other features that would suggest melanoma at least in radial growth phase.

2. Host lymphocytic response. The presence or absence of a host lymphocytic response around the vessels in the papillary dermis underlying the lesion is important because its presence is a prerequisite for the diagnosis. If it is absent then the lesion is not a dysplastic naevus. Usually smaller naevi are the ones that lack a host response. When the host response is very vigorous, even with lymphocytes infiltrating the lesion in the epidermis then a diagnosis of melanoma is more likely.

3. Lentiginous and nesting melanocytic proliferation. The main feature of all naevi is of course the proliferation of melanocytes in the basal layers of the epidermis. The cells may be present singly or in groups, the former described as lentiginous and the latter as nesting proliferation. The type of proliferation is of no other special significance. When melanocytes are seen in the upper layers of the epidermis then it is likely that 'Pagetoid' or 'buck shot' spread may be what is present. This is a feature seen in melanoma rather than in dysplastic naevi.

4. Random cytological atypia (see Fig. 10.10A). A most important criterion is that of cellular atypia. Much time and effort has been expended in recent years on the definition of atypia. Close attention to nuclei and nucleoli is what is required. Cytoplasmic appearances are of little value. To be able to appreciate changes in nuclei and nucleoli it is essential to have well-cut and well-stained thin sections. If the sections are too thick or poorly cut then nuclei detail will not be apparent.

The characteristic feature of a dysplastic naevus is the presence of so-called random cytological atypia. Atypia can be random or non-random. In melanomas the atypia is often non-random in that all of the nuclei are abnormal with enlarged irregular nucleoli. In naevi the nuclei are usually regular with nucleoli that are most usually circular and eosinophilic. In between lies the category of random cytological atypia with changes lying between the two extremes seen in naevus and melanoma.

5. Delicate elongation of rete ridges and fusion of adjacent rete. In association with the proliferation of melanocytes showing random cytological atypia the rete ridges of the epidermis show a curious hyperplasia with exaggeration of the ridges. Adjacent ridges may be fused to form a continuous structure.

6. Narrow elongated spindle-shaped melanocytes orientated horizontally (Fig. 10.9A). When the tips of rete ridges are fused there is often a characteristic appearance of spindle-shaped melanocytes running horizontally to form the major part of the bridge between the adjacent ridges.

7. Lamellar fibroplasia around rete ridges (Fig. 10.9B). The dermal stroma around rete ridges, especially ridges showing nesting hyperplasia, may appear more condensed and eosinophilic than the usual appearance of the collagenous stroma of the papillary dermis.

A junctional or compound naevus without diagnostic features of a dysplastic naevus

Having considered whether or not a particular naevus does or does not satisfy the criteria for classification as a dysplastic naevus many will not fit the bill. Many of these can be appropriately classified as junctional or compound melanocytic naevi. Individual naevi may have one or more of the features of a dysplastic naevus, but strict application of the diagnostic criteria, especially the minimum diameter will allow the correct decision to be made.

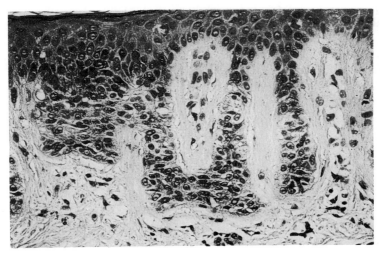

Fig. 10.9A   Dysplastic naevus. A typical example showing basal melanocytic proliferation, elongation of rete ridges and horizontally orientated spindle-shaped melanocytes (H&E).

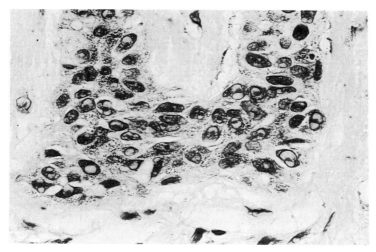

Fig. 10.9B   Dysplastic naevus. High-power view showing spindle-shaped cells and dermal lamellar fibroplasia (H&E).

A naevus of special type, such as a pigmented spindle cell naevus

Occasionally one or other of the variants of melanocytic naevi may be mistaken for a dysplastic naevus on clinical grounds. Of these the pigmented spindle cell naevus is one of the more common examples. A typical spindle cell naevus presents as a darkly pigmented, symmetrically domed lesion on the leg of a young woman. The presence of prominent junctional nests of spindle-shaped melanocytes in a lesion showing radial symmetry and lacking random cytological atypia is the hallmark of the entity. It is entirely benign (Barnhill et al 1991).

Malignant melanoma in radial growth phase (including melanoma in situ; Fig. 10.10B)

The distinction between dysplastic naevus and radial growth phase melanoma is most important and the main reason for most of the biopsies submitted. The criteria for a diagnosis of dysplastic naevus have all been defined above. Radial growth phase melanoma has been described as being in a way a premalignant melanoma in that it is defined as a melanoma 'lacking competence for metastasis'. So although such lesions are called melanoma this is done in the knowledge that the eight-year probability of tumour-free survival is as close to 100% as it is possible to be. Thus both dysplastic naevi and radial growth phase melanoma are clinically benign lesions. The more important clinical distinction is with vertical growth phase melanoma.

Radial growth phase melanoma includes melanoma in situ and is defined as a tumour which goes beyond the changes seen in dysplastic naevi. The

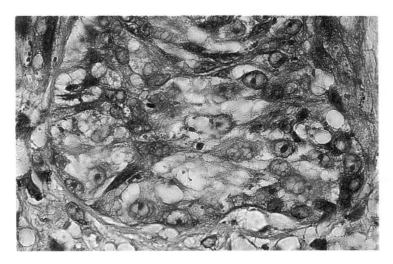

Fig. 10.10A Dysplastic naevus. High-power view showing random cytological atypia, with nucleoli of variable size (H&E, oil immersion × 100 objective).

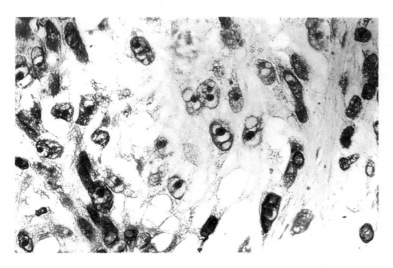

Fig. 10.10B Melanoma in situ. A high-power view showing non-random cytological atypia, with nucleoli of similar size (H&E, oil immersion × 100 objective).

diameter will be more than 5 mm and often more than 8 mm. There will usually be a prominent host lymphocytic response around the vessels in the underlying papillary dermis. Cellular atypia will usually be quite obvious and there will also be easily apparent architectural changes. Pagetoid or 'buck shot' spread of atypical melanocytes will be present.

An important point is that radial growth phase melanoma encompasses both melanoma in situ and some melanomas extending to Clark's level 2 in the papillary dermis. Thus it is not so important to distinguish between tumours with or without a small invasive component. The definition of melanoma in radial growth phase as distinct from melanoma in vertical growth phase calls for two criteria to be satisfied:

1. There should be no melanocytes in mitosis in the dermal component of the tumour, and;
2. The largest intradermal nest of tumour cells should be smaller than the largest intraepidermal nest.

Malignant melanoma in vertical growth phase

The difference between radial and vertical growth phase melanoma is that by definition vertical growth phase melanoma has competence for metastasis whilst radial growth phase melanoma does not. The distinction between the two is relatively straightforward, depending upon the presence of one of two possible features:

1. If there are any melanocytes in mitosis in the dermal component of the tumour then it is in vertical growth phase, or;
2. If the largest intradermal nest of tumour cells is larger than the largest intraepidermal nest then it is in vertical growth phase.

The diagnosis of melanoma in vertical growth phase identifies a lesion with competence for metastasis. The individual prognosis can be further characterized using a model that predicts the eight-year probability of tumour-free survival (Clark et al 1989).

Something completely different

Clinical diagnosis is never infallible and so there will be an inevitable group of biopsies where the clinical diagnosis of a melanocytic proliferation is wide of the mark. Usually it is reasonably straightforward to make the correct diagnosis of lesions such as haemangioma, dermatofibroma, pigmented seborrhoeic wart, lichen planus and others where the clinical impression of a melanocytic lesion is explained by the presence of alternative causes of pigmentation.

CONCLUSION

The histopathological diagnosis of dysplastic naevus can be achieved by the careful application of a combination of diagnostic criteria (Cochran 1994, Shapiro 1992). The diagnosis has a part to play in the understanding of melanoma precursors and the atypical mole syndrome (Cook & Fallowfield 1990). Most frequently the histopathologist will be asked to distinguish between dysplastic naevi and melanoma either in radial or vertical growth phase. This distinction can also be made using the strict application of simple criteria.

REFERENCES

Ackerman, AB, Milde P 1992 Naming acquired melanocytic nevi: common and dysplastic, normal and atypical, or Unna, Miescher, Spitz, and Clark? Am J Dermatopathol 14: 447–453

Barnhill RL, Roush GC 1991 Correlation of clinical and histopathologic features in clinically atypical melanocytic nevi. Cancer 67: 3157–3164

Barnhill RL, Barnhill MA, Berwick M, Mihm MC Jr, 1991 The histologic spectrum of pigmented spindle cell nevus: a review of 120 cases with emphasis on atypical variants. Hum Pathol 22: 52–58

Clark WH Jr, Elder DE, Guerry D et al 1989 Model predicting survival in stage I melanoma based on tumor progression. J Natl Cancer Inst 81: 1893–1904

Clemente C, Cochran AJ, Elder DE et al 1991 Histopathologic diagnosis of dysplastic nevi: concordance among pathologists convened by the World Health Organization Melanoma Programme. Hum Pathol 22: 313–319

Cochran AJ 1994 Commentary: the role of the histopathologist in the diagnosis of dysplastic naevi. Histopathology 24: 589–590

Cook MG, Fallowfield ME 1990 Dysplastic naevi—an alternative view. Histopathology 16: 29–35

Cotton DW, Kirkham N 1991 The use of vernier scales. Histopathology 19: 579

Duncan LM, Berwick M, Bruijn JA et al 1993 Histopathologic recognition and grading of dysplastic melanocytic nevi: an interobserver agreement study. J Invest Dermatol 100: 318S–321S

Duray PH, DerSimonian R, Barnhill R et al 1992 An analysis of interobserver recognition of the histopathologic features of dysplastic nevi from a mixed group of nevomelanocytic lesions. J Am Acad Dermatol 27: 741–749

Elder DE 1985 The dysplastic nevus. Pathology 17: 291–297

Elder DE, Goldman LI, Goldman SC, Greene MH, Clark WH 1980 Dysplastic nevus syndrome: a phenotypic association of sporadic cutaneous melanoma. Cancer 46: 1787–1794

Elder DE, Clark WH Jr, Elenitsas R, Guerry D, Halpern AC 1993 The early and intermediate precursor lesions of tumor progression in the melanocytic system: common acquired nevi and atypical (dysplastic) nevi. Semin Diagn Pathol 10: 18–35

Hastrup N, Hou-Jensen K 1993 Melanocytic lesions in a private pathology practice. Comparison of histologic features in different tumor types with particular reference to dysplastic nevi. Apmis 101: 845–850

Hastrup N, Clemmensen OJ, Spaun E, Sondergaard K 1994 Dysplastic naevus: histological criteria and their inter-observer reproducibility. Histopathology 24: 503–509

Kirkham N, Cotton DW 1984 Measuring melanomas: the vernier method. J Clin Pathol 37: 229–230

Maiweg C, Gartmann H, Lippold A et al 1992 The usefulness of single and combined clinical characteristics for the diagnosis of dysplastic naevi. Melanoma Res 1: 377–383

Shapiro PE 1992 Making sense of the dysplastic nevus controversy. A unifying perspective. Am J Dermatopathol 14: 350–356

11. Fine needle aspiration cytopathology of the thyroid gland

E. McGoogan   K. McLaren

Over the last decade, fine needle aspiration (FNA) of thyroid has become established as a major component in the investigation of solitary nodules or asymmetric thyroid enlargement. It is being used with increasing frequency and now has an important influence on the clinical management of a substantial proportion of patients seen by endocrinologists and surgeons. The literature attests to the contribution of thyroid FNA in the diagnosis and management of thyroid enlargement (see References).

An approach to the investigation of thyroid enlargement, with emphasis on the role of FNA, is illustrated in Fig. 11.1.

In few other clinical situations is there a greater requirement for accurate clinical information than in the approach to thyroid swellings. Age, duration of disease, hyper- and hypofunctional states are all important aspects which must be included in any clinical assessment. The evaluation of the nature of the swelling — diffuse, localized, soft and vascular, nodular and irregular, unilateral, bilateral, cystic, solid — all have bearing on the likely nature of the underlying lesion. Details of thyroid function tests, including thyroid hormone status, thyroid-stimulating hormone (TSH) levels, response of the pituitary to thyrotropin-releasing hormone (TRH) stimulation, thyroid-stimulating immunoglobulins and the presence of antibodies to thyroglobulin, thyroid microsomes and other components of thyroid epithelium, all may contribute to the pursuit of an accurate diagnosis. The nature of the swelling may be evaluated by palpation, plain neck X-ray, thyroid scanning and ultrasound.

Although most apparently solitary nodules represent an exaggerated area in multinodular goitre, it is important to investigate and accurately diagnose the nature of any localized thyroid swelling. Of the truly solitary lesions, approximately 80% will be found to be 'cool' or 'cold' by isotope scanning; the 'hot' nodules, which concentrate the isotope with greater affinity than the surrounding gland, may represent a hyperfunctional follicular adenoma and the patient presents with hyperthyroidism (this is a rare cause of the hyperfunctional state). The non-hyperfunctional adenoma is likely to be solid; the 20% which are cystic may be aspirated, the specimen containing cellular debris, colloid, macrophages, altered blood and occasional simple follicular cells. A cautionary note would remind the cytopathologist of the possibility of a cystic papillary carcinoma whose lining cells may be equally banal but

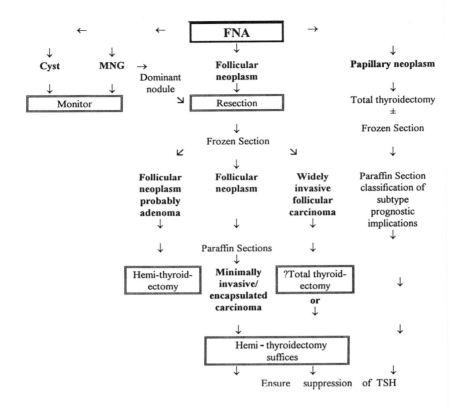

Fig. 11.1A   Investigation of goitre: solitary nodule. MNG, multinodular goitre.

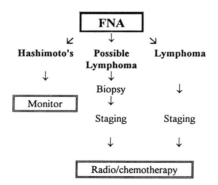

Fig. 11.1B   Investigation of goitre: solitary in diffuse (e.g. Hashimoto's with localized swelling).

should show the nuclear grooves and small nucleoli of a papillary neoplasm. It is important when examining cyst fluid to consider the possibility of a neoplasm — papillary or follicular — with cystic change. Approximately 80% of solid lesions prove to be benign, representing follicular adenomata; the remainder will prove to be malignant.

While FNA of thyroid can often give an accurate diagnosis, there are a number of well-recognized problem areas. These are similar to the difficulties encountered in the histopathological interpretation of thyroid biopsies. While it is possible to identify anaplastic and poorly differentiated follicular carcinomas, benign follicular neoplasms (adenomas) cannot be distinguished from well-differentiated, encapsulated or minimally invasive follicular carcinomas on cytological grounds alone. Therefore the statement 'no malignant cells identified' becomes a meaningless and often misleading comment on thyroid aspirate reports. In addition, it may not be possible to differentiate an adenomatous nodule in a multinodular goitre from a follicular adenoma, particularly where the usual features of multinodular goitre are lacking. Here the best the cytopathologist can do is to give an assessment of which features on balance are more prominent and more in keeping with a multinodular goitre or a follicular neoplasm. Here the statement that 'a neoplasm cannot be excluded' may be helpful.

A common problem area is the identification of lymphoma in Hashimoto's thyroiditis. This should always be considered in aspirates where there has been a recent unexplained change in the gland, particularly an asymmetric change. The picture is often complicated by the presence of pleomorphic Askanazy cells which distract the observer from the background lymphoid cells which often have a more banal appearance. Here immunohistochemical markers are useful in confirming the monoclonality of such an infiltrate as lymphoma.

One cannot overemphasize the importance of correlating the histopathological and cytopathological appearances in thyroid disease. Although not normally aspirated, it is important to be familiar with the appearances of the normal thyroid gland before attempting to report FNA of thyroid lesions. Aspirating fresh tissue sent for frozen section examination is an easy way to gain experience of the range of changes seen in normal and also in diffuse non-neoplastic disease as well as the cytological appearances associated with neoplasms. This practice is recommended to the beginner. The technique allows the accurate correlation of the cytopathological and histopathological appearances from clearly defined sites and lesions within the thyroid gland. It is important that clinicians and cytopathologists work closely together and adopt meaningful terminology in order to develop and maintain confidence in the accuracy of a cytopathology report. Regular clinicopathological review of cases is a useful method of promoting this mutual understanding. With experience it is possible to develop a high degree of accuracy in reporting FNA of thyroid (Table 11.1)

An aspirate from *normal thyroid* should yield blood-stained material containing a few small aggregates of regular follicular cells with fragile cytoplasm and denuded follicular nuclei which resemble lymphocytes (Fig.

Table 11.1   Achievable accuracy of FNA: comparison of FNA
result and subsequent biopsy

Cytopathology	Histopathology
Multinodular goitre	95% Multinodular goitre
	5% Follicular neoplasm
Follicular neoplasm	85% Follicular adenoma
	15% Follicular carcinoma
	100% Carcinoma
Malignant { Follicular / Papillary / Undifferentiated }	
Lymphoma	100% Lymphoma

11.2). Within these follicular clusters, the nuclei frequently overlap, giving a
three-dimensional appearance to the groups. Some small flat sheets of
follicular cells may also be seen. Colloid is thin and scanty. It may be difficult
to distinguish the colloid from the serum accompanying the blood. C cells are
very scanty and not usually recognizable in smears. Inflammatory cells, other
than those in the blood, are not usually present in smears from normal thyroid
but may be increased in number if there has been excessive palpation of the
gland immediately prior to aspiration. Extrathyroidal tissue may be identified
in aspirated material and it is important to recognize skin, adipose tissue,
cartilage, tracheal respiratory epithelium and skeletal muscle when present.
In addition, the lesion aspirated may, either known or unknown to the
clinician, lie outwith the thyroid gland and may represent lymph node,
parathyroid or salivary gland, or thyroglossal, branchial or skin adnexal cyst.

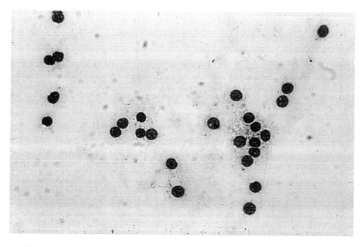

Fig. 11.2   FNA normal thyroid. Regular follicular cells with fragile cytoplasm and some
denuded nuclei resembling lymphocytes. (Papanicolaou stain.)

In the following situations, FNA will prove a reliable component in the investigation.

Localized enlargement

The majority of apparently solitary swellings in fact, represent exaggerated nodularity in a *multinodular goitre*. Here the basic multicellular elements may be seen in aspirated material. Colloid — some thick and cracked, some thin and amorphous with scattered sheets of follicular cells — some of which may be very large — are all typical features (Fig. 11.3). The nuclei of the follicular cells in these sheets are uniform. The cytoplasm is feathery and delicate but some areas may show the well-defined and granular cytoplasm of Hurthle cells. The cytoplasm is often dispersed leaving bare nuclei which resemble lymphocytes. An admixture of foamy macrophages containing iron and finely divided lipid together with degenerating erythrocytes, occasional multinucleated giant cells and fibrous stromal fragments are common.

An area of diagnostic difficulty pertains in the aspiration of a *cellular, dominant nodule* within a multinodular goitre. In this situation, the cellularity is greater. Follicular aggregates varying in size, streaks of denuded follicular nuclei and prominent sheets of uniform follicular cells may be encountered but the regular honeycomb architecture favours a non-neoplastic interpretation.

The aspirate may consist entirely of thin colloid with cholesterol and foamymacrophages suggesting a diagnosis of *simple thyroid cyst*. This can be

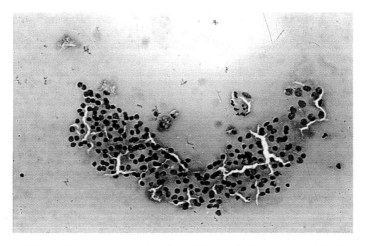

Fig. 11.3 FNA multinodular goitre. Abundant thick, cracked colloid and follicular cells, some forming large sheets. Nuclei are uniform. (Papanicolaou stain.)

managed by regular follow-up and repeat aspiration if fluid re-accumulates. Any tendency for persistence or re-accumulation will warrant resection of the lesion. It is important to bear in mind the possibility of a cystic papillary carcinoma, both within the gland and, if the origin of the aspirate is unclear, in a lateral cervical node. An aspirate consisting entirely of crystal-clear fluid is almost certainly derived from a *parathyroid cyst*. The sample will be virtually acellular and its nature should be confirmed by parathormone estimation of the fluid rather than by microscopy.

FNA may permit a diagnosis of *follicular neoplasm* but will not allow evaluation of its biological growth potential. Since a diagnosis of minimally invasive follicular carcinoma requires the examination of the entire capsule, it is evident that FNA cannot allow recognition of this entity or its distinction from a follicular adenoma. However, surgical resection, probably entailing hemithyroidectomy, is the treatment of choice for both conditions. Such aspirates are cellular and acini or microfollicular clusters are to be expected. The nuclei are enlarged over the normal, contain macronucleoli and may show crowding. There may be some nuclear variation (Fig. 11.4). Colloid is usually scanty or absent but abundant watery colloid may be present in aspirates from a large macrofollicular neoplasm.

On occasion, the cytological appearances alone will denote a *follicular carcinoma*. The aspirate is usually blood-stained and may be highly cellular, the cells showing enlarged, hyperchromatic nuclei, prominent irregular or multiple nucleoli and coarse chromatin. *Hurthle cell tumours* will, on FNA, lack colloid but contain numerous follicular cells showing granular cytoplasm staining orange with Papanicolaou or eosinophilic with haematoxylin and eosin stains. There is often notable nuclear pleomorphism, not pathognomonic of malignancy. It is of interest that the nuclear variation seen may be

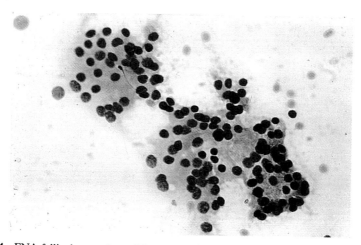

Fig. 11.4 FNA follicular neoplasm. Microfollicular clusters with scanty colloid. The nuclei are larger than normal and show crowding and anisonucleosis. (Papanicolaou stain.)

less than that in the Hurthle (Askanazy) cells of Hashimoto's thyroiditis. Follicular neoplasms, with or without Hurthle cell change, warrant excision.

FNA will permit recognition of the majority of *papillary carcinomata*. The aspirate is cellular containing flat sheets of epithelial cells with a sharp delineating border. This vertical alignment of cells is a useful feature. True papillary fragments in a three-dimensional pattern are a helpful feature but not always present in aspirates. The cell cytoplasm is more solid, resembling that of immature squamous metaplastic cells with distinct cytoplasmic borders. The nuclei contain pale nucleoplasm with a micronucleolus often located on the nuclear membrane. The nuclear membrane is sharply defined and is enfolded, producing nuclear grooves. Intranuclear cytoplasmic protrusions are a typical and useful feature. These nuclear characteristics must be sought but they will be present in most cases (Fig. 11.5). However, an occasional nucleus demonstrating such appearances, in particular the intranuclear protrusion, may be seen in other forms of thyroid neoplasm such as medullary carcinoma. Colloid is scanty and viscous, often pulled out like chewing gum. Psammoma bodies — concentric calcified laminations — when seen, are virtual pathognomonic of papillary carcinoma, but these are infrequently present and care must be taken to distinguish these from the globules of thick colloid.

Though rare, the *medullary carcinoma* of thyroid may be recognized in FNA. The cells are often dispersed and may be round, oval, plasmacytoid or spindle in shape. The cytoplasm is finely granular. Nuclear morphology varies considerably and does not allow specific recognition. If fragments of amyloid are present they can be identified by Congo red staining. Measurement of plasma calcitonin and other appropriate clinical investigations should follow, in an attempt to establish the diagnosis prior to surgery.

The cytological diagnosis of *malignant lymphoma* is usually feasible but, though surgery may be appropriate, preoperative staging is warranted. Since the lymphocytic element of Hashimoto's thyroiditis may exhibit considerable cytological variation, immunohistochemical studies — to demonstrate light change restriction — are necessary. If the cytological impression is suspicious but indefinite, open biopsy with histological and immunohistochemical examination of the tissue will follow and allow diagnosis, classification and grading.

The FNA from an *undifferentiated (anaplastic) carcinoma* may contain polymorphs, fragments of necrotic tissue and pleomorphic cells, often of spindle or giant cell morphology, lying singly or in groups. It may be difficult to distinguish from a true sarcoma or from metastasis to the gland. While there may be no management implications, identification of the epithelial cells by immunohistochemistry may be warranted. Since no therapy is feasible, FNA is a useful method of investigation, preventing unnecessary and often hazardous surgery. In addition, the clinical impression of rapid enlargement of a hard gland may not permit distinction between malignant

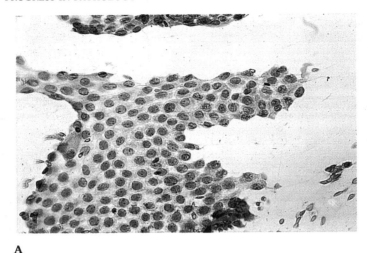

A

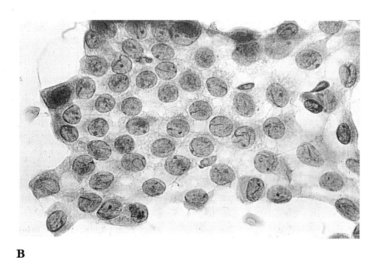

B

Fig. 11.5   FNA papillary carcinoma. **A** Flat sheet of cells with palisaded straight edge, metaplastic-like cell cytoplasm and distinct cytoplasmic borders. (Papanicolaou stain.) **B** The nuclei are pale staining with a micronucleolus often located on the nuclear membrane. The nuclear membrane is sharply defined and enfolded, producing nuclear grooves and intranuclear cytoplasmic protrusions. (Papanicolaou stain.)

lymphoma and undifferentiated carcinoma and, since the prognosis is so different, FNA plays an important role in establishing the correct diagnosis.

Diffuse enlargement

Aspiration cytology plays a role in the diagnosis of the various forms of thyroiditis. In *Hashimoto's thyroiditis*, the smears are cellular with little colloid, abundant lymphocytes, plasma cells and Hurthle (Askanazy) cells (Fig. 11.6). The latter may show considerable nuclear variation. Large lymphoid cells, often derived from germinal centres, and occasional multi-nucleated giant cells may be seen. If the lymphoid component is monomorphic and if the aspirate derives from a localized area of gland enlargement in a patient on adequate replacement thyroxine, then the possibility of lymphoma will be raised. Immunohistochemical pursuit of monotypic light chain expression should follow.

Subacute (de Quervin's) thyroiditis is rare and seldom subject to FNA. However, the aspirate usually contains multinucleated giant cells with small lymphocytes, macrophages and scattered follicular cells, many degenerate, lying in scanty colloid.

In *Riedel's thyroidits*, with its inflammatory and fibrous replacement of the gland, an acellular aspirate is to be expected; occasional fibroblasts may be seen.

The diagnosis of *Graves' disease* is seldom pursued or accompanied by aspiration cytopathology. The product is usually devoid of colloid but may show high cellularity. The follicular cells are enlarged with abundant

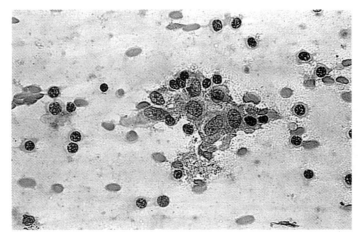

Fig. 11.6   FNA Hashimoto's thyroiditis. Cellular smear with lymphocytes, plasma cells and Askanazy (Hurthle) cells showing marked nuclear variation. (Papanicolaou stain.)

vacuolated cytoplasm and form ring groups. There may be marked variation in nuclear size. A component of lymphocytes is entirely acceptable but makes the condition difficult, in the absence of clinical information, to distinguish from Hashimoto's thyroiditis.

In *dyshormonogenesis*, the gland is highly cellular and may show considerable nuclear pleomorphism. For this reason, a diagnosis of malignant neoplasia will seldom be reached on FNA; indeed, the most strict criteria are required for such a diagnosis in this condition even on histological grounds. Localized benign neoplasia may occur but is more likely to represent focal hyperplasia in a generalized hypercellular gland. If there is localized enlargement in the background of pre-existing dyshormonogenic goitre, examination of an aspirate from the localized area, from elsewhere in that lobe and from the contralateral lobe may be valuable in allowing cytological comparison, but if any concern persists about the nature of the localized swelling, hemithyroidectomy will be warranted.

KEY POINTS FOR CLINICAL PRACTICE

- The typical multicellular elements of a multinodular goitre are usually readily identified in aspirated material but, on occasion, the cytological differentiation between multinodular goitre and follicular neoplasm can be difficult.
- Obtaining fluid with a typical colloid and cholesterol admixture may denote a cystic lesion which, if small, can be managed by regular follow-up, with resection following any repeated re-accumulation of the fluid or growth of the lesion. Care should be taken when reporting cyst fluids to distinguish between multinodular goitre, cystic follicular neoplasm and cystic papillary carcinoma.
- Observing the typical nuclear morphology, in an appropriate background of the papillary carcinoma, provides a high degree of diagnostic accuracy.
- The establishment of the nature, but not the biological potential, of a follicular neoplasm and distinguishing this from the heterogeneous elements of a multinodular goitre, allows appropriate surgical management. Terms such as 'no malignant cells identified' should not be used in the cytopathology report.
- On occasion, the cytological appearances alone will denote a follicular carcinoma. More often, the uniformity of cell morphology, while denoting a follicular neoplasm, does not allow assessment of any invasive element. Surgical resection will follow. Surgical debate may obtain in the management of papillary and follicular carcinoma but standard practice remains that the papillary carcinoma merits total thyroidectomy with removal of only obviously involved lymph nodes. The follicular neoplasm (the adenoma or the encapsulated carcinoma) warrants unilobectomy. A surgical impression of extension outwith the gland will dictate the appropriate surgical management.

REFERENCES

Davidson GH, Campora RG 1991 Thyroid In: Bibbo M (ed) Comprehensive cytopathology. WB Saunders, London, p 649–670

Franklyn JA, Daykin J, Young J et al 1993 Fine needle aspiration cytology in diffuse or multinodular goitre compared with solitary thyroid nodules. Br Med J 307: 240

Kline TS 1988 Thyroid gland. Handbook of fine needle aspiration biopsy cytology. Churchill Livingstone, Edinburgh, Vol 6, p 153

Koss LG 1992 The thyroid. Diagnostic cytology and its histopathologic bases Lippincott, Philadelphia, Vol 2, Ch 29, Part II, p 1268

Koss LG, Zajicek J 1992 Aspiration biopsy. Diagnostic cytology and its histopathologic bases. Lippincott, Philadelphia, Vol 2, Ch 29, p 1234

Koss LG, Woykes S, Olszewski W 1984 The thyroid. Aspiration biopsy. Cytologic interpretations and histologic bases. Igaku-Shoin, Tokyo

Miller TR 1990 Fine needle aspiration of the thyroid gland. In: RW Astarita (ed) Practical cytology. Churchill Livingstone, Edinburgh, Vol 6, p 233

Orell SR, Sterrett GF, Walters MN-I et al 1992 The thyroid gland. Manual and atlas of fine needle aspiration cytology. 2nd edn. Churchill Livingstone, Edinburgh, p 96–128

Sterrett GF 1993 In: JA Young (ed) Fine needle aspiration cytopathology. Blackwells, London, Ch 5, p 31

Zajicek J 1979 Aspiration biopsy cytology. Cytology of supradiaphragmatic organs. Karger, Basel, p 67

12. Clinical audit in histopathology

N. Gibbs   N. Kirkham

'As is your Pathology, so is your Medicine' wrote Osler. Pathology has a vital role to play in determining the overall clinical performance of a hospital. At the same time it has to keep its own house in order. Only by maintaining or improving our own standards can we justify the trust put in us to enquire into disease in the living and the dead. When standards fall then we all suffer.

The report of the enquiry into deficiencies in the cervical cytopathology service at the Inverclyde Hospital near Glasgow in 1993 pointed to a number of deficiencies, including a lack of both internal and external quality controls, together with the problems associated with an individual pathologist working alone and attempting to deal with an excessive workload without undertaking continuing education to keep up to date with developments in the field. All of this was complicated by a lack of communication between the laboratory and the hospital management. A week before this report was published the preliminary report of the enquiry into the bone pathology service in the West Midlands was published. This told a similar story, combining a pathologist working alone and a lack of effective internal or external quality controls.

At the time of writing it was reported that the West Midlands faced a bill likely to be not far short of £30 million in compensation payments to those patients with benign disease who had been given malignant diagnoses and vice versa. The bill would probably have to be settled by raising money from hospital closures. In this chapter we will describe some of the aspects of audit, or quality control, that may help to avoid similar occurrences in the future.

DEFINITION

Quality assurance applies to outcome and the way resources are used to provide a service which will best benefit the patient. *Quality control* relates to the control of laboratory processes and all stages to diagnosis. Correct diagnosis is only part of the process and quality assurance goes beyond this by monitoring the impact of the histopathology report on patient care. Thus timeliness, consultative skill and effective and lucid communication are part of quality assurance, while internal laboratory efficiency is quality control. All these considerations are loosely defined as *audit* and the principles are straightforward and well understood (Lee 1989, Shaw & Costain 1989). Audit

213

is an essential part of *accreditation* (Anonymous 1989) and is reinforced by proposals for the reforms of the National Health Service (Department of Health 1989a, Royal College of Pathologists 1989a). The methods of assessing quality assurance and control are external and internal quality assessment schemes (EQAS and IQAS).

HISTORY AND BACKGROUND

Quality control has always been recognized as an essential part of the regulation of clinical laboratory testing where standardized analytical procedures are the responsibility of non-medical scientific officers and scientists [World Health Organization (WHO) 1981]. The development of the scope of clinical laboratories clearly underlines the necessity for quality control monitoring (Whitehead & Woodford 1981). Peer review of practice is the basis of professional development (Committee of enquiry into competence to practice (Alment Committee) 1975) and attempts at quality control of performance in anatomical pathology laboratories have been mainly by external expert review aimed at accuracy in diagnosis (Owen & Tighe 1975, Rickert 1986). Histopathology, however, is a complex, labour intensive, multifaceted speciality that does not easily lend itself to the discipline of audit, although quality control and quality evaluation have long been recognized as an important objective (Penner 1973, Langley 1978, WHO 1981).

Histopathologists accept a review of technical aspects, but there is resistance to the review of histopathological diagnosis which is regarded by many as a subjective process of experience and judgement that is more an art than a scientific skill and as such may be objectively untestable. It can be accepted that quality assurance in certain difficult areas can be an unattainable ideal but experience has shown that an audit programme can improve the performance of a histopathological department (Morson 1983, Cree et al 1993, Thomas et al 1983). The design of such a system is complicated first by the difficulty of obtaining an acknowledged diagnosis based on an opinion, second by the need for clinical and other pathological data before a diagnosis is reached, and third by variations in terminology.

Owen & Tighe (1975) developed a system of quality evaluation based on consensus diagnosis (peer review). In their scheme the diagnoses made by participants were placed into two categories of major or minor diagnostic differences that could or could not lead to inappropriate treatment. A number of histopathologists since that date have developed in-house systems which have tended to be retrospective, cumbersome and time consuming (Murthy & Derman 1981, Whitehead et al 1984). No general movement towards general audit was made until 1989 when the Department of Health published the background and terms of reference of the EQAS (Lewis & Jennings 1989). In the same year a combined meeting, called 'Laboratory Accreditation and Audit', of the Association of Clinical Pathologists and the Royal College of Pathologists considered audit in all disciplines of pathology and recommended a national programme. This meeting was held in the context of the Department of Health (1989a,b) publications 'Working for patients' and 'Working for patients: medical audit'. In other countries such as Canada, Australia, New Zealand and the USA, audit had developed apace. In the USA, medical audit has expanded at an exponential rate to a nationwide concept of quality assurance for all health care (Hoffman 1989). In 1988 the United States Congress has also proposed federal standards called 'Clinical Laboratory Improvement Amendments 1988'. Whereas the pathologist considers quality an innate part of the work ethic, the government and consumer now expect quantitation of that quality with regard to costs, i.e. 'quality at what cost' instead of 'quality at all costs' (Department of Health and Human Services 1990).

The Advisory Task Force on Standards to the Audit Steering Committee of the Royal College of Pathologists (1991) made the following recommendations which have yet to be brought into practice.

1. All departments should participate in relevant EQAS organized by the clinical pathology accreditation advisory committees.
2. Appropriate quality assurance programmes should be widely published with a regular review of performance.
3. Quality assurance programmes should include clinical audit and should examine access, process, output, outcome and the use of resources.
4. Senior pathology staff should regularly participate in the audit activities of other clinical specialties.

In the USA, the Association of Directors of Anatomic and Surgical Pathology (1992) published their recommendations for the standardization of the surgical pathology report. The majority of their recommendations are part of the general practice of histopathologists in the UK but a number of possible recommendations are relevant.

1. Demographic information should be complete and entered at the top of the report.
2. Surgical pathology number should be placed on the top portion of each page of a report and that each is italicized or underlined.
3. Include a clinical summary.
4. Include a separate section listing 'specimens submitted' in every report so that each can be clearly identified as a separate specimen.
5. Each separately identified specimen should have a gross description and record whether 'part or all' is submitted for microscopic examination.
6. Identify each block with a unique number or letter.
7. Use pictorial records in complicated specimens. These should be included in the report (see Table 12.1).

Table 12.1   Example of complicated report incorporating audit recommendations

---

Surgical identification number (S number)
Surgeon
Biographical data of patient
Computer patient accession number
Computer identity number
Previous relevant accession numbers
Date of receipt of specimen
Clinical information
Date of report
Date of printing
Example of complicated specimen. NB: in small specimens state whether all or part of tissue
is embedded

1. AP excision of rectum, macroscopic description (blocks 1a, b long axis of ca; c, d
   transverse axis; e proximal polyps, 4; f distal line of excision; g lymph glands level 1; h
   lymph glands level 2; i lymph glands level 3; j lymph glands level 4)

2. Polyps removed at colonoscopy from ascending colon, macroscopic description (blocks
   2a(2))

3. Polyps removed at colonoscopy from descending colon, macroscopic description (blocks
   3a(3))

Macroscopic description of 1, 2, 3 can be incorporated in one report or separately as
appropriate.
Microscopic description. Note special stains
SNOMED code

FINAL DIAGNOSIS (STAGING SUMMARY)

A0denocarcinoma of rectum (grade 2, Dukes' C) with lymph gland metastases at level 1.
Maximum tumour thickness (15 mm). Lateral margin spread beyond serosa to adherent
omentum

NB: in referred cases get reports co-signed or alternatively record events, e.g. also seen
by...............
Print the name of junior staff making a report and the consultant checker

---

EXTERNAL AUDIT (EXTERNAL ASSESSMENT SCHEME; EQAS)

Audit in the UK has developed rapidly since 1989 generally by circulations
of slides as an external audit procedure (Klys & Lessels 1992, Sherwood &
Hunt 1984). Slide club circulations between groups of interested pathologists
have been a universal mechanism for spreading experience and keeping up to
date. Slide circulations provide a method of anonymous peer review across a
wide range of material within a defined group of hospitals, over one or more
regions (Klys & Lessels 1992) or even the whole country (Beck et al 1985).
There is the advantage of testing diagnostic skill, albeit with limited clinical
information, perhaps only one histopathological slide and without special
stains. This rather narrow scope can be improved by formalizing the written
reports and including SNOMED codes together with tumour grades and
staging summaries where appropriate. If the diagnosis is uncertain the
possible diagnosis can be listed in descending order of probability, i.e. by
self-marking. Mean scores can be calculated for alternative diagnoses among
the group and compared with individual scores so that criteria of acceptability

can be developed (Furness & Lauder 1993). It is certain that some histopathologists may score badly in some specialist fields where there is no experience or responsibility but allowance can be made for this in the programme. Finally there is the question of whether a diagnosis that is recognized as incorrect matters in the context of patient care (outcome audit) and so an additional score can be given for this item. Alternatively diagnostic accuracy and quality of care can be combined in a stratified scoring system. An example of an external audit programme and grades of scoring is shown in Table 12.2. It should be emphasized that flexibility is important in designing a comprehensive quality assurance programme (Rickert 1986) and an individual audit strategy should be developed for each laboratory (Ramsay 1991).

Anonymity

Anonymity is regarded by some as an essential prerequisite before joining an external audit programme. If the assessment is truly anonymous the identity of pathologists under test will be unknown to their colleagues or reviewers. In this event measures to improve poor scores may be impossible even if considered desirable. Participants are invited to identify their returns by a unique number known only to them with the proviso that the same number must be used in all subsequent circulations. A general report on each slide circulation can be sent to each participant which includes a cumulative list of scores for each unique number leaving individual pathologists to interpret results and hopefully to take any measures that may be necessary to improve performance. However, good and bad performers are not identified by name

Table 12.2 External audit proforma

Name and unique number			
Clinical and pathological information			
Report			10
Diagnosis	If in your opinion there is more than one possible	1	
	diagnosis award yourself marks for each with a total	2	
	of 10 marks to indicate the probability of each	3	
	alternative being correct	Total	10
Staging summary and grade (where appropriate)			(10)
SNOMED CODE			10
Quality of care	a. No clinical significance in the error		10
	b. Intermediate clinical significance		5
	c. Definite or substantial clinical significance		0
or alternative			
	A. No significant change in classification of disease		
	or guidance to clinicians		10
	B. Minor change in diagnosis or guidance		5
	C. Significant change in diagnosis or guidance		0
		TOTAL	60(70)

and only compliant pathologists are tested; refusers are not identified or tested and there is no mechanism for improving low scorers. In practice someone, but not necessarily a histopathologist, should hold the identity codes for all participants. Limited access to identity codes is admissible in circumstances agreed amongst the group in advance.

Advantages

External audit tests diagnostic skill under limited conditions. Schemes can be augmented to evaluate reports and their effects on quality of care. The scoring system may reveal potential deficiencies in practice after several circulations. Action may be desirable in this event. Nevertheless an external audit programme will reveal quite serious inconsistencies in the diagnosis of some lesions which can be evaluated by kappa statistics (Robertson et al 1989, Beck et al 1985, Holman et al 1983). One must not be misled into exaggerating inconsistencies of reporting, as minor nuances of histopathological diagnosis do not stand up to rigorous field testing (Lee 1989).

Disadvantages

Slide circulations are generally composed of interesting or unusual cases which do not test the everyday or banal cases. External audit does not test the pathologist in his laboratory or the efficiency or performance of his histopathological department as a whole.

INTERNAL AUDIT (INTERNAL QUALITY ASSESSMENT SCHEME; IQAS)

An integrated programme in surgical and autopsy pathology must take account of each step in the diagnostic process from the time the surgeon removes the lesion from the patient until the diagnostic report leaves the laboratory (Thomas et al 1991) or perhaps reaches the patient's notes! Delivery services to and from a department were investigated and found wanting in the Royal College of Pathologists pilot scheme in laboratory accreditation (The College Accreditation Steering Committee 1990) which resulted in delays in reporting dispatch for no good reason.

The histopathological report is the final expression of a complex process where responsibility passes step by step from porter, reception clerk, medical laboratory scientific officers, junior and senior pathologists, secretary and data processor, back to the senior pathologist for final checking and signing before dispatch to hospital wards, out-patient or record departments by ward clerks or by post to other hospitals. Standards should be established and targets set to be reached (Ramsay & Gallagher 1992). The timing and content of reports must be suitable and acceptable to surgeons and clinicians in different specialities with different views and requirements. Every pathologist practises market research in some form but may still be the last person to be aware of criticism so no opportunity should be missed to discuss patients and reports with clinicians. Clinical meetings whether formalized or not can identify specific problem areas in diagnosis and provide information regarding diagnostic changes that is unlikely to be available from other sources (McBroom & Ramsay 1993). Reports should be clear and concise and reach clinicians within agreed time limits (Chow & Dilly 1991). Pathologists must answer for what they do and whether it is done well and must be able to convince others that high standards are being maintained (Cowan 1990). Communication skills and timeliness as well as diagnostic acumen are all part of the process and the correct diagnosis is only part of the practice of histopathology. A searching programme of internal audit will also act as a clinical audit by revealing errors and deficiencies in clinical information and documentation and poor performers should be notified (Zuk et al 1991).

Histopathologists' performance by peer review

Considering the natural history of many diseases and the low autopsy rate it is clear that many mistakes in diagnosis may never be discovered. These mistakes may be harmful and influence outcome and must be distinguished from errors which do not threaten or influence outcome (outcome audit). Errors are made unknowingly, so cases for review should be selected at random (random case review) by some suitable scheme such as a random number computer program.

The only exception to random case review is the ongoing review of special procedures, e.g. frozen section, bone marrow biopsy (Cheung & Collins 1992, Bishop et al 1992). Case review should look for accuracy in diagnosis, clarity and timeliness in reports (Murthy & Derman 1981, Herd et al 1992). Above all, reports should be understood by clinicians and set out in such a way that important clinical points are not submerged in descriptive text. The diagnostic summary may be useful in a wide range of reports and it is essential if they are long and complicated. Terminology should be standardized as far as possible or, if not, alternative names for the same condition given with a final diagnosis. Mistakes can be distinguished from differences in interpretation which are not errors but demonstrations of the limitations of the histopathological method. However, in the event of a change in diagnosis subsequent upon a review, a record of any actions should be made. Outside referrals and diagnostic changes which result should be recorded.

Efficiency or the effective use of resources to reach a diagnosis gives a measure of cost efficiency; for example, the average cost per week, month, or year can be calculated within broad limits, bearing in mind the histopathologist must not be regarded as a 'reporting machine' and must be expected to incorporate an element for clinical teaching and research into the routine clinical work.

Turnaround times should as far as possible be standardized within a laboratory, but in general should be no longer than 2 working days for small specimens and 5 working days for larger specimens excluding time unavoidably lost. Employment and training of junior medical staff tends to increase turnaround time. Turnaround times should aim at meeting the requirements of clinical users. The advantage of IQAS is that the whole laboratory process can be audited, but a possible disadvantage is that most medical audits are retrospective.

Organization of internal audit or review

Review should not be carried out by the reporting pathologist but either by a respected pathologist, possibly from a neighbouring laboratory (Stuart & Hicks 1991), or by an audit pathologist appointed for this purpose. The review should aim at a maximum 4% of workload but this would depend on the time available for audit. Thoroughness is more important than volume. Randomly selected cases should include request form, slides, special stains and the final report. A recording sheet should be designed to take account of clinical information, technical performance, pathologist's audit, and subdivisions for the report, reporting time and quality of care and or outcome audit. An example of a recording sheet is shown in Table 12.3.

The role of internal audit in laboratory function

Although internal audit is carried out at the level of pathologists, it includes all laboratory staff whatever their role. It follows that the results of an internal audit should be made available to all. Representatives of the laboratory staff should meet regularly to discuss the results of audit in a formal way (Barr & Williams 1982, Lee 1989). Large laboratories may institute an independent technical audit. Errors and deficiencies should be minuted together with a record of any corrective action that is taken. It is useful to issue an annual report enumerating the results of audit.

Discussion

There is little doubt that even in the best departments where audit can be described as merely the formalization and documentation of best practice, a programme can benefit the efficiency and standards of the laboratory, and has an educational value (Batstone 1992). It also emphasizes team work which is essential for smooth running, and all grades of staff become aware of the importance of their individual role in the production of the final report and its effect on patient care. The advantages are perhaps best seen in big departments where the work may be subdivided into specialist groups with little continuity. Alternatively, small departments in a district environment may become isolated and overburdened with work and find little opportunity

Table 12.3 Scoring sheet for internal and intradepartmental audit

CLINICAL AUDIT	Maximum score	Actual score
Request form		
Biographical data	1	
Specimen information	1	
Clinical history and details	1	
TECHNICAL AUDIT		
Technical performance		
Section quality	1	
Staining quality	1	
Special stains	1	
PATHOLOGIST'S AUDIT		
Report		
Macroscopic description (description of main organ; additional tissues separate from main specimen)	3	
Microscopic report (free text; diagnosis; excision margins; SNOMED coding and staging)	3	
Final diagnosis with grade and staging summary in malignant tumours as required	3	
REPORTING EFFICIENCY AUDIT		
Reporting time (turnover time) based on 3 working days for small specimens; 5 working days for large specimens (excluding special techniques, e.g. decal, EM, markers, etc.)	3	
QUALITY OF CARE AUDIT		
The probable effects of any deficiency or inaccuracy in audit 1–4 inclusive on patient care or outcome	3	
	21	

decal = decalcification; EM = electron microscopy

to discuss wider issues and lapse into idiosyncratic reporting. It is axiomatic that effective management of a histopathology service requires a reliable indicator of the volume of work (Cevill 1988). Overburdened departments should improve staffing levels rather than sacrifice audit procedures.

There have been few reports of internal audit of all histopathology reports in a general histopathology laboratory. A 1-year study of quality assurance with a second pathologist routinely reviewing all surgical pathology reports revealed an error rate of 0.26% with half of the errors affecting clinical care (Safrin & Bark 1993).

Although the advantages of audit seem undeniable, there is little doubt that an effective programme is time consuming and requires organization. It cannot succeed if it is regarded as an irritating irrelevance to normal pratice. Staffing levels in a department should take account of the time element inherent in the audit programme bearing in mind that raising standards requires a review of working practices (Thomas et al 1991). Time should be set aside for meetings on a regular basis and attendance should be *de riguer*.

Dynamic organization of audit is essential to prevent a drift into ineffective bureaucracy.

Additional functions of audit

1. Training audit. Experience and knowledge can be tested and formalized by audit so that the effective use of technical and medical education programmes can be scrutinized by audit methods (Tildsley & Dilly 1991).
2. Autopsy and histology reports have their place in the clinician's audit. The pathologist is an essential member of a clinical audit team (Herd et al 1992).
3. Cancer registries depend on correct information and a histology audit is a valuable means of testing the reliability of registry information (Lapham & Waugh 1992).
4. Central histopathological registry has a role in quality assurance of histopathological diagnosis in certain circumstances (Whitehead et al 1986).

Reaction to audit

Audit is not an end in itself! Deficiencies may be illuminated by audit procedures but laboratories need help in recognizing trends which can lead to improvements in laboratory performance. Changing trends in therapy may require changes in detail and emphasis in histology reports. To this end training courses can be developed for pathologists to take account of therapeutic changes or improvements which may alter the importance of the factual data and thus influence the report as a clinical information system. Regular attendance in such an education structured programme should be recommended. Continuing medical education in the UK is voluntary but in the USA, Canada and New Zealand the situation is different. The American system of credits is attractive for continuing education (Pennington 1989). Certainly medical audit has educational implications (Standing Committee of Postgraduate Medical Education 1990) which must be addressed. The primary objective of medical audit is to improve the overall standard of patient care rather than attempting to identify 'bad apples' (Conference of Medical Royal Colleges 1991).

AUTOPSY AUDIT

Autopsy as an audit procedure can be considered under two main headings. The first is to increase the number of autopsies to a level that is necessary for clinical audit. The second is to plan the autopsy service to make it an effective mechanism for clinical audit.

General considerations

There is a feeling among some clinicians that advances in investigative techniques in all fields have reduced the need for autopsy and this is one of the main factors for decline in rate throughout the world (Harris et al 1993). Certainly lack of clinical interest in autopsy is a factor (Peacock et al 1988). In fact discrepancies between clinical and autopsy diagnosis have remained at around 10%; that is, autopsies have revealed disease which if detected during life would have led to changes in clinical management (Goldman et al 1983, Anderson 1984, Schned et al 1986, Peacock et al 1988, Shanks et al 1991, Mosquera & Goldman 1993). In general autopsies show that deaths due to cardiovascular disease are generally overestimated (Thomas et al 1988, Jamjoom et al 1991, Kendall et al 1993). Furthermore autopsies in patients with malignant disease have shown only 75% agreement that malignancy was the cause of death and that the primary site was correctly identified in only 56% of the cases (Mollo et al 1986). Unsuspected abnormalities were found in 80% of paediatric autopsies (Russell & Berry 1989, Rushton 1991). Mortality statistics which are not supported by autopsy should be viewed with caution. Autopsy is regarded as an essential mechanism for clinical audit and an overall rate of 35% has been suggested as adequate (Yesner et al 1985). Nevertheless there are no studies showing a correlation between an increase in autopsy rate and subsequent decrease in clinicopathological discrepancies, so indisputable proof that autopsy is indispensable for clinical audit is lacking (Battle et al 1987). The report ('The autopsy and audit') of a Joint Working Party of the Royal Colleges (1991) gives detailed consideration to this subject and should be read by pathologists and clinicians alike.

Current position

Autopsies are performed on approximately 1 in 4 people dying in England and Wales, of which 90% are requested by the Coroner (Ashworth 1991). The number of coroners' autopsies has only diminished by 6.6% in the last decade compared with a much greater decline in autopsies performed with the relatives' permission (Anonymous 1991). In spite of the recommendation by the Royal Colleges that a summary of autopsy findings should be despatched within 2 days and a complete report within 3 weeks, it is known that some hospitals fall below these standards (Whitty et al 1991). The Joint Working Party recommend that a complete histopathological examination should be done in all cases but this may not be possible for coroners' autopsies partly because of cost in the market-driven National Health Service or because it is not necessary to establish the cause of death! The view that histopathological examination is essential to prove the cause of death has not been tested in detail although all pathologists know the value of microscopic examination in suspected myocardial infarct for example (Davies et al 1989). Clinicians tend to regard autopsies as unpleasant and suspect that they may carry disease from the mortuary to their patients. For the latter group the installation of facilities such as audiovisual presentation can be regarded as essential.

Autopsy audit in practice

1. Before autopsy can be used as a method of clinical audit it is important that autopsies themselves are performed to agreed standards (Harrison & Hourihane 1989). Guidelines for the investigation of neurological, neurosurgical and psychiatric death as well as sudden and unexpected infant death are available (The College Accreditation Steering Committee 1990, Royal College of Pathologists 1993).
2. Autopsies are not immune from error and the extent of that error needs to be assessed by peer review or other convenient method (Saracci 1991).
3. Autopsies should be selected by random sampling if tests of clinical sensitivity and specificity of clinical diagnosis are to be attempted (Silvestri et al 1988, Sternby 1991).

It is therefore important to separate this random sample from cases selected on 'grounds of interest' or by coroner's direction to avoid distortion of clinical and audit results (Saracci 1991). The use of autopsy as a mechanism for clinical audit needs careful planning and the examination of an unbiased sample of moderate size over years which can be used to compare quantitatively the relative merits of diagnostic methods. An increase of autopsy rate alone will no doubt be a useful educational asset but the raw data so obtained will only give a rough orientation and cannot be used for quantitative comparisons.

CONCLUSION

There is general agreement that the current autopsy rate is too low and that subdivision into two groups of requested autopsies and coroners' autopsies can create problems (Champ et al 1992). Autopsy has a general educational value for clinicians if they attend but a factual report should be available quickly. The use of autopsy as a mechanism for clinical audit still requires evaluation if it is to be used for quantitative comparisons of clinical procedures and diagnostic methods. Autopsies performed to required standards are time consuming and expensive and any major increase in autopsy rate will stretch most laboratories beyond current staffing limits. Initiatives introduced to increase autopsy rate should be planned carefully to secure maximum audit benefit. Only by showing that high standards of diagnosis are being maintained can pathology departments continue to have the support and confidence of their clinical colleagues who use the service.

UPDATE ADDED TO PROOF

Troxel DB and Sabella JD (1994) have reviewed 53 malpractice claims arising in California between 1989 and 1992. During that period the number of claims made against pathologists had risen, whilst the overall rate of claims for all physicians had fallen slightly. Particular problem areas that were identified included failure to diagnose malignant lymphoma; failure to diagnose melanoma; diagnostic problems with breast fine-needle aspiration; diagnostic problems with cervical Pap smears; diagnostic problems with prostate needle biopsy; diagnostic errors by expert consultants and also a mixture of errors in general surgical pathology mainly amounting to random errors. The review presents the issues in detail and makes recommendations to address them. The need to keep original sections in the laboratory file is also emphasized, in case a claim arises.

REFERENCES

Advisory Task Force on Standards to the Audit Steering Committee of the Royal College of Pathologists 1991 J Clin Pathol 44: 798–802

Anderson RE 1984 The autopsy as an instrument of quality assessment. Classification of premortem and postmortem discrepancies. Arch Pathol Lab Med 108: 490–493

Anonymous 1989 Laboratory accreditation and audit. J Clin Pathol 42: 561–566

Anonymous 1991 Statistics of death reported to coroners: England and Wales 1990. Home Office Statistical Bulletin, Issue 5

Ashworth TG 1991 Inadequacies of death certificates: proposal for change. J Clin Pathol 44: 265–268

Association of Directors of Anatomic and Surgical Pathology 1992 Standardisation of the surgical pathology report. Am J Surg Pathol 16: 84–86

Barr WT, Williams E 1982 Value of external quality assessment of the technical aspects of histopathology. J Clin Pathol 35: 1050–1056

Batstone GF 1992 Medical audit in clinical pathology. J Clin Pathol 45: 284–287

Battle RM, Pathak D, Humble CG et al 1987 Factors influencing discrepancies between premortem and postmortem diagnoses. JAMA 258: 339–344

Beck JS and members of the Medical Research Council breast tumour pathology panel associated with the United Kingdom trial of early detection of breast cancer 1985 Observer variability in reporting of breast lesions. J Clin Pathol 38: 1358–1365

Bishop PN, McNally K, Harris M 1992 Audit of bone marrow trephines. J Clin Pathol 45: 1105–1108

Cevill I 1988 Measurement of pathology workload in the United Kingdom. J Clin Pathol 41: 817–819

Champ C, Tyler X, Andrews PS et al 1992 Improve your hospital autopsy rate to 40–50 per cent, a tale of two towns. J Pathol 166: 405–407

Cheung A, Collins RJ 1992 Frozen section diagnosis of ovarian neoplasms. An audit. J Obstet Gynecol 12: 198–201

Chow JW, Dilly SA 1991 Method for auditing turnaround time in histopathology related to user requirements. J Clin Pathol 44: 492–496

Committee of inquiry into competence to practice (Alment Committee) 1975 HMSO, London

Conference of Medical Royal Colleges and their faculties in the United Kingdom 1991 Report. Br Med J 303: 1525

Cowan DF 1990 Quality assurance in anatomic pathology. An information system approach. Arch Pathol Lab Med 114: 129–134

Cree IA, Guthrie W, Anderson JM et al 1993 Departmental audit in histopathology. Pathol Res Pract 189: 453–457

Davies MJ, Bland JM, Hangartner JR et al 1989 Factors influencing the presence or absence of acute coronary artery thrombi in sudden ischaemic death. Br Med J 10: 203–208

Department of Health 1989a Working for patients. HMSO, London

Department of Health 1989b Working for patients: medical audit. Working Paper No. 6. HMSO, London

Department of Health and Human Services 1990 Health care financing administration. Medicare, Medicaid and CLIA programs; regulations implementing the clinical laboratories improvement amendments of 1988 (CLIA '88); proposed rule. Fed Regist 55: 10896–10959

Furness PN, Lauder I 1993 Response analysis in histopathology quality assessment schemes. J Clin Pathol 46: 357–363

Goldman L, Jayson R, Robbins S et al 1983 The value of autopsy in three medical eras. N Engl J Med 308: 1000–1005

Harris A, Ismail I, Dilly S et al 1993 Physicians' attitudes to the autopsy. J R Coll Physicians Lond 27: 116–118

Harrison M, Hourihane DO 1989 Quality assurance programme for necropsies. J Clin Pathol 42: 1190–1193

Herd ME, Cross PA, Dutt S 1992 Histologic audit in acute appendicitis. J Clin Pathol 45: 456–458

Hoffman G 1989 Laboratory accreditation and audit in pathology. J Clin Pathol 42: 562

Holman CDJ, Matz LR, Finlay-Jones LR et al 1983 Interobserver variation in histopathological reporting of Hodgkin's disease. An analysis of diagnostic subcomponents using kappa statistics. Histopathology 7: 399–407

Jamjoom A, Moss T, Jamjoom ZA et al 1991 The value of autopsies in neurosurgery. Acta Neurochir 112: 126–131

Kendall IG, Wynn SM, Quinton DN 1993 A study of patients referred from A&E for coroners post-mortem. Arch Emerg Med 10: 86–90

Klys HS, Lessels AM 1992 External quality assurance in histopathology: experience of the east of Scotland scheme. J Clin Pathol 45: 288–291

Langley FA 1978 Quality control in histopathology and diagnostic cytology. Histopathology 2: 3–18

Lapham R, Waugh NR 1992 An audit of the quality of cancer registration data. Br J Cancer 66: 552–554

Lee FD 1989 External quality assessment in histopathology: an overview. J Clin Pathol 44: 353–357

Lewis SM, Jennings RD 1989 United Kingdom external quality assurance schemes; background and terms of reference. Department of Health, London

McBroom HM, Ramsay AD 1993 The Clinicopathological meeting. A means of auditing diagnostic performance. Am J Clin Pathol 17: 75–80

Mollo F, Bertoldo E, Grandi G 1986 Reliability of death certificates for different types of cancer. An autopsy survey. Pathol Res Pract 181: 442–447

Morson BC 1983 Quality assurance and medical audit in histopathology. J Clin Pathol 36: 1202

Mosquera DA, Goldman MD 1993 Surgical audit without autopsy: tales of the unexpected. Ann R Coll Surg Engl 75: 115–117

Murthy MS, Derman H 1981 Quality assurance in surgical pathology: a personal and peer assessment. Am J Clin Pathol 75 (Suppl): 462–468

Owen DA, Tighe JR 1975 Quality evaluation in histopathology. Br Med J 1: 149–150

Peacock SJ, Machin D, DuBoulay CE et al 1988 The autopsy: a useful tool or an old relic? J Pathol 156: 9–14

Penner DW 1973 Quality control and quality evaluation in histopathology and cytology. Pathol Annu 8: 1–19

Pennington GW 1989 Laboratory accreditation and audit in pathology. J Clin Pathol 42: 561

Ramsay AD 1991 Locally organised medical audit in histopathology. J Clin Pathol 44: 353–357

Ramsay AD, Gallagher PJ 1992 Local audit of surgical pathology. 18 months experience of peer review-based quality assessment in an English teaching hospital. Am J Surg Pathol 16: 476–482

Report of the Joint Working Party of the Royal College of Pathologists, the Royal College of Physicians of London and the Royal College of Surgeons of England 1991 The autopsy and audit. Royal College of Pathologists, London

Rickert RR 1986 Quality assurance in anatomic pathology. Clin Lab Med 6: 697–706

Robertson AJ, Anderson JM, Beck JS 1989 Observer variability in histopathological reporting of cervical biopsy specimens. J Clin Pathol 42: 231–238

Royal College of Pathologists 1989a Comments of the Royal College of Pathologists on the White Paper 'Working for Patients' and the associated Working Papers for England. Bull R Coll Pathol 67: 2–3

Royal College of Pathologists 1989b Codes of practice for pathology departments. Royal College of Pathologists, London

Royal College of Pathologists 1993 Guidelines for post mortem reports. Royal College of Pathologists, London

Rushton DI 1991 West Midlands perinatal mortality survey, 1987. An audit of 300 perinatal autopsies. Br J Obstet Gynaecol 98: 624–627

Russell GA, Berry PJ 1989 Postmortem audit in a paediatric cardiology unit. J Clin Pathol 42: 912–918

Safrin RE, Bark CJ 1993 Surgical pathology signout: routine review of every case by a second pathologist. Am J Surg Pathol 17: 1190–1192

Saracci R 1991 Audit in practice: is necropsy a valid monitor of clinical diagnostic performance. Br Med J 303: 898–900

Schned AR, Mogielnicki RP, Stamffer MA 1986 A comprehensive quality assessment program on the autopsy service. Am J Clin Pathol 86: 113–138

Shanks JH, Anderson NH, McCluggage G et al 1991 Use of the autopsy in Northern Ireland and its value in perioperative deaths. IARC Scientific Publications, Lyon, pp 115–124

Shaw LD, Costain DW 1989 Guidelines for medical audit: seven principles. Br Med J 299: 498–499

Sherwood AJ, Hunt AC 1984 An external quality assessment of clinical laboratories in the United Kingdom. J Clin Pathol 37: 409–414

Silvestri F, Bussani R, Giarelli L 1988 High autopsy rate in Trieste 1901–1985: age associated increase in necropsy rate. Pathologica 80: 523–532

Standing Committee of Postgraduate Medical Education 1990 Medical audit — the educational implications. Postgraduate Medical Federation, London

Sternby NH 1991 The role of the autopsy in cancer registration in Sweden with particular reference to findings in Malmo. In: Riboli E, Delendi M (eds) Autopsy in epidemiology and medical research. IARC Scientific Publications, Lyon, pp 217–222

Stuart J, Hicks JM 1991 Good laboratory management: an Anglo-American perspective. J Clin Pathol 44: 793–797

The College Accreditation Steering Committee 1990 Royal College of Pathologists United Kingdom pilot study of laboratory accreditation. J Clin Pathol 43: 89–91

Thomas AC, Knapman PA, Krikler DM et al 1988 Community study of the causes of 'natural' sudden death. Br Med J 297: 1453–1456

Thomas GD, Dixon MF, Smeeton NC et al 1983 Observer variation in grading of rectal carcinoma. J Clin Pathol 36: 385–391

Thomas JS, Lessells AM, McIntyre ME et al 1991 Prospective study of the quantitative aspects of audit in a large general histopathology laboratory. J Clin Pathol 44: 928–931

Tildsley GJ, Dilly SA 1991 Audit of general surgical pathology experience of histopathology trainees. J Clin Pathol 44: 424–427

Troxel DB, Sabella JD 1994 Problem areas in pathology practice uncovered by a review of malpractice claims. Am J Surg Pathol 18: 821–831

Whitehead ME, Fitzwater JE, Lindley SK et al 1984 Quality assurance of histopathologic diagnoses; a prospective audit of three thousand cases. Am J Clin Pathol 81: 487–491

Whitehead ME, Grieve JH, Payne MJ et al 1986 Quality assurance of histopathologic diagnosis in the British Army: role of the army histopathology registry in completed case reviews. JR Army Med Corps 132: 71–75

Whitehead TP, Woodford FP 1981 External quality assessment scheme for clinical laboratories in the United Kingdom. J Clin Pathol 34: 947–957

Whitty P, Parker C, Prieto-Ramos F et al 1991 Communication of the results of necropsies in North East Thames Region. Br Med J 303: 1244–1246

World Health Organization 1981 External quality assessment of health laboratories. Euro Reports and Studies No. 36. World Health Organization, Copenhagen

Yesner R, Robinson MJ, Goldman L et al 1985 A symposium on the autopsy. Pathol Annu 20: 441–447

Zuk JA, Kenyon WE, Myskow MW 1991 Audit in histopathology: an internal quality assessment scheme with analysis of preliminary results. J Clin Pathol 44: 10–16

13. Pathology literature review

Nigel Kirkham

The well-informed pathologist, whether trainee or consultant, must attempt to keep in touch with the developments described in the literature. The more widespread development of Continuing Medical Education (CME) as a formal activity makes this even more important. The ever increasing number of journals, review journals (and even review books!) being published does not ease the task. Trainees sometimes ask for advice on which journals to choose. It is generally said that one should aim to follow both general and specific journals.

Of the general journals the *British Medical Journal* and *The Lancet* carry a wide range of articles, with the intention of publishing good new material over as wide a range as possible. *The New England Journal of Medicine* also offers good value in this category. For the more scientifically or politically inclined *Nature*, *Science* and *Cell* all publish excellent primary material.

Amongst the journals specifically devoted to pathology *Histopathology*, the *Journal of Clinical Pathology* and the *Journal of Pathology* are the British leaders. They are available at favourable rates to members of the British Division of the International Academy of Pathology (IAP), the Association of Clinical Pathology (ACP) and the Pathological Society of Great Britain and Ireland (Path Soc) respectively. All three of these societies offer reduced rates to trainees. The Royal College of Pathologists publishes detail and policy in its *Bulletin* which is also available to trainees.

In North America there are many excellent journals with the *American Journal of Clinical Pathology*, the *American Journal of Pathology*, the *American Journal of Surgical Pathology* and *Human Pathology* amongst the leaders. There is a further long list of more specialized journals.

In continental Europe there are a variety of journals, some of which are published in English. *Pathology, Research and Practice* is the journal of the European Society of Pathology. *Virchows Archiv*, in its two versions, also publishes many useful papers.

Each individual must make personal decisions about which journals to subscribe to, which should be read in the department or hospital library and which should be scanned from *Current Contents* listings of title pages or from current awareness services provided from the local medical library. It is essential to spend a minimum of 1–2 hours per week reading the journals, preferably to a personal plan. Even better is to form a journal club with colleagues to share the load and sharpen the analysis.

The selection of articles that follows is a personal one based on two different strategies. Firstly, a series of articles are presented that each come from a group led by one of several individuals who have consistently contributed important papers to the literature. The ease with which CD-ROM or on-line searching can be done these days allows you to follow some of the 'stars' more easily as they move around from journal to journal. Secondly, a few topics have been presented with recent articles from all comers, by way of illustrating the range of opinion on these subjects.

LYMPHOMA

This selection of papers has in common the presence of P G Isaacson as one of the authors and illustrates contributions in several areas. The work related to MALT lymphoma at various sites and the developing story of *Helicobacter pylori* and gastric lymphoma are documented here.

Extranodal lymphoma

In a series of papers lymphomas at various extranodal sites are reviewed.

Bobrow LG, Richards MA, Happerfield LC et al. Breast lymphomas: a clinicopathologic review. Hum Pathol 1993; 24: 274-278

Grant JW, Isaacson PG. Primary central nervous system lymphoma. [review]. Brain Pathol 1992; 2: 97–109

Isaacson PG. Pathogenesis and early lesions in extranodal lymphoma. Toxicol Lett 1993; 67: 237–247

Isaacson PG, Spencer J. Malignant lymphoma and autoimmune disease. Histopathology 1993; 22: 509–510

MALT LYMPHOMA

The following papers describe the developing understanding of lymphomas of mucosa-associated lymphoid tissue, in the stomach where they were first recognized, but also at other mucosal sites, including the bladder and conjunctiva.

Isaacson PG. Brief report: a single neoplastic clone in sequential biopsy specimens from a patient with primary gastric-mucosa-associated lymphoid-tissue lymphoma and Sjogren's syndrome. N Engl J Med 1993; 329: 172–175

Diss TC, Peng H, Wotherspoon AC, Pan L, Speight PM, Gould SJ, Isaacson PG. Bronchus-associated lymphoid tissue (BALT) in human fetal and infant lung. J Pathol 1993; 169: 229–234

Hussell T, Isaacson PG, Spencer J. Proliferation and differentiation of tumour cells from B-cell lymphoma of mucosa-associated lymphoid tissue in vitro. J Pathol 1993; 169: 221-227

Hussell T, Isaacson PG, Crabtree JE, Dogan A, Spencer J. Immunoglobulin specificity of low grade B cell gastrointestinal lymphoma of mucosa-associated lymphoid tissue (MALT) type. Am J Pathol 1993; 142: 285-292

Papadaki L, Wotherspoon AC, Isaacson PG. The lymphoepithelial lesion of gastric low-grade B-cell lymphoma of mucosa-associated lymphoid tissue (MALT): an ultrastructural study. Histopathology 1992; 21: 415-421

Pawade J, Banerjee SS, Harris M, Isaacson P, Wright D. Lymphomas of mucosa-associated lymphoid tissue arising in the urinary bladder. Histopathology 1993; 23: 147-151

Wotherspoon AC, Diss TC, Pan LX et al. Primary low-grade B-cell lymphoma of the conjunctiva: a mucosa-associated lymphoid tissue type lymphoma. Histopathology 1993; 23: 417-424

Helicobacter pylori

The recoginition of an association between *Helicobacter pylori* and gastric lymphoma and the more recent contention that some gastric lymphoma can be cured with antibiotic therapy is reported in the following papers.

Wotherspoon AC, Ortiz-Hidalgo C, Falzon MR, Isaacson PG. Helicobacter pylori-associated gastritis and primary B-cell gastric lymphoma. Lancet 1991; 338: 1175-1176

Isaacson PG, Spencer J. Is gastric lymphoma an infectious disease? [editorial]. Hum Pathol 1993; 24: 569–570

Hussell T, Isaacson PG, Crabtree JE, Spencer J. The response of cells from low-grade B-cell gastric lymphomas of mucosa-associated lymphoid tissue to Helicobacter pylori. Lancet 1993; 342: 571-574

Wotherspoon AC, Doglioni C, Diss TC et al. Regression of primary low-grade B-cell gastric lymphoma of mucosa-associated lymphoid tissue type after eradication of Helicobacter pylori. Lancet 1993; 342: 575-577

Isaacson PG. Gastric lymphoma and helicobacter pylori. [editorial]. N Engl J Med 1994; 330: 1310-1311

Techniques

Histopathology has not been left behind in the revolution that has been facilitated by the introduction of the polymerase chain reaction process (PCR). The ability to extract analysable DNA from paraffin blocks of fixed and processed tissue is touched on here, as is the developing application of in-situ hybridization, the use of microwave ovens in immunohistochemistry and the transitory rise of proliferating cell nuclear antigen (PCNA) staining.

Diss TC, Peng H, Wotherspoon AC, Isaacson PG, Pan L. Detection of monoclonality in low-grade B-cell lymphomas using the polymerase chain reaction is dependent on primer selection and lymphoma type. J Pathol 1993; 169: 291–295

Pan L, Happerfield LC, Bobrow LG, Isaacson PG. In situ detection of human Ig light-chain mRNA on formalin-fixed and paraffin-embedded tissue sections using digoxigenin-labelled RNA probes. Histochem J 1993; 25: 57–63

Charalambous C, Singh N, Isaacson PG. Immunohistochemical analysis of Hodgkin's disease using microwave heating. J Clin Pathol 1993; 46: 1085–1088

Schmid C, Isaacson PG. [Proliferating cells in Hodgkin's disease]. Verh D tsch Ges Pathol 1992; 76: 151–154

Schmid C, Sweeney E, Isaacson PG. Proliferating cell nuclear antigen (PCNA) expression in Hodgkin's disease. J Pathol 1992; 168: 1–6

Epstein-Barr virus

It is difficult to avoid Epstein-Barr virus in almost any field of tumour pathology. Here studies are reported of work on infectious mononucleosis and small bowel lymphoma.

Isaacson PG, Schmid C, Pan L, Wotherspoon AC, Wright DH. Epstein-Barr virus latent membrane protein expression by Hodgkin and Reed-Sternberg-like cells in acute infectious mononucleosis. J Pathol 1992; 167: 267–271

Pan L, Diss TC, Peng H et al. Epstein-Barr virus (EBV) in enteropathy-associated T-cell lymphoma (EATL). J Pathol 1993; 170: 137–143

Mantle zone lymphoma

This paper is an attempt to unify the way in which mantle zone lymphoma is described and characterized, from a group of authors from all around the globe.

Banks PM, Chan J, Cleary ML et al. Mantle cell lymphoma. A proposal for unification of morphologic, immunologic, and molecular data. Am J Surg Pathol 1992; 16: 637–640

SOFT TISSUE TUMOURS

The world of soft tissue tumour pathology has been dominated in recent years by the work of C. D. Fletcher and his colleagues. This selection lists recent contributions, including descriptions of newer entities, review of series of established entities and reappraisal of dogma, including the case for abandoning malignant fibrous histiocytoma as a diagnostic entity.

Calonje E, Fletcher CD. New entities in cutaneous soft tissue tumours. [review]. Pathologica 1993; 85: 1–15

Vascular tumours

Fletcher CD, Beham A, Schmid C. Spindle cell haemangioendothelioma: a clinicopathological and immunohistochemical study indicative of a non-neoplastic lesion. Histopathology 1991; 18: 291–301

Chan JK, Frizzera G, Fletcher CD, Rosai J. Primary vascular tumors of lymph nodes other than Kaposi's sarcoma. Analysis of 39 cases and delineation of two new entities. Am J Surg Pathol 1992; 16: 335–350

Beham A, Fletcher CD, Kainz J, Schmid C, Humer U. Nasopharyngeal angiofibroma: an immunohistochemical study of 32 cases. Virchows Archiv A Pathol Anat Histopathol 1993; 423: 281–285

Chan JK, Tsang WY, Pau MY, Tang MC, Pang SW, Fletcher CD. Lymphangiomyomatosis and angiomyolipoma: closely related entities characterized by hamartomatous proliferation of HMB-45-positive smooth muscle. Histopathology 1993; 22: 445–455

Fletcher CD, Tsang WY, Fisher C, Lee KC, Chan JK. Angiomyofibroblastoma of the vulva. A benign neoplasm distinct from aggressive angiomyxoma. Am J Surg Pathol 1992; 16: 373–382

Tsang WY, Chan JK, Lee KC, Fisher C, Fletcher CD. Aggressive angiomyxoma. A report of four cases occurring in men. Am J Surg Pathol 1992; 16: 1059–1065

Calonje E, Fletcher CD, Wilson-Jones E, Rosai J. Retiform hemangioendothelioma. A distinctive form of low-grade angiosarcoma delineated in a series of 15 cases. Am J Surg Pathol 1994; 18: 115–125

Lipoid tumours

Mentzel T, Calonje E, Fletcher CD. Lipoblastoma and lipoblastomatosis: a clinicopathological study of 14 cases. Histopathology 1993; 23: 527–533

Muscle tumours

Gaffney EF, Dervan PA, Fletcher CD. Pleomorphic rhabdomyosarcoma in adulthood. Analysis of 11 cases with definition of diagnostic criteria. Am J Surg Pathol 1993; 17: 601–609

Schmidt D, Fletcher CD, Harms D. Rhabdomyosarcomas with primary presentation in the skin. Pathol, Res Pract 1993; 189: 422–427

Mentzel T, Calonje E, Fletcher CD. Leiomyosarcoma with prominent osteoclast-like giant cells. Analysis of eight cases closely mimicking the so-called giant cell variant of malignant fibrous histiocytoma. Am J Surg Pathol 1994; 18: 258–265

Fibrous tumours

Fletcher CD. Pleomorphic malignant fibrous histiocytoma: fact or fiction? A critical reappraisal based on 159 tumors diagnosed as pleomorphic sarcoma. Am J Surg Pathol 1992; 16: 213–228

Nikolaou I, Barbatis C, Laopodis V, Bekir S, Fletcher CD. Intra-abdominal desmoplastic small-cell tumours with divergent differentiation. Report of two cases and review of the literature. Pathol Res Pract 1992; 188: 981–988

Schofield JB, Krausz T, Stamp GW, Fletcher CD, Fisher C, Azzopardi JG. Ossifying fibromyxoid tumour of soft parts: immunohistochemical and ultrastructural analysis. Histopathology 1993; 22: 101–112

Beham A, Badve S, Suster S, Fletcher CD. Solitary myofibroma in adults: clinicopathological analysis of a series. Histopathology 1993; 22: 335–341

Lee AH, Sworn MJ, Theaker JM, Fletcher CD. Myofibroblastoma of breast: an immunohistochemical study. Histopathology 1993; 22: 75–78

Bittesini L, Dei Tos AP, Doglioni C, Della Libera D, Laurino L, Fletcher CD. Fibroepithelial tumor of the breast with digital fibroma-like inclusions in the stromal component: case report with immunocytochemical and ultrastructural analysis. Am J Surg Pathol 1994; 18: 296–301

Skin tumours

Bass PS, Theaker JM, Griffiths DM, Fletcher CD. Subcutaneous, meningoglial nodule — a novel lesion in the buttock of a neonate. Histopathology 1993; 22: 182–184

Beham A, Fletcher CD, Feichtinger J, Zelger B, Schmid C, Humer U. Synovial metaplasia of the skin. [review]. Virchows Archiv A Pathol Anat Histopathol 1993; 423: 315–318

Calonje E, Wadden C, Wilson-Jones E, Fletcher CD. Spindle-cell nonpleomorphic atypical fibroxanthoma: analysis of a series and delineation of a distinctive variant. Histopathology 1993; 22: 247–254

Mentzel T, Calonje E, Fletcher CD. Dermatomyofibroma: additional observations on a distinctive cutaneous myofibroblastic tumour with emphasis on differential diagnosis. Br J Dermatol 1993; 129: 69–73

Schmidt D, Fletcher CD, Harms D. Rhabdomyosarcomas with primary presentation in the skin. Pathol Res Pract 1993; 189: 422–427

Special techniques

Reeves BR, Fletcher CD, Gusterson BA. Translocation t(12;22) (q13;q13) is a nonrandom rearrangement in clear cell sarcoma. Cancer Genet Cytogenet 1992; 64: 101–103

Kuzu I, Bicknell R, Fletcher CD, Gatter KC. Expression of adhesion molecules on the endothelium of normal tissue vessels and vascular tumors. Lab Invest 1993; 69: 322–328

Dei Tos AP, Doglioni C, Laurino L, Barbareschi M, Fletcher CD. p53 protein expression in non-neoplastic lesions and benign and malignant neoplasms of soft tissue. Histopathology 1993; 22: 45–50

Tos AP, Doglioni C, Laurino L, Fletcher CD. KP1 (CD68) expression in benign neural tumours. Further evidence of its low specificity as a histiocytic/myeloid marker. Histopathology 1993; 23: 185–187

Miettinen M, Fletcher CD, Lasota J. True histiocytic lymphoma of small intestine. Analysis of two S-100 protein-positive cases with features of interdigitating reticulum cell sarcoma. Am J Clin Pathol 1993; 100: 285–292

GASTROINTESTINAL EPITHELIUM

The understanding of cell proliferation in gastrointestinal epithelium in health and disease has been at the centre of the work of N A Wright. The following selection of papers includes original contributions in this area, including the more recent work on trefoil peptides and their importance in relation to peptic ulcers, ulcer healing and related phenomena at other sites in the gut.

Stem cells

Jankowski JA, Wright NA. Epithelial stem cells in gastrointestinal morphogenesis, adaptation and carcinogenesis. Semin Cell Biol 1992; 3: 445–456

Liu KC, Wright NA. The migration pathway of epithelial cells on human duodenal villi: the origin and fate of 'gastric metaplastic' cells in duodenal mucosa. Epithelial Cell Biol 1992; 1: 53–58

Trefoil peptides and ulcers

Levi S, Goodlad RA, Lee CY et al. Non-steroidal anti-inflammatory drugs inhibit the processes of mucosal cell proliferation associated with duodenal ulcer healing. Digestion 1992; 53: 129–133

Wright NA, Poulsom R, Stamp G et al. Trefoil peptide gene expression in gastrointestinal epithelial cells in inflammatory bowel disease. Scand J Gastroenterol Suppl 1992; 193: 76–82

Chinery R, Poulsom R, Elia G, Hanby AM, Wright NA. Expression and purification of a trefoil peptide motif in a beta-galactosidase fusion protein and its use to search for trefoil-binding sites. Eur J Biochem 1993; 212: 557–563

Hanby AM, Poulsom R, Elia G, Singh S, Longcroft JM, Wright NA. The expression of the trefoil peptides pS2 and human spasmolytic polypeptide (hSP) in 'gastric metaplasia' of the proximal duodenum: implications for the nature of 'gastric metaplasia'. J Pathol 1993; 169: 355–360

Hanby AM, Poulsom R, Singh S et al. Hyperplastic polyps: a cell lineage which both synthesizes and secretes trefoil-peptides and has phenotypic similarity with the ulcer-associated cell lineage. Am J Pathol 1993; 142: 663–668

Hauser F, Poulsom R, Chinery R et al. hP1.B, a human P-domain peptide homologous with rat intestinal trefoil factor, is expressed also in the ulcer-associated cell lineage and the uterus. Proc Natl Acad Sci USA 1993; 90: 6961–6965

Poulsom R, Chinery R, Sarraf C et al. Trefoil peptide gene expression in small intestinal Crohn's disease and dietary adaptation. J Clin Gastroenterol 1993; 17 Suppl 1: S78–S91

Wright NA. Trefoil peptides and the gut. Gut 1993; 34: 577–579

Wright NA, Poulsom R, Stamp G et al. Trefoil peptide gene expression in gastrointestinal epithelial cells in inflammatory bowel disease. Gastroenterology 1993; 104: 12–20

Jankowski JA, Goodlad RA, Wright NA. Maintenance of normal intestinal mucosa: function, structure, and adaptation. [review]. Gut 1994; 35: S1–S4

REPRODUCTIVE PATHOLOGY

For many years now the names of H Fox, R E Scully and R H Young have been synonymous with all that is new in reproductive pathology. Constant monitoring of the journals is required to keep up with the torrent of new entities and reappraisals of established entities that flow from these authors and their associates.

Cervix

Hale RJ, Buckley CH, Fox H, Williams J. Prognostic value of c-erbB-2 expression in uterine cervical carcinoma. J Clin Pathol 1992; 45: 594–596

Hale RJ, Buckley CH, Gullick WJ, Fox H, Williams J, Wilcox FL. Prognostic value of epidermal growth factor receptor expression in cervical carcinoma. J Clin Pathol 1993; 46: 149–153

Mitchell KM, Hale RJ, Buckley CH, Fox H, Smith D. Cathepsin-D expression in cervical carcinoma and its prognostic significance. Virchows Arch A Pathol Anat Histopathol 1993; 422: 357–360

Young RH, Scully RE. Minimal-deviation endometrioid adenocarcinoma of the uterine cervix. A report of five cases of a distinctive neoplasm that may be misinterpreted as benign. Am J Surg Pathol 1993; 17: 660–665

Endometrium

Young RH, Scully RE. Uterine carcinomas simulating microglandular hyperplasia. A report of six cases. Am J Surg Pathol 1992; 16: 1092–1097

Clement PB, Scully RE. Endometrial stromal sarcomas of the uterus with extensive endometrioid glandular differentiation: a report of three cases that caused problems in differential diagnosis. Int J Gynecol Pathol 1992; 11: 163–173

Dickersin GR, Scully RE. Role of electron microscopy in metastatic endometrial stromal tumors. [review]. Ultrastructural Pathology 1993; 17: 377–403

Huntsman DG, Clement PB, Gilks CB, Scully RE. Small-cell carcinoma of the endometrium. A clinicopathological study of sixteen cases. [review]. Am J Surg Pathol 1994; 18: 364–375

Products of conception

Fox H. Histological classification of tissue from spontaneous abortions: a valueless exercise? Histopathology 1993; 22: 599–600

Suresh UR, Hale RJ, Fox H, Buckley CH. Use of proliferation cell nuclear antigen immunoreactivity for distinguishing hydropic abortions from partial hydatidiform moles. J Clin Pathol 1993; 46: 48–50

Ovary

Small cell carcinoma

Eichhorn JH, Bell DA, Young RH et al. DNA content and proliferative activity in ovarian small cell carcinomas of the hypercalcemic type. Implications for diagnosis, prognosis, and histogenesis. Am J Clin Pathol 1992; 98: 579–586

Eichhorn JH, Young RH, Scully RE. Primary ovarian small cell carcinoma of pulmonary type. A clinicopathologic, immunohistologic, and flow cytometric analysis of 11 cases. Am J Surg Pathol 1992; 16: 926–938

Eichhorn JH, Young RH, Scully RE. Nonpulmonary small cell carcinomas of extragenital origin metastatic to the ovary. Cancer 1993; 71: 177–186

Dickersin GR, Scully RE. An update on the electron microscopy of small cell carcinoma of the ovary with hypercalcemia. Ultrastructural Pathology 1993; 17: 411–422

Kleinman GM, Young RH, Scully RE. Primary neuroectodermal tumors of the ovary. A report of 25 cases. Am J Surg Pathol 1993; 17: 764–778

Scully RE. Small cell carcinoma of hypercalcemic type. Int J Gynecol Pathol 1993; 12: 148–152

Matias-Guiu X, Prat J, Young RH et al. Human parathyroid hormone-related protein in ovarian small cell carcinoma. An immunohistochemical study. Cancer 1994; 73: 1878–1881

Other ovarian pathology

Fox H. The pathology of premature ovarian failure. J Pathol 1992; 167: 357–363

Fox H. Pathology of early malignant change in the ovary. Int J Gynecol Pathol 1993; 12: 153–155

Young RH. Sertoli-Leydig cell tumors of the ovary: review with emphasis on historical aspects and unusual variants. Int J Gynecol Pathol 1993; 12: 141–147

Young RH, Gersell DJ, Roth LM, Scully RE. Ovarian metastases from cervical carcinomas other than pure adenocarcinomas. A report of 12 cases. Cancer 1993; 71: 407–418

Young RH, Kozakewich HP, Scully RE. Metastatic ovarian tumors in children: a report of 14 cases and review of the literature. Int J Gynecol Pathol 1993; 12: 8–19

Bell DA, Scully RE. Early de novo ovarian carcinoma. A study of fourteen cases. Cancer 1994; 73: 1859–1864

Peritoneum

Clement PB, Young RH. Florid mesothelial hyperplasia associated with ovarian tumors: a potential source of error in tumor diagnosis and staging. Int J Gynecol Pathol 1993; 12: 51–58

Clement PB, Young RH, Hanna W, Scully RE. Sclerosing peritonitis associated with luteinized thecomas of the ovary. A clinicopathological analysis of six cases. Am J Surg Pathol 1994; 18: 1–13

Testis

Ferry JA, Harris NL, Young RH, Coen J, Zietman A, Scully RE. Malignant lymphoma of the testis, epididymis, and spermatic cord. A clinicopathologic study of 69 cases with immunophenotypic analysis. Am J Surg Pathol 1994; 18: 376–390

Prostate

Simons BD, Morrison AS, Young RH, Verhoek-Oftedahl W. The relation of surgery for prostatic hypertrophy to carcinoma of the prostate. Am J Epidemiol 1993; 138: 294–300

Bladder

Young RH, Eble JN. Unusual forms of carcinoma of the urinary bladder. Hum Pathol 1991; 22: 948–965

Chor PJ, Gaum LD, Young RH. Clear cell adenocarcinoma of the urinary bladder: report of a case of probable mullerian origin. Mod Pathol 1993; 6: 225–228

Jones EC, Clement PB, Young RH. Inflammatory pseudotumor of the urinary bladder. A clinicopathological, immunohistochemical, ultrastructural, and flow cytometric study of 13 cases. Am J Surg Pathol 1993; 17: 264–274

MESOTHELIOMA

The problems that many pathologists have in making a confident diagnosis of malignant mesothelioma on the basis of an often inadequate pleural biopsy has led to many attempts to find other ways of supporting the diagnosis.

Mayall FG, Gibbs AR. 'Pleural' and pulmonary carcinosarcomas. J Pathol 1992; 167: 305–311

Mayall FG, Goddard H, Gibbs AR. Intermediate filament expression in mesotheliomas: leiomyoid mesotheliomas are not uncommon. Histopathology 1992; 21: 453–457

Mayall FG, Goddard H, Gibbs AR. p53 immunostaining in the distinction between benign and malignant mesothelial proliferations using formalin-fixed paraffin sections. J Pathol 1992; 168: 377–381

Mayall FG, Goddard H, Gibbs AR. The frequency of p53 immunostaining in asbestos-associated mesotheliomas and non-asbestos-associated mesotheliomas. Histopathology 1993; 22: 383–386

Mayall FG, Goddard H, Gibbs AR. The diagnostic implications of variable cytokeratin expression in mesotheliomas. J Pathol 1993; 170: 165–168

OPERATION DESERT STORM

Many of the troops who served in the Gulf war have developed complications since returning home. Some of these complications are due to infections such as Leishmaniasis that are well known in the area. Others have a variety of problems, some of which remain to be evaluated in detail. As is so often the case with new diseases and rapidly moving events the *N Engl J Med* has been the first to publish much of this material

Anonymous. Viscerotropic leishmaniasis in persons returning from Operation Desert Storm — 1990–1991. MMWR 1992; 41: 131–134

Gasser RA, Jr., Magill AJ, Oster CN, Tramont EC. The threat of infectious disease in Americans returning from Operation Desert Storm. N Engl J Med 1991; 324: 859–864

Hyams KC, Malone JD, Kapikian AZ et al. Norwalk virus infection among Desert Storm troops [letter]. J Infect Dis 1993; 167: 986–987

Killick-Kendrick R, Peters W. Leishmaniasis and 'Desert Storm' [letter]. Trans R Soc Trop Med Hyg 1992; 86: 698

Korenyi-Both AL, Molnar AC, Fidelus-Gort R. Al Eskan disease: Desert Storm pneumonitis. Milit Medi 1992; 157: 452–462

Magill AJ, Grogl M, Gasser RA, Jr., Sun W, Oster CN. Visceral infection caused by Leishmania tropica in veterans of Operation Desert Storm. New Engl J Med 1993; 328: 1383–1387

Malone JD, Paparello S, Thornton S, Mapes T, Haberberger R, Hyams KC. Parasitic infections in troops returning from Operation Desert Storm [letter; comment]. N Engl J Med 1991; 325: 1448–1449

Ohl CA, Hyams KC, Malone JD, Oldfield E. Leishmaniasis among desert storm veterans: a diagnostic and therapeutic dilemma. Milit Med 1993; 158: 726–729

Oster CN, Sanford JP. Febrile illness in a Desert Storm veteran. Hosp Pract (Off) 1992; 27: 145–148, 151, 155–160

ORAL PATHOLOGY

Oral pathology is often kept within the province of a small band of highly specialized pathologists mainly centred in dental hospitals and dental schools, but deserves wider attention. A selection of recent papers is listed here.

Carcinoma

Oral carcinoma, often associated with a history of tobacco smoking and alcohol drinking remains a very common problem. The following series of papers charts some of the variants and describes studies that have been performed to gain a greater understanding of the events taking place in the development of carcinoma in the mouth.

Hogewind WF, van der Kwast WA, Van der Waal I. Oral leukoplakia, with emphasis on malignant transformation. A follow-up study of 46 patients. J Craniomaxillofac Surg 1989; 17: 128–133

Kratochvil FJ, Cioffi GA, Auclair PL, Rathbun WA. Virus-associated dysplasia (Bowenoid papulosis?) of the oral cavity. Oral Surg Oral Med Oral Pathol 1989; 68: 312–316

Rajendran R, Sugathan CK, Augustine J, Vasudevan DM, Vijayakumar T. Ackerman's tumour (Verrucous carcinoma) of the oral cavity: a histopathologic study of 426 cases. Singapore Dent J 1989; 14: 48–53

High AS, Hume WJ, Dyson D. Atypical fibroxanthoma of oral mucosa: a variant of malignant fibrous histiocytoma. Br J Oral Maxillofac Surg 1990; 28: 268–271

Massa MC, Greaney V, Kron T, Armin A. Malignant transformation of oral lichen planus: case report and review of the literature. Cutis 1990; 45: 45–47

Bryne M, Nielsen K, Koppang HS, Dabelsteen E. Grading of nuclear pleomorphism in oral carcinomas. Higher prognostic value than stereological assessment of nuclear volume. Acta Pathol Microbiol Immunol Scand 1991; 99: 333–339

Damm DD, O'Connor WN, White DK, Drummond JF, Morrow LW, Kenady DE. Intraoral sebaceous carcinoma. Oral Surg Oral Med Oral Pathol 1991; 72: 709–711

Takata T, Ito H, Ogawa I, Miyauchi M, Ijuhin N, Nikai H. Spindle cell squamous carcinoma of the oral region. An immunohistochemical and ultrastructural study on the histogenesis and differential diagnosis with a clinicopathological analysis of six cases. Virchows Archiv A Pathol Anat Histopathol 1991; 419: 177–182

Bryne M, Koppang HS, Lilleng R, Kjaerheim A. Malignancy grading of the deep invasive margins of oral squamous cell carcinomas has high prognostic value. J Pathol 1992; 166: 375–381

Colmenero CM, Patron M, Burgueno M, Sierra I. Polymorphous low-grade adenocarcinoma of the oral cavity: a report of 14 cases. J Oral Maxillofac Surg 1992; 50: 595–600

Milian A, Bagan JV, Vera F. Epidermoid carcinoma of the oral cavity: a histopathological study of 85 cases. [French]. Bull Group Int Rech Sci Stomatol Odontol 1992; 35: 131–139

Gaillard-Perera H, Gaillard A. Carcinoma of the oral cavity independent of tobacco and alcoholic beverages. Apropos of 23 cases in elderly persons. [French]. Rev Stomatol Chir Maxillofac 1992; 93: 58–59

de Araujo VC, Biazolla ER, Moraes NP, Furuse TA, Melhado RM. Basaloid squamous carcinoma of the oral cavity. Report of a case. Oral Surg Oral Med Oral Pathol 1993; 75: 622–625

de Araujo VC, Pinto Junior DS, de Sousa SO, Nunes FD, de Araujo NS. Vimentin in oral squamous cell carcinoma. Eur Arch Otorhinolaryngol 1993; 250: 105–109

Jones AC, Freedman PD, Kerpel SM. Oral adenoid squamous cell carcinoma: a report of three cases and review of the literature. J Oral Maxillofac Surg 1993; 51: 676–681

Noguchi M, Kohama G, Hiratsuka H, Sekiguchi T. Clinical significance of laminin deposition and T-cell infiltration in oral cancer. Head Neck 1993; 15: 125–132

Ogden GR, Chisholm DM, Adi M, Lane EB. Cytokeratin expression in oral cancer and its relationship to tumor differentiation. J Oral Pathol Med 1993; 22: 82–86

Ogden GR, Lane EB, Hopwood DV, Chisholm DM. Evidence for field change in oral cancer based on cytokeratin expression. Br J Cancer 1993; 67: 1324–1330

Scully C, Burkhardt A. Tissue markers of potentially malignant human oral epithelial lesions. J Oral Pathol Med 1993; 22: 246–256

Kaposi's sarcoma

Kaposi's sarcoma is a moderately common finding in patients with HIV/AIDS. Interpretation of oral biopsies may not be straightforward, with other reactive changes including epithelial hyperplasia masking the tumour cells. The patients may also not be HIV-positive.

Regezi JA, MacPhail LA, Daniels TE, DeSouza YG, Greenspan JS, Greenspan D. Human immunodeficiency virus-associated oral Kaposi's sarcoma. A heterogeneous cell population dominated by spindle-shaped endothelial cells. Am J Pathol 1993; 143: 240–249

Beckstead JH. Oral presentation of Kaposi's sarcoma in a patient without severe immunodeficiency. Arch Pathol Lab Med 1992; 116: 543–545

Melanocytic lesions

Melanoma may occur as a primary tumour in the mouth. This, and its relationship to underlying or associated benign pigmentary or melanocytic disorders and naevi has been studied in the following series of papers.

Bucci E, Lo Muzio L, Mignogna MD, Troncone G. Pigmented lesions of the oral cavity. I. Classification and etiopathogenesis. [Italian]. Minerva Stomatol 1989; 38: 369–378

Buchner A, Leider AS, Carpenter WM, Littner MM. Melanocytic nevi of the oral mucosa — a clinicopathologic study of 60 new cases. Dent Med 1990; 8: 3–8

Modica LA, Youngberg GA, Avila FO. Melanocyte colonization of an oral carcinoma. Histopathology 1990; 17: 477–478

Barrett AW, Beynon AD. A histochemical study on the distribution of melanin in human oral epithelium at six regional sites. Arch Oral Biol 1991; 36: 771–774

Ohashi K, Kasuga T, Tanaka N, Enomoto S, Horiuchi J, Okada N. Malignant melanomas of the oral cavity: heterogeneity of pathological and clinical features. Virchows Archiv Pathol Anat Histopathol 1992; 420: 43–50

Oral hairy leukoplakia

This condition is one of the complications of HIV infection and seems to be very uncommon in the experience of histopathologists. Nevertheless some studies of its nature have been performed.

Greenspan JS, Greenspan D. Oral hairy leukoplakia: diagnosis and management. Oral Surg Oral Med Oral Pathol 1989; 67: 396–403

Reichart PA, Langford A, Gelderblom HR, Pohle HD, Becker J, Wolf H. Oral hairy leukoplakia: observations in 95 cases and review of the literature. J Oral Pathol Med 1989; 18: 410–415

Andersen L, Philipsen HP, Reichart PA. Macro- and microanatomy of the lateral border of the tongue with special reference to oral hairy leukoplakia. J Oral Pathol Med 1990; 19: 77–80

Fernàndez JF, Benito MA, Lizaldez EB, Montanes MA. Oral hairy leukoplakia: a histopathologic study of 32 cases. Am J Dermatopathol 1990; 12: 571–578

Kratochvil FJ, Riordan GP, Auclair PL, Huber MA, Kragel PJ. Diagnosis of oral hairy leukoplakia by ultrastructural examination of exfoliative cytologic specimens. Oral Surg Oral Med Oral Pathol 1990; 70: 613–618

Ficarra G, Gaglioti D, Di Pietro M, Adler-Storthz K. Oral hairy leukoplakia:

clinical aspects, histologic morphology and differential diagnosis. Head Neck 1991; 13: 514–521

Schulten EA, Snijders PJ, ten Kate RW et al. Oral hairy leukoplakia in HIV infection: a diagnostic pitfall. Oral Surg Oral Med Oral Pathol 1991; 71: 32–37

Williams DM, Leigh IM, Greenspan D, Greenspan JS. Altered patterns of keratin expression in oral hairy leukoplakia: prognostic implications. J Oral Pathol Med 1991; 20: 167–171

Greenspan D, Greenspan JS. Significance of oral hairy leukoplakia. Oral Surg Oral Med Oral Pathol 1992; 73: 151–154

Oral lymphoma

Both Hodgkin's disease and non-Hodgkin's lymphomas are uncommon in the mouth. When these tumours do occur there is often an association with some other underlying factor, such as HIV or Epstein-Barr virus infection. The following series of articles describes some examples.

Green TL, Eversole LR. Oral lymphomas in HIV-infected patients: association with Epstein-Barr virus DNA. Oral Surgery Oral Medicine Oral Pathology 1989; 67: 437–442

Mathews FR, Appleton SS, Wear DJ. Intraoral Hodgkin's disease. J Oral Maxillofac Surg 1989; 47: 502–504

Soderholm AL, Lindqvist C, Heikinheimo K, Forssell K, Happonen RP. Non-Hodgkin's lymphomas presenting through oral symptoms. Int J Oral Maxillofac Surg 1990; 19: 131–134

Takahashi H, Fujita S, Okabe H, Tsuda N, Tezuka F. Immunophenotypic analysis of extranodal non-Hodgkin's lymphomas in the oral cavity. Path Res Pract 1993; 189: 300–311

Takahashi H, Tsuda N, Tezuka F, Okabe H. Primary extranodal non-Hodgkin's lymphoma of the oral region. J Oral Pathol Med 1989; 18: 84–91

MELANOMA

The understanding of the mechanisms underlying prognosis and metastatic behaviour of melanoma is at the centre of any possible future developments in therapy. D J Ruiter has worked consistantly in this area for a number of years. Current work includes studies of angiogenesis and of markers of tumour progression.

Denijn M, Ruiter DJ. The possible role of angiogenesis in the metastatic potential of human melanoma. Clinicopathological aspects. Melanoma Res 1993; 3:5–14

Weterman MA, van Muijen GN, Ruiter DJ, Bloemers HP. Thymosin beta-10 expression in melanoma cell lines and melanocytic lesions: a new progression marker for human cutaneous melanoma. Int J Cancer 1993; 53: 278–284

Danen EH, van Muijen GN, ten Berge PJ, Ruiter DJ. Integrins and melanoma progression. Recent Results Cancer Res 1993; 128: 119–132

Ruiter DJ, Brocker EB. Immunohistochemistry in the evaluation of melanocytic tumors. Semin Diagn Pathol 1993; 10: 76–91

Danen EH, van Muijen GN, van de Wiel-van Kemenade E, Jansen KF, Ruiter DJ, Figdor CG. Regulation of integrin-mediated adhesion to laminin and collagen in human melanocytes and in non-metastatic and highly metastatic human melanoma cells. Int J Cancer 1993; 54: 315–321

de Wit PE, Moretti S, Koenders PG et al. Increasing epidermal growth factor receptor expression in human melanocytic tumor progression. J Invest Dermatol 1992; 99: 168–173

Brocker EB, Reckenfeld C, Hamm H, Ruiter DJ, Sorg C. Macrophages in melanocytic naevi. Arch Dermatol Res 1992; 284: 127–131

Ruiter DJ. Clinical and pathologic diagnosis, staging and prognostic factors of melanoma and management of primary disease. Curr Opin Oncol 1992; 4: 357–367

Weterman MA, Stoopen GM, van Muijen GN, Kuznicki J, Ruiter DJ, Bloemers HP. Expression of calcyclin in human melanoma cell lines correlates with metastatic behavior in nudemice. Cancer Res 1992; 52: 1291–1296

DEATH

The Dutch Government, anxious to address the issues relating to euthanasia, but not without adequate data, commissioned a study of medical attitudes and experience in the area. This work was led by Professor van der Maas and his colleagues. The concept of informing political debate with clear relevant data is one that could readily be considered by other national governments anxious to move the agenda in health care provision.

van der Maas PJ, van Delden JJ, Pijnenborg L, Looman CW. Euthanasia and other medical decisions concerning the end of life. Lancet 1991; 338: 669–674

Pijnenborg L, van der Maas PJ, van Delden JJ, Looman CW. Life-terminating acts without explicit request of patient. Lancet 1993; 341: 1196–1199

Index

Page numbers in *italic* indicate figures or tables.